# STATE
## OF THE
# HEART

The Practical Guide to Your Heart and Heart Surgery

# ABOUT THE AUTHORS

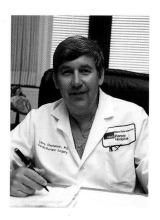

Larry W. Stephenson, M.D., is the Ford-Webber professor of surgery and chief of the Division of Cardiothoracic Surgery for Wayne State University in Detroit, Michigan. He is also chief of Cardiothoracic Surgery at the Detroit Medical Center and Harper Hospital. Besides having a busy clinical practice, he has authored or co-authored more than 270 scientific articles and book chapters and three medical books. Dr. Stephenson was born in Appleton, Wisconsin, and attended college and medical school at Marquette University in Milwaukee. He completed his general surgical residency at the University of Alabama, where he also did a cardiovascular research fellowship. Next he did his cardiothoracic surgical residency at the University of Pennsylvania, where he stayed on the faculty. Previously, he was a cardiothoracic surgeon at the Children's Hospital of Philadelphia and at the Hospital of the University of Pennsylvania. While at the University of Pennsylvania, he rose through the faculty ranks to professor of surgery and was awarded the prestigious J. William White Professorship in Surgery. Dr. Stephenson is a retired colonel, U.S. Army Medical Corps, with more than 20 years of service in the U.S. Army Reserves. He has held numerous command positions and was on active duty at Walter Reed Army Medical Center in Washington, D.C., during Operation Desert Storm.

Jeffrey L. Rodengen, president and CEO of Write Stuff Enterprises, Inc., is the author of the acclaimed and award-winning Legend series of coffee-table books. With more than 40 books to his name, he is the country's foremost biographer of American industry and technology, including comprehensive works on such global organizations as Pfizer, Inc, Boston Scientific Corp., Cessna Aircraft Co., Advanced Micro Devices, Inc., The Stanley Works, Chris-Craft Industries, Inc., and Ashland Inc. Throughout his remarkable career, Jeff has interviewed thousands of scientists, CEOs, business and national leaders, and celebrities. Before beginning his career in publishing, Rodengen enjoyed a 15-year career in Hollywood as a writer, producer and director. He has written or produced nearly 30 films, network television specials (including six for Arnold Schwarzenegger), Las Vegas revues and Broadway productions. Jeff has degrees in psychology and post-graduate degrees in engineering. He lives in Fort Lauderdale with his wife Karine, award-winning photographer, and their twin children.

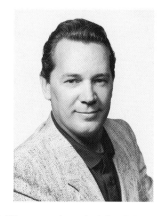

# STATE

## —— OF THE ——

# HEART

The Practical Guide to Your Heart and Heart Surgery

**Larry W. Stephenson, M.D.**

with
Jeffrey L. Rodengen

Edited by Jon VanZile
Design and layout by Sandy Cruz

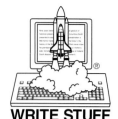

**WRITE STUFF**

Write Stuff Enterprises, Inc.
1001 South Andrews Avenue, Second Floor
Fort Lauderdale, FL 33316
**1-800-900-Book** (1-800-900-2665)
(954) 462-6657
www.writestuffbooks.com
www.stateoftheheartbook.com

## Publisher's Cataloging in Publication

Rodengen, Jeffrey L.
    State of the heart /Jeffrey L. Rodengen.
— 1st ed.
    p. cm.
    Includes bibliographical references and index.
    ISBN 0-945903-26-X — hardbound cover
    ISBN 0-945903-63-4 — softbound cover

    1. Heart — Diseases — Popular works.
2. Cardiologists — Interviews. I. Title.

    RC682.R64 1999       616.1'2
                    QBI98-928

Library of Congress
Catalog Card Number 98-61623

ISBN 0-945903-26-X Hardbound Cover
ISBN 0-945903-63-4 Softbound Cover

Completely produced in the
United States of America
10 9 8 7 6 5 4 3 2 1

## In Remembrance

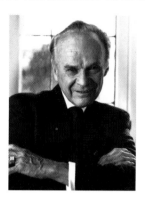

C. Walton Lillehei, M.D., Ph.D.
October 23, 1918–July 5, 1999
Heart Surgery Pioneer

*"I would like to think that
I've left the world of cardiovascular surgery
better than when I found it.
That would be a suitable epitaph."*

— *C. Walton Lillehei, 1995*

### Notice to Readers

# TABLE OF CONTENTS

Reader's Tip: The ♥ icon denotes a section that is of historical significance in the development of heart surgery.

## Chapter Eleven: Advanced Heart Failure: Transplants, Heart Assist Devices, and the Future . . . . . . . . . . . . . . . . . . . . . . . . . . . . .**178**

## Chapter Twelve: Arrhythmias, Pacemakers, and Defibrillators . . . . . . . . . . .**204**

TABLE OF CONTENTS

# FOREWORD

## BY
## C. EVERETT KOOP, M.D.
### FORMER SURGEON GENERAL OF THE UNITED STATES

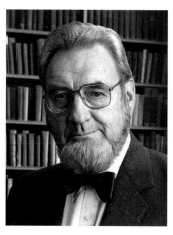

I KNEW I WANTED TO BE A DOCtor when I was five. I knew I wanted to be a surgeon when I was six. At the time, pediatric surgeons didn't exist — so I couldn't say I envisioned working with children and their families. Later, during my training, I wish I could say I had the great foresight to recognize that pediatrics was the field needing the most help. But that's not the case.

In 1946, I had my mind set to move into the field of cancer surgery when my chief, Doctor I.S. Ravdin, who was professor and chairman of surgery at the University of Pennsylvania and had been a brigadier general in the U.S. Army Medical Corps during World War II, asked me if I'd like to be surgeon-in-chief of the Children's Hospital of Philadelphia. I accepted the job and the requisites that came with it. It required me to go to Boston Children's Hospital for training and to give up the practice of adult surgery. Finally, he told me that I had to devote my attention to developing the country's finest academic training program for child surgery.

When I set out to create this training program, there was no true competition. The closest thing was the program in Boston run by Dr. William E. Ladd, under whom I was supposed to train. Ladd, however, retired just before I moved to Boston and had no immediate successor. As a result, I spent about seven months working with Dr. Robert E. Gross.

I learned several important lessons right away. I learned that children cannot be treated as small adults. They have a different tolerance for surgery, and dealing with their families is a completely different matter from dealing with adults.

I also saw that many of the mortal congenital defects at that time were basically untreatable. These defects — conditions like abdominal organs outside the body in the umbilical cord, or a hole in the diaphragm and all the internal abdominal organs up in the chest where a healthy lung should have developed — often had mortality rates as high as 95 percent in 1946. It was not at all uncommon to have a two-and-a-half–pound or three pound youngster brought to the hospital with one of these defects.

We made our contribution to pediatric surgery very quickly. We went from a 95 percent mortality rate in 1946 to a 95 percent survival rate for many of the most serious conditions in about a decade. I've always considered this a remarkable accomplishment for a bunch of doctors in a new specialty.

Cardiac surgery has followed a similar upward path. Just like pediatric surgery, open heart surgery was a thing of the future in the 1940s. There were only a few cardiac surgical procedures available: ligation of the patent ductus arteriosus, repair of coarctation of the aorta, and atrial wells to aid in the repair of an interatrial septal defect, but many doctors thought cardiac conditions were surgically untreatable.

Within a few years, just as my pediatric practice was gaining momentum, the heart-lung machine progressed to the point where open heart surgery became possible. In fact, at about that time I built a heart-lung machine that we used successfully in the laboratory with $6,000 of my own money. I had to make a decision at that time. I had an extraordinarily busy practice — for some time, I was the only pediatric surgeon south of Boston and east of Chicago. I had to decide whether I was going to continue what I was doing in pediatric surgery and add open heart surgery or whether I would just do the cardiac surgery. I didn't believe I could do both and do them well. I felt that I should continue doing what I was doing.

Since then, the field of cardiac surgery has been up there with the greatest strides in modern medicine. Every portion of the heart can be reached, and almost any conceivable operation has already been done. It's been a very exciting time, especially when heart transplantation came along. Consider all the things that can be done today, especially on newborns where we can even correct certain defects in utero.

Some problems we haven't thoroughly corrected are related to the heart's electrical system, but that will come. The research with angiogenesis, which deals with growing new blood vessels in the heart, is another frontier yet to be conquered. People say, "Oh, you can't fiddle around with those." Well, of course they say that, but they said that 10 years ago about other things. I've learned that you never say, "That's not going to happen."

Many of the other hurdles we face in medicine are not actual treatment hurdles but due to society and the changing nature of medical care. Transplantation, for instance, is a viable option for thousands of patients, yet that surgery is underutilized. We need to improve the organ donation program in this country. We've got to change our basic approach and reverse our thinking in this matter. Currently, we assume that no one wants their organs given for transplantation unless they had said so before their death. In France, doctors assume everybody wants to donate organs unless they specifically object. I'm sure there are some people there who don't want their organs taken but never get around to saying no — and some of these people may have their organs taken.

But even with this unfortunate consequence, lives are saved. It's terrible to be in a children's hospital and see the kind of emotional stress that develops. Two parents will be waiting for a liver, and in comes a child who doctors don't think is going to live. They question how soon the child is going to die, and which one of the kids is going to get the liver. The enmities and the hostilities are terrible. Doctors feel defeated by death, and many surgeons are not anxious to talk to those families about organ donation.

Hospitals that have gone to a donor program, with a special health educator acting as the organ procurement specialist probably do better. It's too hard for doctors to face the fact that in order to have one patient survive, they've got to lose another. That's part of the reason I think it ought to be taken out of doctors' hands and put in a donor specialist's.

A federal donor program would help tremendously with organ procurement. As surgeon general, I thought we were on the way to developing one. It was an uphill issue on a national level because doctors usually want donated organs to stay in their area and object to a heart, for instance, traveling across the country to benefit another patient. We sponsored workshops on organ donation and transplantation and brought people in from all over the world who taught us a great deal. We also funded the start-up of the ACT, the American Council on Transplantation, which helped us come to grips with trading organs from one procurement agency in Richmond to another in Florida and so forth.

I think public awareness may be the problem. I never fail to compliment the press on the fact that when AIDS came along, a most complicated disease, they kept it in the headlines for eight years and made it understandable to the average person. If we had that kind of effort for transplantation, I think we would get state laws that said if you die in an accident, your organs are available for transplantation unless you specifically object or carry a warrant on you that says, "Do not take my organs."

In greater society, I am also concerned about the way medical care is delivered. The old system is changing, and I'm concerned that my great grandchildren won't have as good pediatric surgical care, for example, as my grandchildren. That may sound strange, but the same may apply for cardiovascular surgery.

It takes a lot of practice and experience to become adept at dealing with a three-pound baby and get a survivor. We may be training too many pediatric surgeons and pediatric surgical specialists, thus not allowing doctors to develop their expertise in a greater volume of cases. In the most complicated operations, there is a danger of producing so many surgeons that they will never get enough experience to become as adept as the Denton Cooleys, John Kirklins and the Michael DeBakeys.

I've been fortunate enough to have experienced a very exciting period in medicine through my career, and have served as Surgeon General of the United States for eight years. Undoubtedly, in the future, many of the things that people are excited about now, like minimally invasive medicine, will be tested. In the operating rooms, doctors will successfully attack even more complicated conditions. Over the years, I've learned to think that almost anything is possible.

# ACKNOWLEDGEMENTS

THE AUTHORS WOULD LIKE TO THANK THE people who contributed to this book. A project of this size involved the creative efforts of many people, including the artists who provided illustrations and photographs. Medical illustrators Kelly Moore at the University of Miami and Denis Lee, formerly at the University of Michigan, provided the color and black and white illustrations, while Bill Loechel and Dr. Frank Shannon graciously donated additional color illustrations.

Much of the photography is the work of Ben True, the staff photographer at Harper Hospital in Detroit. We are especially grateful also to Dr. Harris B. Shumacker, Jr., distinguished professor of surgery, emeritus, Indiana University, himself a pioneer and major contributor to the field of cardiovascular surgery, for generously allowing use of numerous photographs from his collection. Likewise, in addition to their contributions, Stephen Westaby and Earl Bakken graciously allowed us to use photos from their collections.

Photography and artwork were also obtained from Medtronic for the pacemaker chapter, St. Jude Medical, Inc., for pages 153, 156, 159, 160 and 165, and Sulzer Carbomedics, Inc., for pages 224 and 225. In addition, artwork was kindly donated by Charles C. Thomas, Publisher, Ltd., Thomas Jefferson University Archives, Scott Memorial Library, the Baylor College of Medicine, W.L. Gore and Associates, Inc., Rick Bielaczyc, the University of Pennsylvania Medical School and by many of the contributors, who opened up their collections for our use.

In addition, material for a graph in chapter seven was adapted from *Heart Disease: A Textbook of Cardiovascular Medicine*, edited by Eugene Braunwald and published by W.B. Saunders.

We would like to thank the members of Dr. Stephenson's staff and his family and friends, who reviewed the chapters and made helpful suggestions, including: Laura Archer, Walter Frasher, P.A.-C., Jim and Nancy Gram, Phyllis Grissom, Donna Hammond, Vicky Hass, P.A.-C., Ken Jackson, P.A.-C., Donald Kossick, P.A.-C., Thomas McGarry, P.A.-C., Darcy Sibilia, P.A.-C., Helen Smith, R.N., Jennifer and William Stephenson, Melissa Stuckey, R.N., and Leah and Stephen Vartanian.

A special debt of gratitude is also extended to Carol Stephenson, who reviewed the manuscript and provided invaluable support throughout the project.

Thanks are also due to the scores of physicians, including cardiologists, cardiothoracic surgeons and others, who reviewed this material in progress and made innumerable contributions of fact and accuracy. They include:

Dimitrious Apostolou, M.D., Agustin Arbulu, M.D., Pierre Atallah, M.D., Frank Baciewicz, M.D., Joseph Bassett, M.D., Martin Blank, M.D., Gerald Cohen, M.D., Marcelo DiCarli, M.D., Maria Dan, M.D., Lingareddy Devireddy, M.D., Michael Ebstein, M.D., Steven Gellman, M.D., James Glazier, M.D., Gary Goodman, M.D., Narshima Gottam, M.D., Narsingh Gupta, M.D., Richard Harris, M.D., Robert Higgins, M.D., Antoine Khoury, M.D., Ronald Kline, M.D., Jay Kozlowski, M.D., Marvin Kronenberg, M.D., Steven Lavine, M.D., Edward Malinowski, M.D., David Martin, M.D., Arthur Mcunu, M.D., Hassan Nemeh, M.D., John O'Connell, M.D., Samuel Perov, M.D., Katherine Pitone-Lipkin, D.O., Kevin Radecki, M.D., Peter Rossi, M.D., Paul Ruble, M.D., Paul Sabotka, M.D., Chanderdeep Singh, M.D., Renata Soulen, M.D., J. Richard Spears, M.D., Joseph Talbert, M.D., Mark Taylor, M.D., Deepak Thatai, M.D., Gregory Thomas, M.D., Henry Walters, M.D., Bruce Washington, M.D., Clifford Weldon, M.D., and Alkis Zingas, M.D.

Finally, the staff at Write Stuff worked diligently for two years to produce this book. Medical proofreader Ellen Kurek and proofreader Bonnie Freeman provided meticulous and accurate proofreading, while transcriber Mary Aaron worked quickly and efficiently to transcribe the many interviews with pioneering heart surgeons. Indexer Erika Orloff assembled the comprehensive index. Executive assistants to Mr. Rodengen Colleen Azcona and Amanda Fowler scheduled interviews and coordinated travel. Thanks are also extended to the editorial, administrative and design staff, including Jon VanZile, principal editor; Alex Lieber, executive editor; and Melody Maysonet, associate editor; Sandy Cruz, senior art director; Jill Apolinario and Rachelle Donley, art directors; Fred Moll, production manager; Marianne Roberts, office manager; Mike Monahan, director of sales, promotion and advertising; Bonnie Bratton, director of marketing; Rafael Santiago, logistics specialist; and Karine Rodengen, project coordinator.

# CONTRIBUTORS' LIST

**HEART SURGERY PIONEERS**

**Nikolay M. Amosov**, M.D.
Academician
Formerly Director of the Insitute of
Cardiovascular Surgery
Kiev, Ukraine
Formerly Deputy, Supreme Soviet, U.S.S.R.

**Earl E. Bakken**, B.S., E.E.
Founder and Former Chairman of the Board
Medtronic, Inc.
Minneapolis, Minnesota

**Christiaan N. Barnard**, M.D., Ph.D.
Former Head of the Department of Cardiothoracic
Surgery
University of Capetown
Capetown, South Africa

**Brian G. Barratt-Boyes**, K.B.E., M.B., Ch.M.
Professor of Surgery (Hon.)
Formerly Surgeon-in-Charge
Cardiothoracic Surgical Unit
Greenlane Hospital
Auckland, New Zealand

**Alain F. Carpentier**, M.D., Ph.D.
Professor, Université de Paris VI
Chief, Department of Cardiovascular Surgery and
Organ Transplantation
Hôpital Broussais
Paris, France

**Denton Cooley**, M.D.
Surgeon-in-Chief, Texas Heart Institute
Chief, Cardiovascular Surgery
St. Luke's Episcopal Hospital

Clinical Professor of Surgery
University of Texas
Houston, Texas

**Michael E. DeBakey**, M.D.
Formerly Chairman, Department of Surgery and
formerly Chancellor
Baylor College of Medicine

Olga Keith Weiss Professor and
Distinguished Professor of Surgery
Baylor College of Medicine
Houston, Texas

**Wenner Dudley Johnson**, M.D.
Associate Clinical Professor,
Department of Cardiothoracic Surgery
Medical College of Wisconsin

Chairman, Department of Cardiovascular Diseases
St. Mary's Hospital
Milwaukee, Wisconsin

**Adrian Kantrowitz**, M.D.
Clinical Professor of Surgery
Wayne State University School of Medicine

Formerly Chief, Section of
Cardiovascular Surgery
Sinai Hospital
Detroit, Michigan

**John W. Kirklin**, M.D.
Formerly Professor and Chairman
Department of Surgery
University of Alabama
Birmingham, Alabama

Formerly Professor and Chairman, Department of
Surgery
Mayo Clinic and Mayo Foundation
Rochester, Minnesota

**Willem J. Kolff**, Ph.D., M.D.
Distinguished Professor of Medicine and Surgery
University of Utah

Formerly Director of Institute for
Biomedical Engineering and
Director Division of Artificial Organs
University of Utah
Salt Lake City, Utah

Formerly Scientific Director
Artificial Organs Program
Cleveland Clinic Foundation
Cleveland, Ohio

**C. Walton Lillehei**, Ph.D., M.D.
*(deceased July 5, 1999)*
Professor of Surgery, Emeritus
University of Minnesota
Minneapolis, Minnesota

Fomerly Louis Atterbery Stimson Professor of
Surgery and Chairman, Department of Surgery
The New York Hospital-Cornell Medical Center

Formerly Professor of Surgery
University of Minnesota Medical School
Minneapolis, Minnesota

**Bruce A. Reitz**, M.D.
Chairman, Cardiothoracic Surgery,
Stanford University Medical Center
Palo Alto, California

Formerly Cardiac Surgeon-in-Charge,
Johns Hopkins Hospital
Baltimore, Maryland

**Donald Nixon Ross**, B.Sc., M.B., Ch.B.
Formerly Director of the Department of Surgery
National Heart Hospital
London, England

**Ake Senning**, M.D.
Formerly Professor of Surgery and Director
University Surgical Clinic
Zurich, Switzerland

**Albert Starr**, M.D.
Director
Heart Institute of St. Vincent Medical Center
Portland, Oregon

Formerly Professor and Chief
Division of Cardiopulmonary Surgery
The Oregon Health Sciences University
Portland, Oregon

**CONTRIBUTING ESSAYISTS**

**Michael A. Acker**, M.D.
Associate Professor of Surgery
Division of Cardiothoracic Surgery
University of Pennsylvania
Philadelphia, Pennsylvania
*Cardiomyoplasty and Aortomyoplasty*

**Cary W. Akins**, M.D.
Clinical Professor of Surgery
Harvard University

Visiting Surgeon
Massachusetts General Hospital
Boston, Massachusetts
*Strokes, Carotid Arteries and Heart Surgery*

**Morrison C. Bethea**, M.D.
Clinical Professor of Surgery
Tulane University School of Medicine

Chief of Thoracic Surgery
Memorial Medical Center-Baptist Campus
New Orleans, Louisiana
*Nutrition for a Healthy Heart*

**Charles R. Bridges**, M.D., D.Sc.
Assistant Professor of Surgery
Division of Cardiothoracic Surgery
University of Pennsylvania
Philadelphia, Pennsylvania
*Building a Heart Pump from
Your Back Muscle*

**Randolph Chitwood**, M.D.
Professor and Chairman of
Department of Surgery
East Carolina University School of Medicine
Greenville, North Carolina
*Robotic Heart Valve Surgery:
Is This Reality or Fantasy?*

**Sary Aranki**, M.D.
Associate Professor of Surgery
Harvard Medical School
Boston, Massachusetts
and
**Lawrence H. Cohn**, M.D.
Professor of Surgery
Harvard Medical School
Boston, Massachusetts
and Chief, Cardiothoracic Surgery
Brigham and Women's Hospital
Boston, Massachusetts
*Transmyocardial Laser Revascularization*

**James L. Cox**, M.D.
Professor and Chairman, Cardiovascular and
Thoracic Surgery Surgical Director
Georgetown University
Cardiovascular Institute
Georgetown University Medical Center
Washington, D.C.
*Surgery for the Irregular Heartbeat*

**C.B. Dhabuwala**, M.D.
Professor of Urology
Wayne State University
Detroit, Michigan
*Viagra, Male Impotence*

**R. Curtis Ellison**, M.D.
Professor of Medicine and Public Health
Boston University School of Medicine
Boston, Massachusetts
*Wine, Alcohol and Your Heart*

**O. Howard Frazier**, M.D.
Professor of Surgery
University of Texas
and Surgeon
Texas Heart Institute
Houston, Texas
*Mechanical Heart Assist Devices*

**A. Marc Gillnov**, M.D.
Cardiothoracic Surgeon
The Cleveland Clinic Foundation
Cleveland, Ohio
and
**Delos M. Cosgrove**, M.D.
Chief, Cardiothoracic Surgery
The Cleveland Clinic Foundation
Cleveland, Ohio
*Minimally Invasive Heart Valve Surgery*

**Pamela Gordon**, M.D., F.A.C.C.
Associate Professor, Internal Medicine
Division of Cardiology
Wayne State University
Detroit, Michigan
*What You Should Know About
Your Heart During Pregnancy*

**Renee S. Hartz**, M.D.
Professor of Cardiothoracic Surgery
Tulane University
New Orleans, Louisiana
*Women and Coronary Artery Surgery*

**Nicholas T. Kouchoukos**, M.D.
Cardiothoracic Surgeon
Missouri Baptist Hospital
St. Louis, Missouri

Former Cardiac Surgeon-in-Charge
Jewish Hospital of St. Louis
Shoenberg Professor of Surgery
Washington School of Medicine
St. Louis, Missouri
*Surgery for the Thoracic Aorta*

**Michael Mack**, M.D.
Assistant Clinical Professor of Surgery
University of Texas SW Medical School
Dallas, Texas
*Minimally Invasive Direct Coronary Artery Bypass
Surgery — MIDCAB*

**James Marsh**, M.D.
Professor of Medicine and Chief
Division of Cardiology
Wayne State University
Detroit, Michigan
*Dissolving Blood Clots During Heart Attacks*

**John Mayer**, M.D.
Professor of Surgery
Harvard Medical School, and
Senior Associate in Cardiac Surgery
Boston Children's Hospital
Boston, Massachusetts
*Tissue Engineering of Cardiac Valves and Arteries*

**Patrick McCarthy**, M.D.
Cardiothoracic Surgeon
Cleveland Clinic Foundation
Cleveland, Ohio
*The Batista Procedure*

**Marc D. Meissner**, M.D.
Associate Professor of Internal Medicine
Cardiac Electrophysiologist and Cardiologist
Detroit Medical Center and Wayne State University
Detroit, Michigan
and
**Randy A. Lieberman**, M.D.
Assistant Professor of Internal Medicine
Cardiac Electrophysiologist and Cardiologist
Detroit Medical Center and Wayne State University
Detroit, Michigan
*Management of Atrial and Ventricular Arrhythmias*

**D. Craig Miller**, M.D.
Thelma and Henry Doelger Professor of
Cardiovascular Surgery
Stanford University
Stanford, California
*Aortic Endovascular Stents*

**John B. O'Connell**, M.D.
Professor and Chairman
Department of Medicine
Wayne State University
Physician-in-Chief
Detroit Medical Center,
Detroit, Michigan
*Your Visit to the Cardiologist*

**Todd Rosengart**, M.D.
Associate Professor of Surgery
Cornell University
New York, New York
*Gene Therapy for Heart Failure*

**Julie Swain**, M.D.
Professor of Surgery
Gill Heart Institute
University of Kentucky
Lexington, Kentucky
*How to Choose a Cardiac Surgeon*

**Stephen Westaby**, BSc, M.S., F.R.C.S.
Oxford Centre
John Radcliffe Hospital
Oxford University
Oxford, United Kingdom
*The Future in Artifical Heart Technology*

**Terrence M. Yau**, M.D., M.Sc.
Assistant Professor
Department of Surgery
University of Toronto
Toronto, Ontario, Canada
and
**Ren-Ke Li**, M.D., Ph.D.
Associate Professor
Department of Surgery
University of Toronto
Toronto, Ontario, Canada
and
**Donald A.G. Mickle**, M.D.
Professor
Department of Laboratory Medicine and Pathology
University of Toronto
Toronto, Ontario, Canada
and
**Richard Weisel**, M.D.
Professor of Surgery
University of Toronto
Toronto, Ontario, Canada
*Heart Cell Transplantation for the Failing Heart*

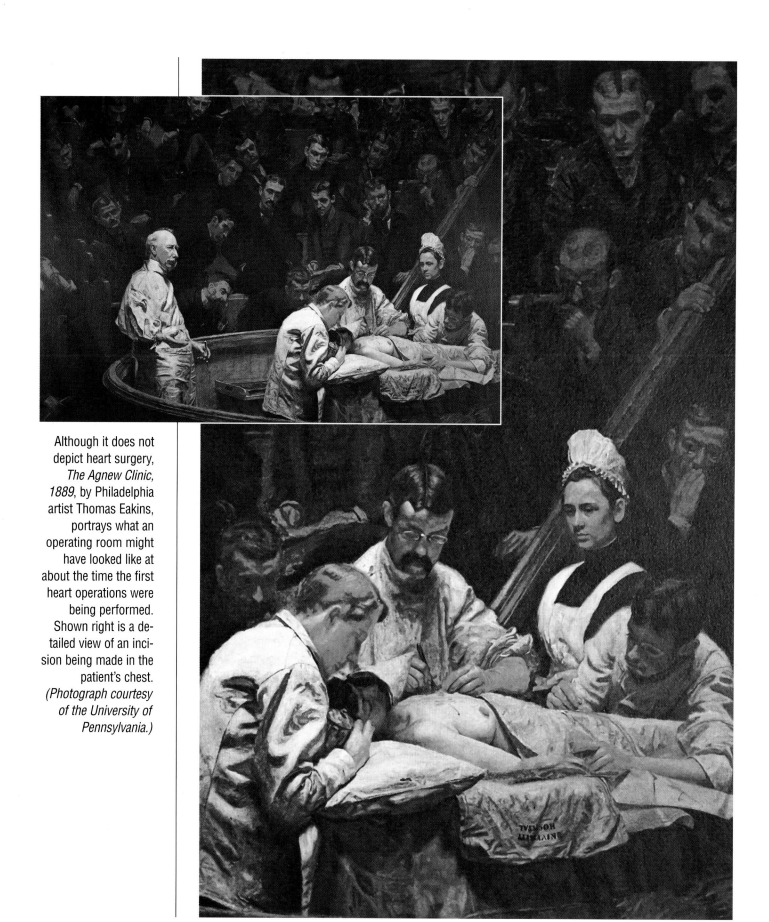

Although it does not depict heart surgery, *The Agnew Clinic, 1889*, by Philadelphia artist Thomas Eakins, portrays what an operating room might have looked like at about the time the first heart operations were being performed. Shown right is a detailed view of an incision being made in the patient's chest. *(Photograph courtesy of the University of Pennsylvania.)*

## CHAPTER ONE

# ♥THE DAWN OF OPEN HEART SURGERY

FOR MANY YEARS, DOCTORS HAD assumed the heart was too important to interfere with and too fragile to be operated on. In those days, cardiac problems often meant death. During the last fifty years, however, our understanding of the complicated cardiac system has increased greatly, and doctors now routinely perform surgeries that were once beyond the furthest reaches of medical imagination.

### The Early Days

The development of major surgery was retarded for centuries by a lack of knowledge and technology. Significantly, general anesthetics like ether and chloroform weren't developed until the middle of the nineteenth century. They made major surgical operations possible, which led to an interest in repairing wounds to the heart, and the first simple heart operations were soon reported in the medical literature.

On July 10, 1893, Dr. Daniel Hale Williams, an African-American surgeon from Chicago, successfully operated on a twenty-four-year-old man who had been stabbed in the heart during a fight. The patient was admitted to Chicago's Provident Hospital on July 9 at 7:30 P.M. The stab wound was slightly to the left of the breast bone (sternum) and dead center over the heart. Initially, the wound was thought to be superficial, but during the night there was persistent bleeding, pain, and pronounced symptoms of shock. Williams decided to operate. He opened the patient's chest and tied off an artery and a vein that had been injured inside the chest wall, possibly causing the blood loss. Then he noticed a tear in the pericardium (sack around the heart) and a puncture wound of the heart "about one-tenth of an inch in length."

The wound itself, in the right ventricle, was not bleeding, so Williams did not place a stitch through the heart wound. He did, however, stitch closed the hole in the pericardium. The patient recovered. Williams went on to report this case in a medical journal four years later. This is the first successful operation involving a documented stab wound to the heart.

At the time, Williams' surgery was considered bold and daring, but he never received the credit he deserved, probably because he did not actually place a stitch through the wound in the heart. Yet his treatment seems to have been appropriate

Daniel Hale Williams

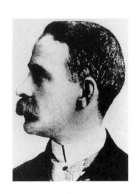

under the circumstances and most likely saved that patient's life.

The first stitch closure of a human heart wound was performed by Dr. Ansel Cappelen in Norway on a twenty-four-year-old man stabbed in the left chest. Upon arrival at the hospital, the victim was unconscious, pale, and pulseless. The operation began at 1:30 A.M. on September 5, 1894. A tear of the ventricle was closed with catgut stitches. Unfortunately, the patient's condition remained poor, and he died four days later.

Two years later, Dr. Ludwig Rehn, a surgeon in Frankfurt, Germany, performed what many consider the first successful heart operation. On September 7, 1896, a twenty-two-year-old man was stabbed in the heart and collapsed. The police found him pale, covered with cold sweat, and extremely short of breath. His pulse was irregular, and his clothes were soaked with blood. On September 9, his condition was worsening.

With his patient in profound shock and near death, Rehn opened the chest and found blood and a blood clot inside the pericardium, in addition to a wound in the right ventricle that was actively bleeding (it probably started to bleed again when Rehn removed the blood clot). Rehn placed three silk stitches through the heart wound, and the bleeding stopped. The patient made a full recovery.

In his official report to a medical journal, Rehn wrote, "Today the patient is cured. He looks very good. His heart action is regular.... This proves the feasibility of cardiac suture repair without a doubt. I hope this will lead to more investigations regarding surgery of the heart. This may save many lives." Ten years after Rehn's initial heart repair, he had accumulated a series of 124 patients who had undergone suture repair of heart wounds with a survival rate of 40 percent.

On September 14, 1902, the first successful stitching of a human heart in America happened under circumstances that would be hard to comprehend by modern day heart surgeons. Henry Myrick, a thirteen-year-old boy, was stabbed by another youth earlier that day. The boy was already in profound shock when the local country doctor arrived. The doctor remembered that Dr. Luther Hill from nearby Montgomery, Alabama, had spoken on the repair of cardiac wounds at a medical society meeting. Hill was sent for and arrived sometime after midnight with his brother, who was also a physician, and five other physicians.

The surgery took place on the patient's kitchen table in a run-down shack. Since it was night, the doctors borrowed two kerosene lamps from a neighbor. Luther Hill's brother administered chloroform anesthesia, and the doctors located the stab wound in the left ventricle. About forty-five minutes later, they had stitched the heart wound shut with two catgut stitches.

Although the early postoperative course was stormy, Henry made a complete recovery. He eventually moved to Chicago, where, in 1942 at the age of fifty-three, he got into a heated argument and was stabbed in the heart again, very close to the original stab wound. This time, Henry was not so lucky and died from the wound.

### The Heart-Lung Machine

From these early operations into the twentieth century, the development of heart surgery did not move very quickly until a single innovation, the heart-lung machine, ushered in the age of modern heart surgery. Before the invention of the heart-lung machine, surgeons confronted a very simple yet seemingly insurmountable problem. If the heart was stopped and opened so the surgeon could see it directly, the patient died. The heart-lung machine finally allowed physicians to stop the beating heart yet keep their patients alive.

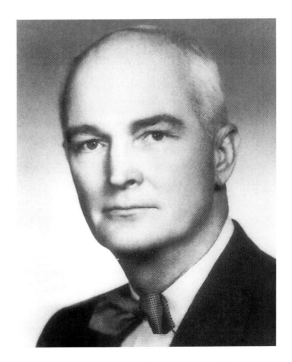

The solution to this great riddle came in the years after World War II. Teams of doctors at major hospitals enlisted the help of teams of engineers, in some cases at the country's largest corporations, and the race was on to develop a heart-lung machine that could support circulatory function while doctors stopped the heart.

The effort involved many doctors, yet from a research point of view, a young doctor named Dr. John Gibbon contributed more to the development of the heart-lung machine than anyone else. His interest began one October night in 1930 while at Massachusetts General Hospital in Boston. A patient was suffering from a blood clot in the lungs and was in shock. Gibbon was supposed to record blood pressure every fifteen minutes until either the patient recovered or her condition deteriorated to the point at which a high-risk operation would have to be attempted to remove the blood clot. Her condition worsened, and the operation was performed. Unfortunately, the patient did not survive the operation, but Gibbon learned an important lesson. He realized that if there were a way to keep the blood oxygenated while the surgeon operated on

the lung, many people suffering from this condition might be saved.

Three years later, while he was a research fellow in surgery at Harvard Medical School, Gibbon began experimental work on the heart-lung machine. His wife, Mary, was his research assistant. His research continued at the University of Pennsylvania in Philadelphia when he became the Harrison Fellow in Surgical Research in 1936.

By 1937, he was able to demonstrate that life could be maintained with an artificial heart and lung and that an animal's own heart and lungs could later resume function when the machine was turned off. In his first demonstration, however, only three animals resumed breathing adequately after he used a primitive heart-lung machine to bypass their hearts and lungs, and even these animals died within a few hours.

His work steadily progressed, however, and by 1939, Gibbon reported at the annual meeting of the American Association for Thoracic Surgery that three cats whose circulation had been totally supported by the heart-lung machine had survived more than nine months after the surgery. Dr. Clarence Crafoord, chief of thoracic surgery at the prestigious Karolinska Institute in Stockholm, said Gibbon's report was "a pinnacle of success in the progress of surgery." Dr. Leo Eloesser, a prominent chest surgeon from San Francisco, said the work reminded him "of Jules Verne's dreamlike visions, regarded as impossible at the time but later actually accomplished."

Gibbon's work was interrupted in 1942 by World War II but resumed after the war ended and he was appointed professor of surgery and director of the surgical research laboratory at Jefferson Medical College in Philadelphia. During his tenure there, Gibbon met Thomas Watson, chairman of International Business Machines (IBM) Corporation. Watson was fascinated by Gibbon's research and promised to help

In the 1930s, Dr. John Gibbon was among the first doctors to begin building a heart-lung machine. His first device served as a model for later, successful cardiopulmonary bypass machines.

him. Shortly afterward, a team of IBM engineers arrived at Thomas Jefferson University and built a heart-lung machine based on knowledge gained from Gibbon's earlier machine. It contained a rotating oxygenator apparatus and a modified rotary blood pump. The pump was based on one developed earlier by Dr. Michael DeBakey.

Gibbon successfully used the new IBM heart-lung machine for the repair of heart defects in small dogs and had several long-term survivors. The blood oxygenator, however, was too small for humans. The team soon developed a larger oxygenator that IBM engineers incorporated into a new machine.

By 1949, Gibbon's mortality in animals was 80 percent (meaning that only 20 percent survived the surgery), but it was improving, and he was ready to move to human patients. His first human patient was a fifteen-month-old girl with severe heart failure. She didn't survive the procedure; at autopsy, an unexpected congenital heart malformation was found.

Gibbon's second patient was an eighteen-year-old woman also with heart failure due to a congenital defect. On May 6, 1953, Gibbon successfully repaired the defect with the Gibbon-IBM heart-lung machine. The woman recovered, and several months later, the defect repair was confirmed repaired by cardiac catheterization. Unfortunately, Gibbon's next two patients did not survive operations using the heart-lung machine.

# THE ROLLER PUMP

DURING DR. JOHN GIBBON'S work on the heart-lung machine, he turned to a pump developed by Dr. Michael DeBakey while DeBakey was still a medical student at Tulane University in New Orleans.

In those early days, DeBakey worked as a technician in the medical lab and remembered his first exposure to blood pumps:

*"I didn't get paid very much, but I liked the work. The faculty member I was working with wanted a pump in the laboratory because he was interested in the pulse wave so he asked me to get a pump for him. I went to the library to learn something about pumps, and I didn't find a great deal in the med-*

An early roller pump that was used to move blood through the first heart-lung machines.

*ical school library. A friend of mine who was a college mate and went into engineering said, 'You know, you ought to go to the Engineering School library. They have a lot of articles on hydraulics.'*

*"I went to the Engineering School and found a wonderful bibliographic record of pumps going back to Archimedes, two thousand years ago. There was an article about rubber tubing, which came into being in the middle of the last century, being used to pump fluid by compressing it. That's what gave me the idea for my roller pump, which John Gibbon adapted, and that's how I contributed to the development of the heart-lung machine."*

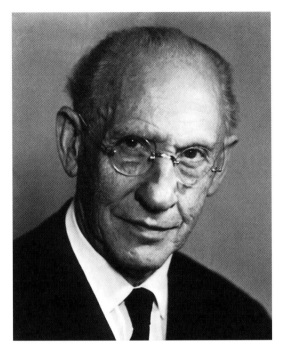

These failures upset Gibbon, who declared a one-year moratorium on use of the machine in humans until more work could be done to solve the problems.

Meanwhile, other groups were working to develop a heart-lung machine. They included those led by Crafoord at the Karolinska Institute in Stockholm, Sweden; Drs. S.S. Brukhonenko and N.N. Terebinsky in Moscow, Russia; Dr. J. Jongbloed at the University of Utrecht in Holland; Dr. Clarence Dennis at the University of Minnesota; Dr. Mario Dogliotti at the University of Turino in Italy; and Dr. Forrest Dodrill in Detroit, Michigan.

### The Dodrill Pump

At Harper Hospital in Detroit, Dr. Forrest Dodrill and colleagues used a mechanical blood pump on a forty-one-year-old man on July 3, 1952. The pump had been developed in conjunction with engineers at General Motors. It was used to substitute for the left ventricle, the heart's main pumping chamber, for fifty minutes while a defective heart valve was surgically repaired.

This was the first time the human left ventricle had been successfully bypassed. For his first human patient, Dodrill used the patient's own lungs to oxygenate the blood.

In an interview twenty-seven years later, the patient recalled seeing dogs romping on the roof of a nearby building from his hospital room. He later learned those dogs had been used in the final test of the Dodrill-General Motors mechanical heart machine.

Several months after its first demonstration in a human, Dodrill and associates used their machine on a sixteen-year-old boy with a narrowed pulmonary heart valve. They were able to open the valve as they viewed it directly while the patient's right ventricle, which pumps blood to the lungs, was supported by the Dodrill-General Motors blood pump. This operation was also successful, and the patient was alive and well forty-six years later.

During the same period, other innovative methods were being tested to close abnormal holes inside the heart without having to use a heart-lung machine. One technique used hypothermia. The patient's body temperature was lowered using an ice bath until the heart stopped. The hole in the heart was repaired, and the patient was rewarmed. The cold body temperature protected the patient from oxygen starvation by decreasing the metabolic rate and the body's consumption of oxygen.

### Lillehei's Cross-Circulation

The heart-lung machine, in its various forms, was not considered the only practical way to bypass the circulation. A young surgeon named Dr. C. Walton Lillehei and colleagues at the University of Minnesota studied a technique they called cross circulation, which did not use a bypass machine at all. Using this technique, the cir-

Dr. Clarence Crafoord started a research team in Sweden that worked toward developing an open-heart program. However, he became best known for a pioneering operation that corrected a defect in the aorta called coarctation of the aorta.

culation of one dog was used to support that of another dog while the second dog's heart was temporarily stopped and opened. After a simulated heart repair in the second dog, the circulations of the two animals were disconnected and they were allowed to recover.

But this technique was fraught with ethical issues. Lillehei himself remarked that "clinical cross circulation for intracardiac surgery was an immense departure from the established surgical practice.... This thought of taking a normal human to the operating room to serve as a donor circulation (with potential risk, however small) even temporarily was considered by critics at that time to be unacceptable, even immoral."

Others were "quick to point out that this proposed operation was the first in all of surgical history to have the potential for a 200 percent mortality."

Moreover, there were practical problems with the technique, including blood type. Cross circulation would work only for people with the same blood type. There was also a problem with blood volume — how much work would the nonsurgical patient's heart have to do?

In spite of these obstacles, Lillehei wrote, "The continued lack of any success in the other centers around the world that were working actively on heart-lung bypass made the decision to go ahead (with cross circulation) inevitable. I felt the technique was ready to use in a human; however, even in such a progressive and primary medical school as the University of Minnesota, there was opposition to the idea. Dr. Owen Wangensteen, chairman of the Department of Surgery, was a tremendous help. He was well aware of these experiments and wholeheartedly supported them. Where there seemed a possibility that the first clinical operation might be canceled the night before because of opposition, I left a note for Dr. Wangensteen, 'Is our case still on in the morning?' His answer: 'Dear Walt: By all means, go ahead.'"

During cross circulation for repair of a congenital defect in a child, a major artery and vein in the parent's groin were

# C. WALTON LILLEHEI'S LEGACY

C. Walton Lillehei

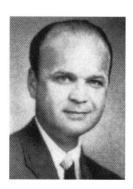

OPEN-HEART SURGERY WAS NOT possible when Dr. C. Walton Lillehei completed his surgical training. Indeed, Lillehei had only switched into medical school at the last minute, veering away from pre-dentistry at the University of Minnesota. As did a select group of surgeons around the world, Lillehei spent much of his early career trying to find a practical way to conduct open-heart surgery. This led him to the novel idea of cross circulation, or using one person's circulation to support that of another, while heart surgery was performed.

For his first patient, he selected "an infant who was about one year of age and had been in the hospital most of his life," Lillehei remembered in a 1999 interview.

Around the same time, ninety miles away, Dr. John Kirklin and his team at the Mayo Clinic were working on a machine that would support patients during cardiopulmonary bypass — and the competition between the teams was fierce.

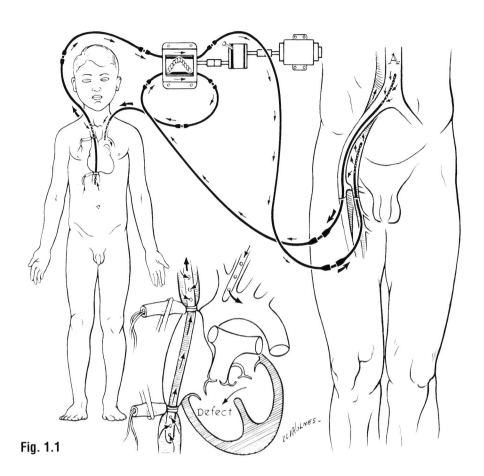

**Fig. 1.1**

**Fig. 1.1:**
Dr. C. Walton Lillehei (opposite page), working at the University of Minnesota, developed a novel technique of cardiopulmonary bypass called cross circulation, in which the circulation of one person is used to support that of another during an open-heart operation. It was used successfully in sick children.

"There was significant competition, obviously," Lillehei commented during a 1999 interview. "Kirklin knew the schedule that we were going on, and we didn't operate on Saturday, and they did. So our team was inclined to go down to the Mayo Clinic on Saturday and see what was going on!"

Before long, both teams were using different forms of bypass successfully, and, for more than a year, they were the only ones in the world performing open-heart surgeries. Throughout this time, doctors traveled from all over the world to see the first open-heart operations and their incredible results.

With Kirklin's success with the machine, however, Lillehei began a slow transition away from cross circulation and toward a heart-lung machine of his own design. In the beginning, Lillehei used the heart-lung machine for the simpler, more straightforward cases and continued using cross-circulation, with which he was more familiar, for the more serious cases.

Along with his own pioneering work, Lillehei, who passed away on July 5, 1999, had another lasting effect. Beginning in 1952, he was involved in the training of more than 150 cardiac surgeons at the University of Minnesota. These young physicians came from the U.S., Canada, and thirty-nine other countries, and many have become preeminent in their field and have gone on to make important contributions in their own rights.

# JOHN KIRKLIN'S INSPIRATION: HOW WE WOULD FIX THE INSIDE OF THE HEART

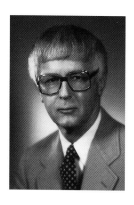

John Kirklin

**Ductus Arteriosus:**
A tube connecting the pulmonary artery to the aorta. After birth, when the lungs begin to function, this tube normally closes. If it stays open, the condition is known as patent ductus arteriosus. Over time, this can cause problems such as heart failure and may need to be surgically closed.

D R. JOHN KIRKLIN, WHO WAS more interested in football than medicine in his undergraduate days, remembers clearly the moment he became a cardiac surgeon. He was enrolled in the medical school at Harvard University when Dr. Robert Gross, a Boston surgeon, visited to give a lecture. It was the 1930s, and heart surgery was almost nonexistent — except for Gross, who had become "the only world-famous cardiac surgeon" by successfully closing a patent **ductus arteriosus** a few months before.

"On this Saturday morning, into this lecture hall, down on the ground level, walked this man," Kirklin said in a 1999 interview. "He was very young,

connected through tubes to the child's circulation, and the heart of the parent pumped enough oxygenated blood to also support the circulation of the small child (Fig. 1.1). A mechanical pump was used to control the interchange of blood between the patient and the donor.

On March 26, 1954, Lillehei and associates used the cross-circulation technique at the University of Minnesota to correct a ventricular septal defect, or a hole in the wall between the heart's two pumping chambers, in a twelve-month-old infant.

The patient had been hospitalized ten months for uncontrollable heart failure and pneumonia. During the operation, the child's circulatory system was connected to his father's. The procedure was a success, and the patient seemed to be making a good recovery until death on the eleventh postoperative day from an infection of the trachea. At autopsy, the hole between the pumping chambers was confirmed closed. Two weeks later, and only three days apart, the second and third patients with ventricular septal defect underwent successful heart surgery. Both

became long-term survivors with normal heart function.

A year later, Lillehei published a report on thirty-two children with various types of cardiac malformations that had undergone surgical repair. Although Lillehei had met with fairly good success with his technique, it would not become established. After its use in forty-five patients during 1954 and 1955, it was discontinued. Although its clinical use was short lived, cross circulation was an important stepping stone in the development of cardiac surgery.

### Kirklin's Heart-Lung Machine

At the same time Lillehei was working on cross circulation, Dr. John W. Kirklin announced he was launching an open-heart program at the Mayo Clinic, only ninety miles away from Lillehei's operating room. Kirklin and his team had developed their own heart-lung machine, basing it on the Gibbon-IBM machine, but with their own modifications.

At that time, there were perhaps fewer than a dozen laboratory research programs, very neat, with slicked-back hair. He was a good-looking man in a blue suit. He walked in and looked around that amphitheater with a slightly haughty look and said he was giving a lecture on wound healing. At that moment, 110 cardiac surgeons came into existence, of which a few of us stayed in business."

Over the next years, Kirklin remembers sitting with colleagues filling notebooks "about how we would fix the inside of the heart if we could get there. We couldn't, of course, but being young, you dream!" The obstacles to overcome in creating an open heart surgery program were awesome. Doctors on the Mayo team thought they were only months from performing the procedure on their first patient when a prominent pathologist, having observed a practice run with the heart-lung machine, said it was impractical and would never work. This pathologist happened to be in charge of the blood bank and declared it would not be possible to supply enough fresh blood to prime the machine for an ongoing open heart surgery program.

Kirklin's development program at the Mayo Clinic did, in fact, overcome the obstacles, resulting in a successful heart-lung machine that finally gave him the opportunity to realize those early ambitions. He was first to have a series of patients successfully undergo heart surgery using the heart-lung machine.

At the Mayo Clinic, Dr. John Kirklin used Gibbon's basic design to build the Mayo-Gibbon heart-lung machine. Pictured below is the screen oxygenator, which was responsible for infusing the blood with oxygen much like a lung does. This model was used in 1955 during the first open-heart operations.

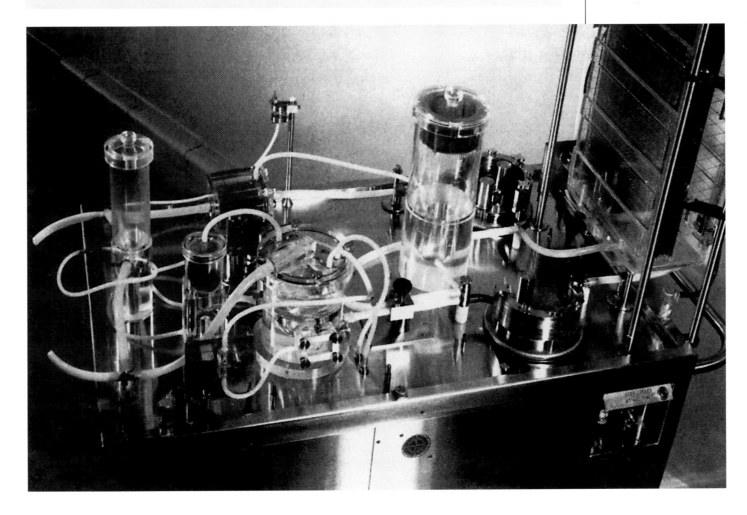

including Kirklin's and Lillehei's, focusing on open heart surgery in the world. Of them all, these two were among the most promising, and, because of their proximity to each other, the competition between the two teams of doctors was fierce, yet remained focused on the goal. Medicine appeared to be on the brink of open cardiac surgery, and doctors from around the world visited the developing programs.

The implications for a major improvement in the treatment of heart birth defects were enormous, and it was an extraordinarily exciting time in the development of medicine. Remembering this period, Kirklin later wrote:

*"Dr. Earl Wood, a great physiologist and my coworker, and I went back to his office ... and decided that either we would either have to be content with cardiac surgery as a rather minor specialty, limited to passing instruments into the heart, or we would need a heart-lung machine.... 'It's the oxygenator that is the problem,' said Wood.*

*"We investigated and visited the groups working intensely with the mechanical pump oxygenator. We visited Gibbon in his laboratories in Philadelphia and Dodrill in Detroit, among others. The Gibbon pump oxygenator had been developed and made by International Business Machines Corporation and looked quite a bit like a computer. Dodrill's heart-lung machine had been developed and built for him by General Motors, and it looked a great deal like a car engine. We came home, reflected, and decided to try to persuade the Mayo Clinic to let us build a pump oxygenator similar to the Gibbon machine but somewhat different.*

*"Most people were very discouraged with the laboratory progress. The American Heart Association and the National Institutes of Health had stopped funding any projects for the study of heart-lung machines because it was felt that the*

*problem was physiologically insurmountable. Dr. David Donald and I undertook a series of laboratory experiments lasting about a year and a half, during which time the engineering shops at the Mayo Clinic constructed a pump oxygenator based on the Gibbon model....*

*"Of course a number of visitors came our way, and some of them came to the laboratory to see what we were doing. One of those visitors was Dr. Ake Senning (from Stockholm, Sweden). I still remember one day when he was there and one of the connectors came loose, and we ruined his beautiful suit as well as the ceiling of the laboratory by spraying blood all around the room."*

*"The electrifying day came in the spring of 1954 when the newspapers carried an account of Walt Lillehei's successful open-heart operation on a small child. Of course, I was terribly envious, and yet I was terribly admiring at the same moment. That admiration increased exponentially when a short time later a few of my colleagues and I visited Minneapolis and observed one of what was now a series of successful open-heart operations with controlled cross-circulation. Walt then took us on rounds, and it was absolutely exciting to see small children recovering from these miraculous operations. However, it was also a difficult time for me. Some of my colleagues at the Mayo Clinic, and some of my influential ones, indicated to me that we had wasted much time and money. After all, this young fellow in Minneapolis was successful with a very simple apparatus and did not even require an oxygenator....*

*"However, in the winter of 1954 and 1955, we had nine surviving dogs out of ten cardiopulmonary bypass (heart-lung machine) runs. With my wonderful colleague and pediatric cardiologist, Dr. Jim DuShane, we had earlier selected eight patients for intracardiac repair. Two had to be put off because two babies with*

*very serious congenital heart disease came along, and we decided to fit them into the schedule.*

*"We did our first open heart operation on a Tuesday in March 1955. That evening, I had a telephone call from Dr. Dick Varco in Minneapolis who indicated that Sir Russell Brock (a prominent chest surgeon from England) was visiting their cardiac surgical program at the University of Minnesota. Walt Lillehei and Dick Varco indicated to Sir Russell that we had done an operation earlier that day, and they called to see if he could come to Rochester the next day to see the patient, to which I said 'Certainly.' "*

Kirklin later remembered that he was worried Sir Russell would ask to sit in on another surgery, which he did. "So I sort of said yes, but imagine it," Kirklin said.

*"It was one of the world's great surgeons saying to some kid, 'May I come and visit?' He was a very imperious, tough guy with a bad reputation, which I think he totally did not deserve. I asked him if he'd like to be on the operating team. 'No. No,' he said, 'I wouldn't. I don't want to be a problem. I just want to watch. Do you have a gallery? I'll sit in the gallery.'*

*"The next morning, I walked in to do the second case. He was already in the gallery, but in a place that I knew he wouldn't be able to see very well. I suggested that he might want to move, but he said, 'I'll be in your field of vision and I don't want you to be distracted by my presence.' He didn't move and that was a great, great man, a world-famous man with a bad reputation who was wonderful to me."*

By this time, he and Lillehei "were on parallel but intertwined paths," Kirklin later wrote. "I am extremely grateful

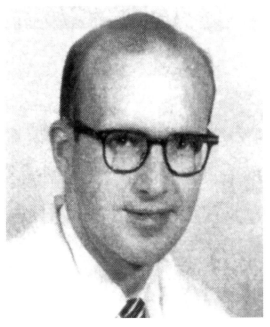

Dr. Richard DeWall helped develop the bubble oxygenator that eventually replaced the screen oxygenator and became a standard in heart-lung machines.

to Walt Lillehei and am very proud for the two of us that during that twelve- to eighteen-month period when we were the only surgeons in the world performing open intracardiac operations with cardiopulmonary bypass and surely in intense competition with each other, we shared our gains and losses with each other. We continued to communicate, and we argued privately in nightclubs and on airplanes rather than publicly over our differences."

In Kirklin's first group of eight patients, four survived the surgery. He was able to lower his open-heart mortality rate to 20 percent the following year and 10 percent the year after that.

During 1955, Lillehei began to gradually switch over from cross circulation to a heart-lung machine of his own team's design. With a colleague, Dr. Richard DeWall, they developed a "bubble" type of oxygenator that, with modifications made by Dr. Denton Cooley in Houston, Texas, became popular. The concept is still used today.

Kirklin's heart-lung machine, which was known as the Mayo-Gibbon heart-lung machine, was the accepted standard in those early days. By this time,

# DENTON COOLEY: INVENTOR AND PIONEER SURGEON

DR. DENTON COOLEY, ONE OF heart surgery's most noteworthy pioneers, originally planned on becoming a dentist and taking over his father's practice.

Although he was interested in medicine, he was worried that the academic track to a medical degree was too difficult. This fear was put to rest when he achieved the highest grades in his college fraternity. Soon after, Cooley transferred into medicine and eventually graduated from Johns Hopkins Medical School. During World War II, he also interned at Johns Hopkins, training under Dr. Alfred Blalock, where he was present at the world's first "blue baby" operation.

"There was a great superstition about the heart at the time," Cooley remembered during a recent interview, "and whether one could operate inside of the heart with expectation of survival. I went through what I called the closed era, when we operated on the surface of the heart, to the open era, when we were actually inside the heart doing much more extensive types of repairs."

The open era of heart surgery is credited to the heart-lung machine, an exciting innovation that Cooley studied in development. His laboratory re-

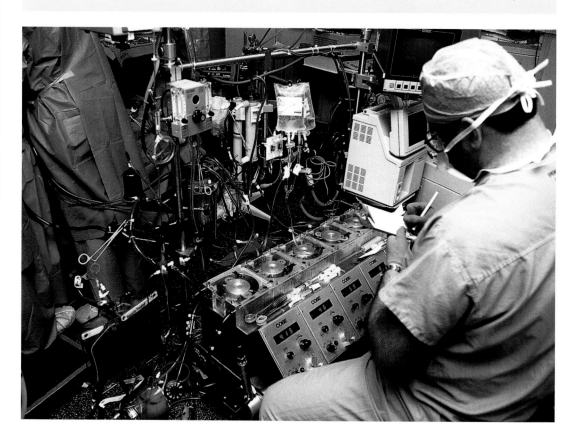

A modern heart-lung machine.

search in this area started in 1952 and was initially slow, causing him to visit Minnesota.

*"I had gone up to Minnesota to visit Lillehei in Minneapolis and then Kirklin over at Rochester. There, within the space of two or three days, I got to see what could be done. Lillehei was using cross circulation, which seemed to work well but obviously could not be used safely in adult patients. Then I saw Kirklin, who had a very elaborate machine, modeled after what Gibbon had devised, but it was very complex. From that experience, I decided I was going to go with the bubble oxygenator and pump."*

Cooley felt that a bubble oxygenator, which Lillehei and DeWall had just developed, was simpler than the oxygenator Kirklin was using, and he began developing a reusable bubble oxygenator made of stainless steel.

His first chance to use it in a human came when a desperately ill forty-nine-year-old man was referred to him. The patient had a ruptured ventricular septum caused by a heart attack. Cooley successfully repaired the hole in the ventricular septum on April 6, 1956. This marked the beginning of open-heart surgery in Texas. In time, other patients began to follow.

"Within an eight-month period, I had done ninety-five open-heart operations, which far exceeded what anyone else had done anywhere in the world," Cooley said. "At that time, we enjoyed almost a monopoly on open-heart surgery in that there were only two other institutions that were really active in the field, and they were both in Minnesota [at the University of Minnesota and the Mayo Clinic]."

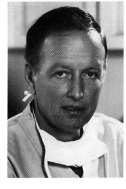

Dr. Denton Cooley began performing open-heart operations in the mid-1950s, soon after the heart-lung machine had been developed. He helped develop the bubble oxygenator.

many university groups around the world had developed open heart programs, and the modern era of cardiac surgery had begun. With their greatest obstacle overcome, teams of surgeons began to tackle ever-more-complex cardiac problems in both children and adults. Right after the introduction of the heart-lung machine, the pace of advance was so rapid that by the 1960s, surgeons were treating coronary artery disease, congenital heart defects, cardiac injuries, heart valve problems, and diseased or damaged major arteries in the chest.

As the field became more specialized, the role of the heart surgeon became more narrowly focused, and pediatric congenital heart surgery separated from adult heart surgery into a specialty of its own. For the most part, cardiac surgery in the adult addresses acquired heart disease. Nevertheless, a close connection between adult and pediatric heart surgery continues because advances in one subspecialty usually are applicable in the other, and this kinship will probably remain for the foreseeable future.

Currently, almost one million cardiac operations are performed each year worldwide with the use of the heart-lung machine. In most cases, the operative mortality is quite low, approaching 1 percent for some operations. Today, hundreds of thousands of physicians, scientists, and engineers are involved in a broad and deep effort to develop new and safer operations and procedures, new valves, new biomaterials, new heart substitutes, and new life-support systems. These efforts are supported by a vigorous infrastructure of basic science, biology, medicine, chemistry, pharmacology, engineering, and computer technology.

# NIKOLAY AMOSOV: HEART SURGEON AND PUBLIC SERVANT IN THE U.S.S.R.

THE INITIAL DRIVE TO DEVELOP heart surgery was a worldwide effort, with doctors in North and South America, Europe, the U.S.S.R., and elsewhere all pushing towards open heart surgery and techniques to correct many forms of heart disease. In the former Soviet Union, Dr. Nikolay Amosov became one of the leading surgeons of his day. In a recent interview, Amosov remembered his introduction to medicine and his early days as a surgeon.

"I had been interested in medicine since my childhood," Amosov said. "However, I happened to choose the only post-graduate degree available in the medical school in Arkhangelsk, and this was military surgery. There I began my surgical career. I spent only one year in post-doctoral training and went to the city of Cherepovets, where I worked as a surgeon for a year before World War II broke out. They were recruiting to the military field hospital in Cherepovets, where there was a need for a chief surgeon. I was offered the spot and served in this hospital throughout the war."

Amosov's workload was enormous. His two-hundred-bed hospital with only five doctors treated forty thousand wounded Russian soldiers throughout the war.

By 1953, after additional, non-wartime surgical experience in Moscow, Amosov moved to the Ukrainian capital of Kiev and became chairman of the Department of Surgery in the Kiev State Medical School. Like other surgeons around the world, he performed heart operations such as opening narrowed mitral valves and placing the Blalock-Taussig shunt for **tetralogy of Fallot**. These operations did not require a heart-lung machine.

"Of course, I had never been out of the country and had never seen heart surgery done by someone else," he said. "Mostly, I used books to educate myself. It was very difficult to start."

In 1957, Amosov traveled with a group of Russian surgeons — including Dr. Boris Petrovsky, a prominent pioneer chest surgeon and minister of health of the U.S.S.R. for sixteen years — to the Mexico International Congress of Surgeons. There, for the first time, he saw an operation performed with a heart-lung machine.

**Tetralogy of Fallot:** A congenital heart defect that consists of four different abnormalities: 1. An abnormal opening between the right and left ventricles; 2. An abnormal position of the aorta so that it partially overrides the right and left ventricular hole; 3. Obstruction of blood flow to the lungs; 4. An abnormal thickening of the right ventricle.

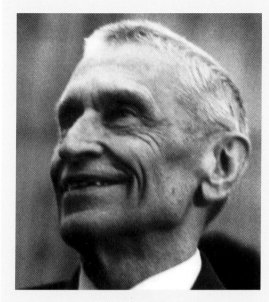

"When we came back, I wanted to start that kind of surgery, but I did not have the opportunity to buy a heart-lung machine. But, because in addition to medical school, I also had a degree in engineering, I created a heart-lung machine myself in 1958. A local factory built it. In 1959, we did our first case of tetralogy of Fallot using our own heart-lung machine."

Slowly, Amosov and his team advanced into more complicated cases. Nevertheless, their surgical results were very good, and in 1962, his team in Kiev was the first in the U.S.S.R. to replace a mitral valve with nylon leaflets. Interestingly enough, he used nylon from a shirt he had bought in the United States.

Throughout his career, Amosov was widely recognized for his standing as a world-class heart surgeon. Even the Communist Party leadership admired the doctor, who had never been a member of the Communist Party, and named him to the Supreme Soviet.

"It was important for the Party bosses to have somebody in the Supreme Soviet who was popular in the public eye," he said. "People supported me, and I was elected unanimously. But then, everyone was elected unanimously. I was not attracted to being a deputy in the Supreme Soviet, but you could not refuse this kind of offer. You might lose your job. The Supreme Soviet had its sessions biannually. Every vote was unanimous. Debates were not too long. I made a speech once. I spoke about health care and was very critical. In 1979, after seventeen years on the Supreme Soviet of the Soviet Union, my services there came to an end."

By the late 1980s, the volume at the Institute of Cardiovascular Surgery in Kiev grew to about five thousand surgical cases a year, making it one of the busiest cardiovascular centers in the world.

"In 1988, when I became seventy-five, I decided it was inappropriate for me to continue as director of the Cardiovascular Institute. An election was held at the Institute, and Dr. Gennady Knyshov was elected my successor. And then I made one more call to public service in 1989. Everyone had so much enthusiasm that our country would be a democracy. Employees of our institute nominated me. Elections were held, but on a democratic basis and without interference. On election day, 60 percent of the ballots were cast for me. This time when I was elected to the Supreme Soviet, it was organized like a real parliament. However, all my hopes to improve the health care system never succeeded.

"In December 1992, the Soviet Union ceased to exist. With its demise, my public service ended."

*This text was based on an interview conducted for this book by Dr. Gennady Knyshov, director, Cardiovascular Institute, Kiev, Ukraine, and translated by Dr. Vitaly Piluiko.*

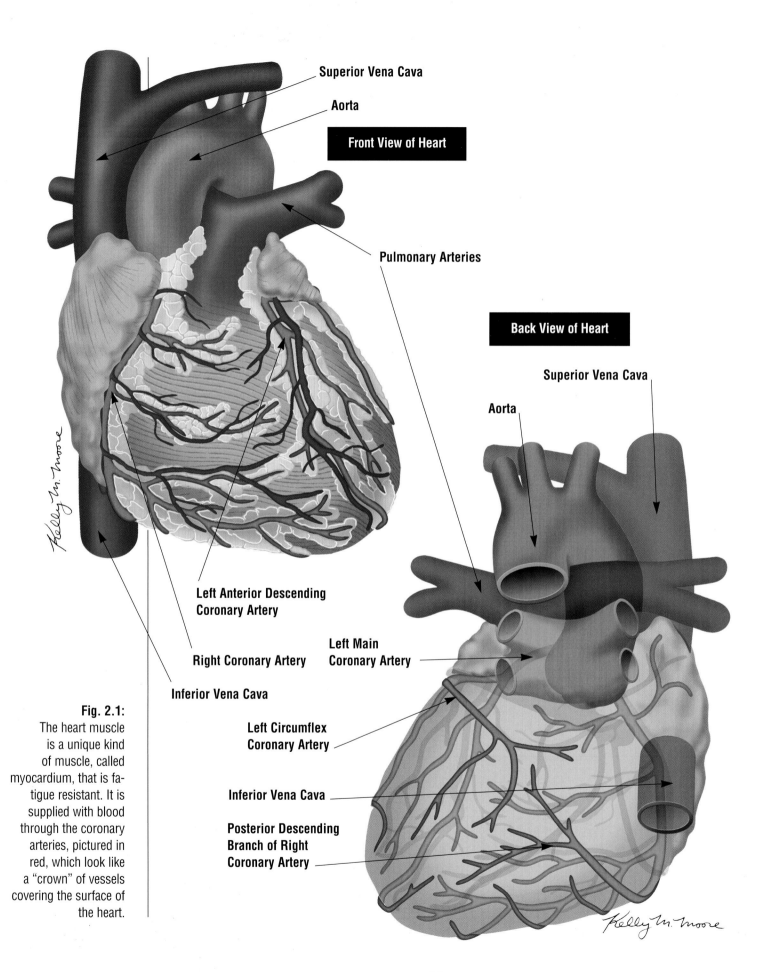

**Superior Vena Cava**

**Aorta**

**Front View of Heart**

**Pulmonary Arteries**

**Back View of Heart**

**Superior Vena Cava**

**Aorta**

**Left Main**
**Coronary Artery**

**Left Anterior Descending**
**Coronary Artery**

**Left Circumflex**
**Coronary Artery**

**Right Coronary Artery**

**Inferior Vena Cava**

**Inferior Vena Cava**

**Posterior Descending**
**Branch of Right**
**Coronary Artery**

**Fig. 2.1:**
The heart muscle
is a unique kind
of muscle, called
myocardium, that is fa-
tigue resistant. It is
supplied with blood
through the coronary
arteries, pictured in
red, which look like
a "crown" of vessels
covering the surface of
the heart.

## CHAPTER TWO

# THE NORMAL HEART

THE HEART SITS AT THE CENTER of the incredible network of **arteries** and **veins** whose job it is to nourish your organs and tissues with blood. Of all your muscles, your heart is perhaps the most durable — it is expected to perform continuously without missing a beat for your entire life. Imagine your heart as a very efficient machine. It helps convert the food you eat into mechanical energy, which is then used to pump blood first through the lungs, where it receives oxygen, and then throughout the rest of the body.

Your heart is about the size of your fist and rests slightly to the left of center under your breastbone or sternum. It has four chambers: the two upper chambers are filling chambers, or atria, and the two lower chambers are powerful pumping chambers called ventricles. The ventricles are separated by a common wall called the interventricular **septum**, and the atria are separated by the atrial septum. These common walls, like the rest of the heart, are composed of heart muscle called myocardium.

### The Right Side of the Heart

Blood begins its journey toward the heart in millions of tiny blood vessels called **capillaries** throughout the body. Capillaries are the smallest elements of the circulatory system and are where the transfer of oxygen and nutrients from blood to the body's tissues occurs. After the blood gives off the oxygen in the capillaries, it turns a dark red to purple color. The red blood cells in the capillary then pick up the carbon dioxide molecules that are the byproducts of cell and tissue function.

Capillaries feed into small veins, which in turn feed into larger veins as blood moves closer to the heart. The veins from the abdomen and lower body drain into the inferior vena cava. This large vein is about the same diameter as your thumb and drains directly into the right atrium. The blood returning from the chest and upper body drains into the superior vena cava, also about the diameter of your thumb. It, too, drains into the right atrium (Fig. 2.1).

When the unoxygenated blood reaches the right atrium, it flows through the tricuspid valve into the right ventricle (Fig. 2.2). Like the other three heart valves, the tricuspid valve is a one-way valve and does not allow blood to flow backwards (Fig. 2.3).

After the right ventricle fills with blood, it begins to contract, forcing blood out

**Artery:**
A blood vessel that carries blood from the heart to the body or from the heart to the lungs.

**Vein:**
A vessel that channels blood from the capillaries back to the heart.

**Septum:**
A wall that separates two chambers, such as two chambers of the heart.

**Capillaries:**
The smallest elements of the circulatory system. Capillaries are where the transfer of oxygen and nutrients from blood to the body's tissues occurs.

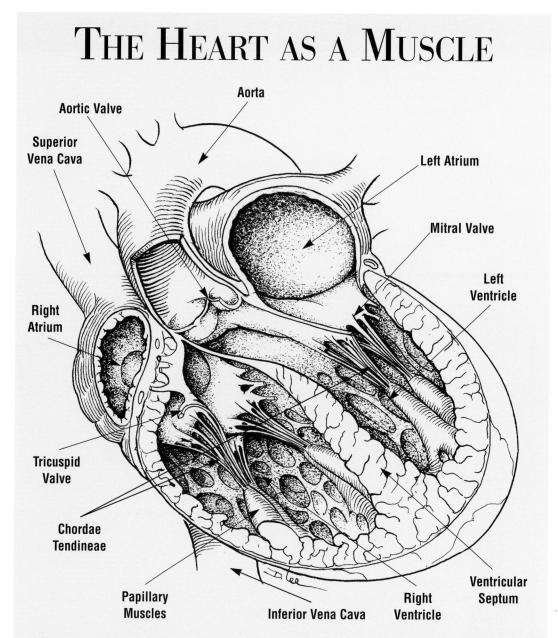

# THE HEART AS A MUSCLE

Aorta

Aortic Valve

Superior
Vena Cava

Left Atrium

Mitral Valve

Left
Ventricle

Right
Atrium

Tricuspid
Valve

Chordae
Tendineae

Ventricular
Septum

Papillary
Muscles

Right
Ventricle

Inferior Vena Cava

**Fig. 2.2:**
The heart is a
remarkably resilient
muscle. Shown in
a cut-away view, the
chambers and valves,
with their chordae
tendineae, are
clearly visible.

THE BODY CONTAINS THREE types of muscles, one of which is cardiac muscle, or myocardium. The heart is mainly composed of myocardium, which has unique properties that make it able to meet the demands placed on it.

Unlike other types of muscle, myocardial muscle is relatively fatigue-resistant. In an adult, the heart beats about seventy times a minute, or more than one hundred thousand times in a single day. Incredibly, it never gets tired. The heart pumps about five to seven quarts of blood a minute. Over a lifetime, the heart of a person at rest pumps enough fluid to fill a super-tanker ship with a million barrels. Since the heart pumps much more blood when a person is active, the actual amount of fluid pumped during a life would be even greater.

through the pulmonary valve into the pulmonary artery. Pulmonary means "lung related," and arteries are responsible for carrying blood away from the heart. The pulmonary artery carries blood into the lungs. The pulmonary arteries are a unique element of the circulatory system because the pulmonary arteries carry unoxygenated blood, whereas the rest of our arteries carry oxygenated blood.

In the lung, carbon dioxide molecules are given off by the red blood cells. These tiny molecules travel through the capillary wall into small air sacs called **alveoli** (Fig. 2.4). In turn, the oxygen that we breathe in moves through the alveoli wall and is taken up by the blood. The newly oxygenated blood next passes into the pulmonary veins, which carry the oxygenated blood back to the heart. This oxygenated blood is bright red.

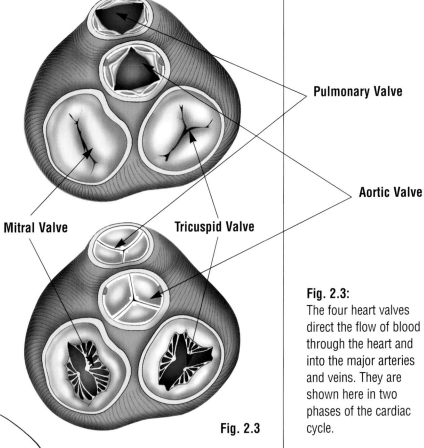

**Pulmonary Valve**

**Aortic Valve**

**Mitral Valve**  **Tricuspid Valve**

**Fig. 2.3:**
The four heart valves direct the flow of blood through the heart and into the major arteries and veins. They are shown here in two phases of the cardiac cycle.

**Fig. 2.3**

**Fig. 2.4**

**Pulmonary Artery**

**Lung**

**Alveoli**

**Alveolus**

O₂

CO₂

O₂

O₂

CO₂

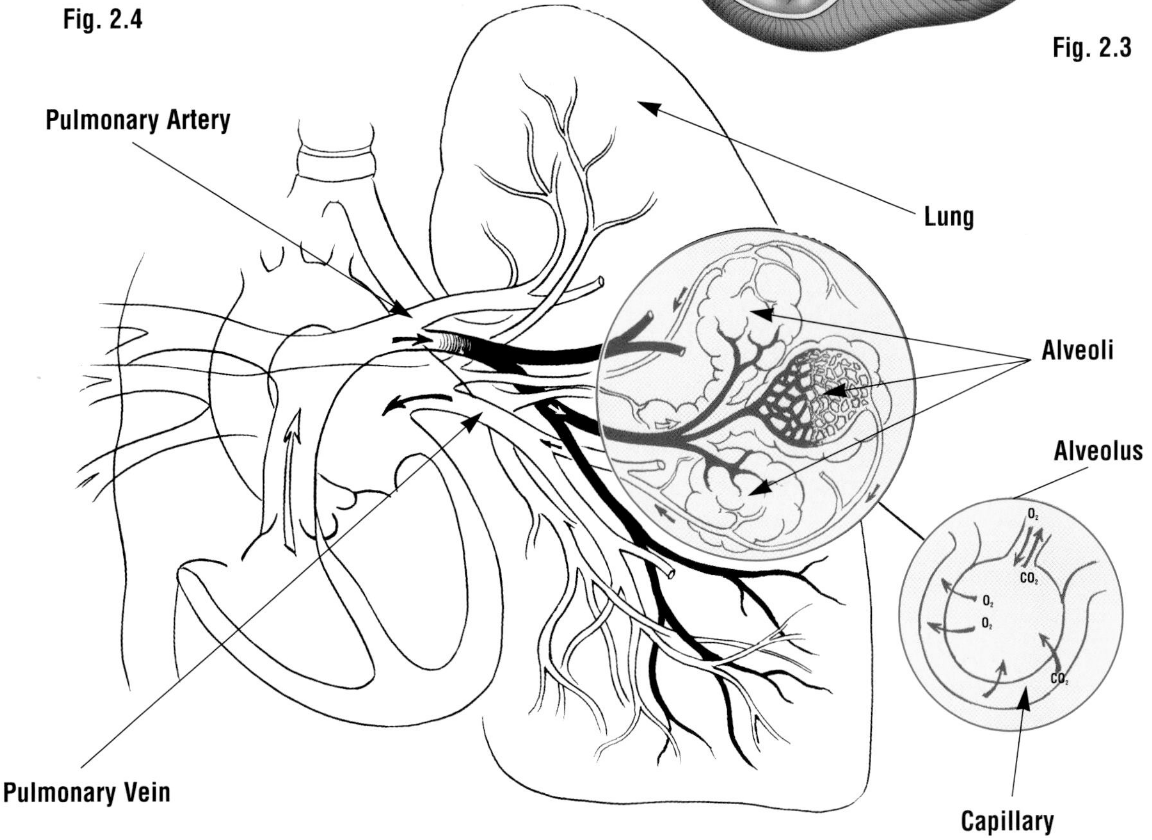

**Fig. 2.4:**
Oxygen transfer takes place in the lungs through the thin membranes of the **alveoli**. When the blood vessels release carbon dioxide, it passes back through the alveoli and is exhaled during respiration.

**Pulmonary Vein**

**Capillary**

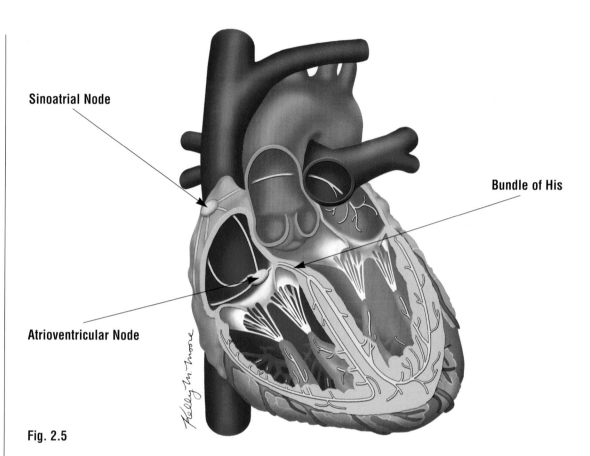

Sinoatrial Node

Bundle of His

Atrioventricular Node

**Fig 2.5:**
The heart's beat is caused by an electrical impulse that travels from the S-A, or sinoatrial, node to the A-V, or atrioventricular, node and through the specialized heart muscle.

**Fig. 2.5**

**Systole:**
Means the heart is contracting. It usually means the ventricles are contracting, but it can also refer to atrial contraction.

**Diastole:**
The portion of the cardiac cycle in which the heart is relaxed.

### The Left Side of the Heart

Blood returning through the pulmonary veins empties into the left atrium. Some of the oxygen is contained in fluid, or plasma, but most is contained in the red blood cells, which are designed to carry oxygen. Once in the left atrium, blood flows through another one-way valve called the mitral valve into the left ventricle.

The left ventricle is the heart's main pumping chamber. As the left ventricle contracts, the mitral valve closes and the aortic valve opens. Blood is forced through the one-way aortic valve into the aorta, which is the main artery of the body and somewhat larger than your thumb.

The aorta first heads upward toward the neck, then makes a U-turn at the top of the chest just before the neck and heads down through the chest and into the abdomen toward the pelvis. It divides into two arteries, known as iliac arteries, which supply the pelvis and legs with oxygenated blood. In the chest and abdomen, the aorta gives off numerous branches to supply blood to the brain, the heart muscle itself, and other organs, muscles, and tissues.

### Blood Pressure

The heart forces blood into the aorta under pressure, which can be measured and is called your blood pressure. Blood pressure depends on the strength of the heart's contraction and the number of beats per minute. It also depends on the volume of blood in the heart and blood vessels and the elasticity of the arteries.

There are two phases of blood pressure. When the heart is contracting, the highest pressure generated in the heart and arteries is known as **systolic pressure**. As the heart relaxes, blood pressure declines, and the lowest pressure level is known as **diastolic pressure**. For example, if blood pressure is recorded as "120 over

# THE BLOOD

BLOOD IS A VERY COMPLEX fluid that both feeds and cleanses the body. It is the means by which oxygen, tiny food particles, and other nutrients are delivered to tissue and, conversely, waste products are removed and eventually discarded by the lungs, liver, and kidneys.

The blood consists of plasma, which is a straw-colored solution, and three formed elements suspended in the plasma: red blood cells, white blood cells, and platelets. Blood travels through an immense network of arteries and veins. Arteries typically carry bright red, oxygenated blood from the heart to the tissues, whereas veins carry dark purple, unoxygenated blood back to the heart. The tiniest blood vessels linking the two kinds of vessels are called capillaries. Capillaries are so small that blood cells travel through some capillaries in single file. The diameter of a capillary can be as small as three or four microns — and there are approximately twenty-five thousand microns in an inch!

The amount of blood in your body depends on your size and some other factors. A person of 160 pounds has about five quarts of blood.

Plasma is mostly water but contains hundreds of other substances, including proteins, digested food, waste products, and electrolytes, which are mainly minerals in solution. There are substances in blood that cause clotting in response to injury. There are also dissolved gases and chemical transmitters called hormones. Hormones, which originate in various glands, activate or deactivate certain bodily functions.

Serum is a term often confused with plasma. Serum is plasma that has had the clotting elements removed.

Each of the three formed elements in blood has a specific function. Red blood cells are produced in the bone marrow and are also called erythrocytes. One ounce of blood contains billions of red blood cells. Their main job is to carry oxygen from the lungs to the body and to carry carbon dioxide from the tissues to the lungs.

White blood cells are also called leukocytes and help protect the body against disease and infection. They are somewhat larger than the red blood cells and are also produced in the bone marrow. There are several types of white blood cells, each with a different function. There are millions of white blood cells per ounce of blood.

Platelets are disk-shaped structures produced in the bone marrow. They are much smaller than red or white blood cells. They are responsible for helping to stop bleeding if a blood vessel is damaged. They clump or stick together around the edges of a damaged blood vessel. As they pile up, they form a seal that helps to start the blood-clotting process so a permanent plug can form.

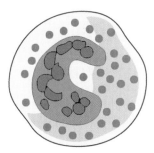

**White Blood Cell**

**Red Blood Cell**

**Platelet**

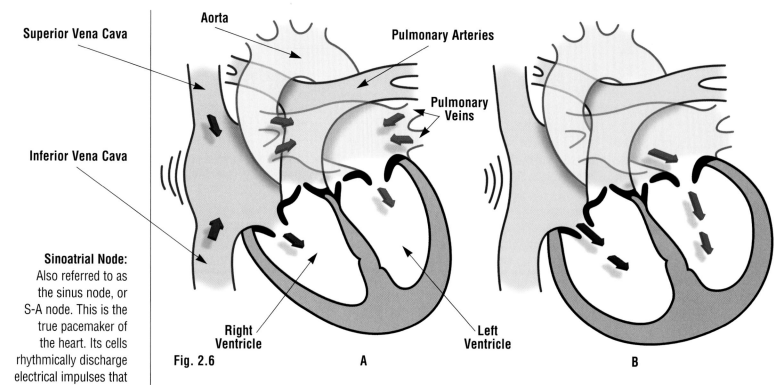

**Fig. 2.6**                  **A**                                      **B**

**Sinoatrial Node:**
Also referred to as the sinus node, or S-A node. This is the true pacemaker of the heart. Its cells rhythmically discharge electrical impulses that cause the heart to contract. These impulses also travel to the A-V node.

**Atrioventricular Node:**
A specialized nerve-type tissue located in the wall of the right ventricle, also called the A-V node. It receives electrical impulses from the sinoatrial node that cause it to relay electrical impulses that cause the heart to contract.

**Bundle of His:**
A special nerve-type tissue extending from the atrioventricular node (A-V node) along the ventricular septum. It helps conduct electrical impulses from the A-V node through the ventricles.

80 mmHg," the highest pressure in the artery measured during systole is 120 and the lowest pressure, recorded in your arteries while the heart is relaxing, is 80.

When you visit your doctor's office, the doctor or nurse will use a device placed around your right or left arm to measure your pressure. This blood pressure cuff and the device it is attached to are called a sphygmomanometer. Its reading is valuable because it can tell your doctor various things about the condition of your heart and arteries.

### The Electrical Conduction System

Heart muscle has another unique quality. The fibers that make up the heart muscle are connected by electrical conduction mechanisms called intercalated disks. These allow current to flow from one muscle-fiber cell to another so if one part of the heart is stimulated, the current will flow through all of the heart muscle, causing the entire heart to contract.

The heart has its own natural "pacemaker" system to regulate your heartbeat (Fig. 2.5). The main pacemaker for the heart is located at the junction of the right atrium and superior vena cava. It is called the **sinoatrial node** or S-A node. This S-A node sets the rhythm of heart beats.

Its electrical impulse spreads through the atrium to a second area of conducting tissue located between the atria and the ventricles known as the **atrioventricular node** or A-V node. The electrical impulse travels through the A-V node along a main bundle of special nerve-type fibers called the **bundle of His** (pronounced "hiss") and from there throughout the ventricles.

This electrical impulse moves through the heart with blinding speed, causing the heart to contract as a single unit. If something happens to the S-A node, such as disease or traumatic injury, the A-V node can take over as the heart's pacemaker.

### The Cardiac Cycle

There are different phases to a healthy heartbeat, or cardiac cycle. During the first phase, the heart is relaxed and blood

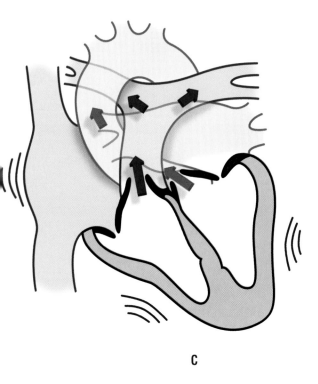

C

flows from the venae cavae into the right atrium and from the pulmonary veins into the left atrium. The tricuspid and mitral valves open, then blood flows from the atria into the ventricles (Fig. 2.6A).

In the next phase, the atria contract and force more blood through the tricuspid and mitral valves, which "tops up" the ventricles. This is called atrial systole (Fig. 2.6B).

Next, the right and left ventricles contract. This is called ventricular systole. The mitral and tricuspid valves shut and the pulmonary and aortic valves open as blood travels into the pulmonary artery and the aorta (Fig. 2.6C).

When the ventricles complete their contraction phase, the pulmonary and aortic valves close. The atria expand again and fill with blood. The ventricles relax

and the tricuspid and mitral valves open, completing one cardiac cycle and beginning another. If the heart is beating sixty times per minute, all of this is accomplished in one second.

In an adult at rest, a heart rate of seventy beats per minute is fairly typical. If you're exercising, such as running, weightlifting, swimming, or playing tennis, your heart rate increases to supply more blood to your muscles, which need more oxygen and nutrients as they work.

**The Coronary Arteries**

As the heart rate increases and more blood is required by the body, the heart muscle itself needs more oxygen. Coronary arteries are the arteries that supply the heart muscle with oxygenated blood. Typically, there are two coronary arteries that branch off the aorta (Fig. 2.1). The right coronary supplies blood to the right ventricle and usually a portion of the interventricular septum. The left coronary or left main coronary immediately divides into two large branches, the left anterior descending coronary and the left circumflex coronary, which supply blood to the left ventricle.

Unoxygenated blood is drained from the heart muscle by a network of coronary veins. Most of these gather in a larger vein called the coronary sinus, which empties the unoxygenated blood into the right atrium.

Much of the heart disease in the United States is caused by blockages of the coronary arteries, and therefore maintaining healthy coronary arteries is a major means of preventing this type of heart disease.

**Fig. 2.6:**
During the phases of a single heartbeat, or cardiac cycle, blood flows into the atria (A), through the tricuspid and mitral valves into the ventricles (B), and then is ejected forcefully into the pulmonary artery and aorta (C). A typical heartbeat takes less than a second.

# WHAT YOU SHOULD KNOW ABOUT YOUR HEART DURING PREGNANCY

By

Pamela R. Gordon, M.D., F.A.C.C.

Associate Professor of Internal Medicine
Division of Cardiology
Wayne State University
Detroit, Michigan

and

a Mother of Three

PREGNANCY POSES A SPEcial challenge to the mother's cardiovascular system. Unlike other vital organs such as the brain or the kidneys, the mother's heart must increase the amount of blood pumped to provide blood to the growing fetus and placenta. The increase is tremendous during the pregnancy and becomes intense during labor and delivery.

Pregnancy is also associated with symptoms that mimic heart disease. Pregnant women often complain of chest pain, leg swelling, and shortness of breath. In women who are not pregnant, these may signal an underlying cardiac problem.

For the woman born with heart disease or who develops heart disease in young adulthood, pregnancy-related risks may increase from the extra demands on the heart. Pregnancy may also unmask a previously undiagnosed heart problem. However, with few exceptions, the majority of women, even those with heart disease, are able to safely com-

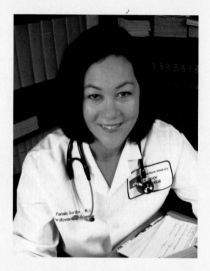

plete their pregnancy with proper, specialized prenatal care.

## Cardiovascular Physiology

In the first three months of pregnancy, a woman's blood volume rises rapidly. This increase continues into mid-pregnancy, then slows down. The average overall increase in blood volume is 50 percent but varies among individuals and is connected to fetal weight, placental size, and maternal weight gain. As a result, larger increases are seen in multiple pregnancies (twins or more).

The number of red blood cells, however, does not increase as fast as the circulating blood volume, which explains why many women develop a relative anemia — the "physiologic anemia of pregnancy." In a woman with normal hemoglobin before conception, a slight drop is average and inconsequential. For the woman who begins her pregnancy with anemia, iron supplementation may help correct a major drop.

Along with the increased blood volume, one of the more dramatic changes that occurs in pregnancy is an increase in cardiac output — that is, the amount of blood pumped from the heart each minute. This is due to the raised blood volume and faster heart rate (an average increase of ten to twenty beats per minute). The maximum increase in cardiac output occurs by approximately twenty-four weeks after conception, after which it plateaus.

On average, the increase in cardiac output during pregnancy is 50 percent for a single pregnancy and increases with multiple fetuses. It is estimated that with triplets, the heart at least doubles its output. Therefore, a heart that before pregnancy pumped six quarts each minute would be pumping twelve quarts each minute in the fifth month of pregnancy!

This rise in blood volume and cardiac output, which increases the work of the heart as it supplies oxygen-rich blood to a greater body mass, is partly counterbalanced by lowered blood pressure. Hormonal changes early in pregnancy relax blood vessels, which in turn lowers blood pressure so the heart doesn't have to work quite so hard. This decrease is greater in the diastolic pressure (the bottom number of the blood pressure measurement). Later in pregnancy, the growth of blood supply to the uterus and placenta further contributes to this decrease.

A common problem in an otherwise uncomplicated pregnancy is high blood pressure, or pregnancy-induced hypertension. This condition is thought to occur from inadequate uteroplacental blood flow and, if untreated, is associated with low birth weight and serious maternal consequences. Fortunately, it can be treated by the use of low-dose aspirin.

**The Last Trimester**

The majority of these changes occur in the first six months and stabilize in the last three months. At that point, body position becomes an important factor. The enlarged uterus exerts pressure on the veins of the pelvis and lower extremities, decreasing blood return to the heart, which results in decreased cardiac output. This is most pronounced when the mother is lying on her back. In up to 10 percent of women, there may be a profound drop in blood pressure and heart rate, causing the woman to pass out. Referred to as the Supine Hypotensive Syndrome of Pregnancy (SHSOP), it is promptly relieved by rolling onto the side, which restores normal blood return. This is the major reason for recommending that late-term women sleep on their left sides.

This posture-dependent decrease in blood return in the third trimester may also reduce the heart's ability to increase output during strenuous exercise.

**Labor and Delivery**

Labor places additional demands on the heart. A single strong contraction forces an extra pint of blood into the circulation. Blood pressure increases substantially, especially while pushing, and is influenced by pain and anxiety. The amount of oxygen consumed by a woman in labor increases three-fold. Pain relief and anesthesia reduce these effects of labor and may be especially helpful in the woman with underlying heart disease.

After delivery, complete return to normal cardiovascular status requires weeks. However, there is an immediate and large increase in blood volume soon after delivery as blood shifts from the uterus back to circulation and pressure on the veins is relieved. Cardiac output falls substantially and nearly to normal within twenty-four hours.

**The "Symptoms" of Pregnancy, and Warning Signs of Cardiac Disease**

The pregnant woman often comes to the doctor's office complaining of symptoms that mimic those of heart disease. Although an examination may reveal signs of abnormal cardiac anatomy or function, it is essential that the physician know the normal signs and symptoms of pregnancy, as well as conduct a thorough history and physical exam. If questions remain after the exam, additional testing or consultation may be necessary.

There are many normal signs of pregnancy. Pregnant women are typically tired. Early in pregnancy, an increase in the hormone progesterone leads to sleepiness. Later in pregnancy, anemia and weight gain contribute to fatigability. The majority of women also complain of shortness of breath, or "dyspnea," by the third trimester. This may be only a "hyperawarenes" of breathing rather than true breathlessness or air hunger. It is normal to hyperventilate in pregnancy, again an effect of progesterone. There is also restriction of the diaphragm, which is the muscle used for breathing, by the enlarged uterus, especially when lying down. This may cause the patient to complain of "orthopnea," or difficulty breathing when lying down that improves in the upright position. Any of these symptoms requires careful questioning, and, if excessive, conditions such as heart failure or low cardiac output need to be evaluated further.

Chest pain, the hallmark of coronary artery disease, is a common complaint during pregnancy. Fortunately, pregnant women are in an age group with a low risk of atherosclerotic coronary disease. More likely causes of chest pain include esophageal reflux (heartburn) or pressure on the rib cage. Typical angina pectoris, the type of chest pain caused by blocked coronary arteries, can be easily distinguished from other causes by history alone.

Many women feel their heart beating during pregnancy. It is usually an exaggerated awareness of the heart beating due to the extra blood volume and perhaps a higher heart rate. During pregnancy, the heart is displaced upward and closer to the chest wall, which also may add to the sensation. Only when the

palpitations are coupled with extreme elevations in heart rate, or with lightheadedness, fainting, or chest pain, should a potentially dangerous heart rhythm be suspected. Outpatient heart rhythm monitoring can rule out an abnormality and reassure both patient and physician. If an abnormality is detected and treatment is considered, there are multiple available and safe therapies.

Lightheadedness and fainting are not unusual during pregnancy. Nausea from early hormonal changes may trigger dizziness. Also, the uterine pressure on the veins causes pooling of the blood in the legs. The pregnant woman may not easily adjust to movement because venous return to the heart is limited. If fainting occurs unrelated to body position or after exercise, additional investigation is warranted.

Also typical during pregnancy, evaluation with a stethoscope

of the increased cardiac output will reveal new sounds. Flow through the enlarged mammary arteries to the breasts, known as the "mammary soufflé," may also be heard. Veins throughout the body, especially in the neck, may appear full or engorged. Leg swelling (edema) eventually develops in most women because of the increased pressure on the veins of the legs and pelvis. This "dependent" edema should improve with leg elevation (above the level of the heart) and should not involve the face and arms.

### Safe Tests during Pregnancy

If there are concerns about heart disease based on symptoms or physical findings, diagnostic tests may be performed that are safe for the developing fetus. An electrocardiogram can diagnose abnormal heart rhythm. A twenty-four-hour monitor or "loop recorder" over weeks may detect an abnormal heart rhythm. A chest x-ray can be performed with proper shielding to protect the fetus.

The most useful test is cardiac ultrasound, or echocardiography, which provides information with regard to cardiac size, function, and structure, as well as blood flow patterns. An echocardiogram can evaluate heart valve abnormalities, causes of heart failure, and a multitude of other cardiac problems. Exercise stress testing and even cardiac catheterization may be performed, if necessary, without serious risks to the fetus. Only cardiac testing that uses radionuclides (e.g., thallium) should always be avoided.

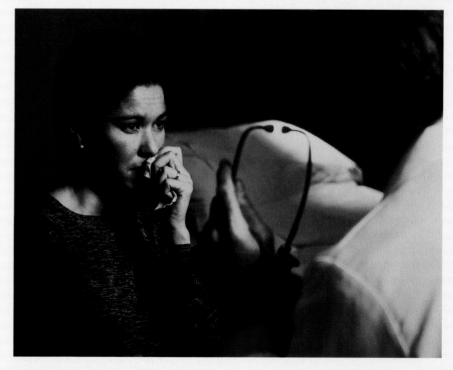

## Pregnancy in the Woman with Heart Disease

Before becoming pregnant, a woman may have a congenital heart defect or acquired heart disease. Many congenital defects can now be surgically repaired in infancy, and the first generation of these patients has only recently reached childbearing age. They represent a new kind of patient for obstetricians and cardiologists.

Acquired heart disease in pregnant women includes primarily rheumatic disease involving heart valves, heart failure, and coronary artery disease. Because many women are now delaying pregnancy until they are older, acquired heart disease is somewhat more common in pregnant women than earlier in this century.

When considering pregnancy in the presence of heart disease, the most important factor is the severity of the heart-related symptoms. In general, patients without symptoms or those only slightly symptomatic enjoy a good outlook for both mother and fetus.

In the moderately or severely symptomatic patient, both maternal and fetal health are at high risk. Thorough evaluation by history, physical examinations, and diagnostic testing will allow the physician to assess the risk of pregnancy to mother and fetus. For the patient who requires drug therapy, consideration of risk to the fetus is especially important. Fortunately, many cardiac drugs can be safely administered during pregnancy.

In some cases, intervention such as coronary artery angioplasty (balloon dilatation of a coronary artery) or surgical repair of a valve may be necessary for maternal survival and cannot be delayed until after delivery. Although risk to the fetus is increased, many of these procedures have been successfully performed with a good outcome for both mother and fetus.

Heart disease in adults generally develops later in life. Although heart disease is not completely preventable, there are many things that can be done to help enjoy a healthy, longer life free from heart disease.

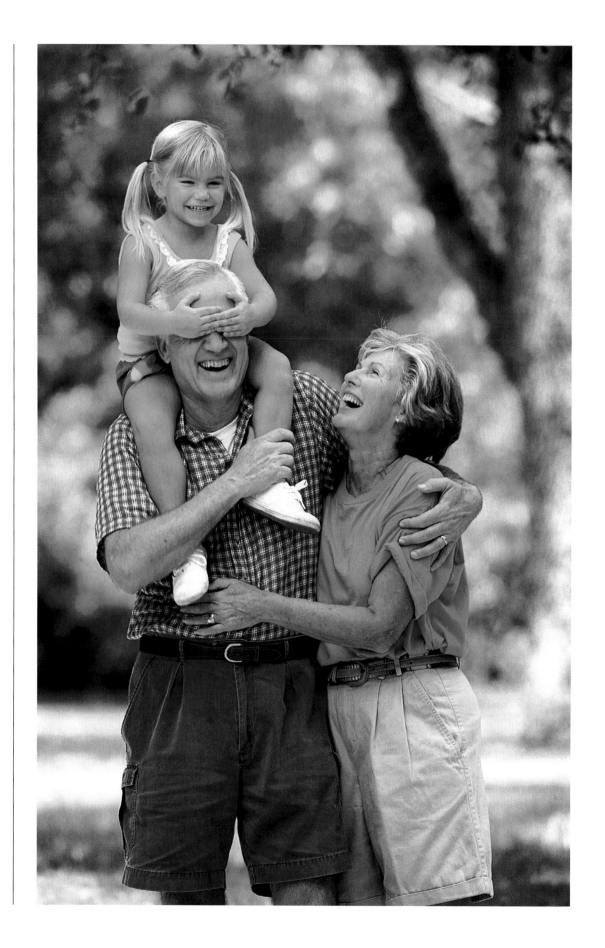

## CHAPTER THREE

# STAYING HEALTHY

HEART DISEASE IN ADULTS IS usually acquired, meaning that it develops or is caused later in life. It can be brought about by **rheumatic fever**, as in the case of some heart valve diseases. Many physicians believe that genetics may play a role in the susceptibility to heart disease.

Obviously, some risk factors cannot be controlled. However, when physicians talk about "preventing" heart disease, they are talking about addressing certain other risk elements that are known to contribute to the development and progression of heart disease — especially **atherosclerosis**, the condition most often underlying coronary artery disease.

### Smoking

People who smoke cigarettes should stop. Smoking is bad for the lungs, other organs and the heart. The chemicals in tobacco smoke increase stress on the heart and accelerate the atherosclerotic process in the blood vessels throughout the body.

Quitting smoking is not easy, but it is very important and has wide-ranging health and lifestyle benefits. There are stop-smoking support groups, and friends and family are often willing to help. Medications can also be prescribed to help smokers quit.

### High Blood Pressure (Hypertension)

High blood pressure (hypertension) is dangerous. If blood pressure is high, the heart has to work harder to pump the same amount of blood, which puts a great stress on the cardiovascular system. Patients with high blood pressure are more prone to heart attacks, heart failure, kidney failure, and strokes. Fortunately, blood pressure can be controlled with appropriate medications and lifestyle modifications, greatly reducing the risk of complications.

Some measures that help to control high blood pressure include stopping smoking, losing excess weight, avoiding excessive salt, and exercising at least three to four times a week.

### High Cholesterol

**Cholesterol** contributes to atherosclerosis, which narrows and blocks blood vessels and can result in heart attack and strokes. Many doctors believe that the ideal cholesterol level for American adults should be less than

**Rheumatic Fever:**
Associated with streptococcus infections, although not actually an infection itself. It usually appears weeks after the infection and may be an allergic reaction to the infection. It can affect the heart, the heart valves, the joints, and the nervous system.

**Atherosclerosis:**
Lipids, cholesterol, and other fatty deposits located on the inner surface and wall of the artery. It can cause coronary blockages and heart attacks.

**Cholesterol:**
A fat-like substance, both produced in the body and present in certain types of foods that are made from animals.

**Low-density Lipoprotein (LDL):** Although it is necessary for the body to function, it is considered the bad type of cholesterol. An excess amount makes a person more prone to developing coronary artery disease and other types of atherosclerotic diseases.

200 milligrams per deciliter (mg/dl) of blood. Studies of large groups of people have shown that when a person's cholesterol level is more than 240 mg/dl, the risk of heart attack is double that of those people with a cholesterol level less than 200 mg/dl. What is an acceptable cholesterol level may actually vary from one person to another. For example, when a person has no risk factors for cardiovascular disease — is not obese, is not diabetic, is a nonsmoker, and has no family history of heart disease — the doctor may be comfortable in regularly reevaluating such a patient with a cholesterol level in the 240 mg/dl range without prescribing cholesterol-lowering medication. On the other hand, when a patient has numerous risk factors or known atherosclerotic heart disease, a doctor will work with the patient to decrease the total cholesterol level to less than 200 mg/dl.

One subtype of cholesterol, **low-density lipoprotein** (LDL), can be dangerous if its level in the blood is excessively elevated. It is desirable to keep the LDL level less than 130 mg/dl. Patients with a level of more than 160 mg/dl are at significantly greater risk of developing heart attacks and other problems related to atherosclerosis. From a practical standpoint, LDL serves as the most important cholesterol-related guide to the risk of heart disease and other atherosclerosis-related diseases.

In patients with known heart disease, such as post–coronary bypass patients, this level should be kept to less than 100 mg/dl. In patients who are not actually known to have coronary heart disease but are at high risk of developing heart disease, such as patients with high blood pressure and diabetes, a positive family history of coronary disease, a history of smoking, and obesity, this level should be less than 130 mg/dl.

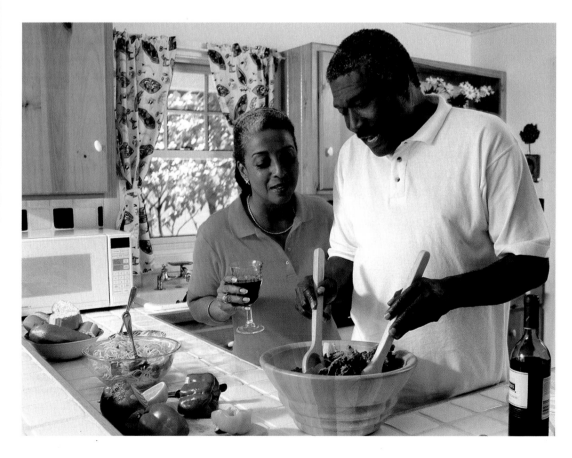

Cholesterol levels are affected by diet. Diets rich in vegetables and fruits — and even including moderate amounts of alcohol — have been shown to help prevent heart disease.

Lowering of the cholesterol level should first be attempted by diet and exercise. If these interventions alone are not successful in obtaining satisfactory levels, a number of very effective medicines can be used. Most of them belong to a class of drugs called the **statins**. These drugs can usually be used safely but require monitoring by a physician with periodic blood tests because certain side effects and complications sometimes occur when these drugs are taken.

It is important to know that not all cholesterol subtypes are harmful. **High-density lipoprotein**, or HDL, is considered the good or protective type of cholesterol. It is desirable to have an HDL level of thirty-five mg/dl or higher, and ideally of more than forty-five. If the HDL level is less than thirty-five, one is at higher risk for heart attacks and strokes.

After your physician checks your serum cholesterol level and cholesterol subtypes (LDL, HDL), he or she will recommend which foods to avoid and medicines to take, if necessary.

**Vitamin E and the Heart**

Vitamin E is an antioxidant found in vegetable oil, wheat germ, leafy vegetables, egg yolks, margarine, and legumes (beans).

A number of recent studies have attempted to determine whether taking vitamin E supplements lowers the risk of atherosclerotic heart disease and heart attacks by inhibiting low-density lipoprotein (LDL, the bad type of cholesterol). In the early 1990s, three studies found no correlation between the naturally occurring level of vitamin E in the blood and heart attacks or cardiovascular deaths. In a randomized, double-blind study, a relatively low dose of vitamin E was tested for lung cancer prevention effects. No effect on cardiovascular mortality was found.

Subsequently, the British conducted a study known as the Cambridge Heart Anti-Oxidant Study (CHAOS). One thousand thirty-five patients were assigned to receive vitamin E in relatively large doses (400 to 800 IU), and 960 patients received an identical placebo. All of the patients in the study had coronary atherosclerosis proven by **coronary angiogram**. The patients were studied for about eighteen months.

There were fourteen nonfatal heart attacks in the group receiving vitamin E and forty-one in the placebo group. However, there were actually more cardiovascular deaths in the vitamin E group (twenty-seven versus twenty-three). The authors published their paper in the prestigious British medical journal *Lancet* in 1996 and concluded that vitamin E supplements substantially reduced the rate of nonfatal heart attacks.

More recently, the August 7, 1999, issue of *Lancet* contained an article by a group of Italian doctors who reported their findings about vitamin E in a group of 11,324 patients. All of their patients had suffered heart attacks and were randomized to receive vitamin E and/or another drug or no drug treatment. The patients were studied for about three and a half years. When the doctors compared the group that had been treated with vitamin E against those patients who had been given no treatment, they could find no cardiovascular benefit in the vitamin E–supplemented group.

In another recent *Lancet* article, Drs. Andy Ness and George Davey-Smith reviewed updated CHAOS data as well as information from a number of other published trials with vitamin E supplements and concluded, "On the basis of all available data, we believe that vitamin E supplements cannot be recommended for patients with coronary heart disease."

In that same issue, Dr. Malcolm J. Mitchinson, on behalf of the CHAOS investigators, replied to Ness and Davey-Smith with the comment, "Their facts seem substantially correct." He went on to state, "No

**Statins:**
A group of lipid-lowering drugs.

**High-Density Lipoprotein:**
This is known as the good type of cholesterol. A higher HDL level is good and indicates one is less likely to suffer a heart attack.

**Coronary Angiogram:**
An x-ray movie of a coronary artery.

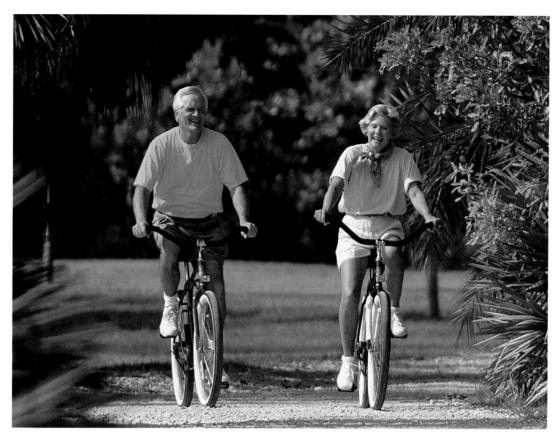

Light exercise like bike riding is recommended for both heart patients and people with no heart disease. It is recommended that people exercise at least three times a week for twenty minutes per session.

one would dissent from the express conclusion that CHAOS alone cannot justify a policy of prophylactic supplementation by vitamin E."

Nonetheless, Mitchinson remains optimistic about vitamin E and its potential cardiac health benefits, and he thinks that cardiovascular benefits will eventually be shown with longer follow-up of the CHAOS patients.

The bottom line is that vitamin E is an extremely important vitamin, and we can't live without it. At this point, however, studies of the use of vitamin E supplements to prevent or lessen the effects of cardiovascular disease have not decisively shown a benefit.

However, more studies are underway, and people who are considering taking vitamin E should check with their healthcare professionals, who are continually updated on this research through medical journals and national meetings.

### Exercise

Exercise is important. This does not mean you have to run the New York Marathon, but you should try to exercise for at least twenty minutes, three to five times a week. Examples include swimming, walking, bicycling, running, and canoeing. Vigorous exercise is not recommended for some older heart patients.

### Stress

Stress and mental attitude can contribute to heart attacks and possibly strokes. Stress can cause elevation of blood pressure. It is caused by many things, including work, school, and relationships.

Lowering stress levels can be very difficult. Learning to relax isn't easy for many people. Sometimes it is a matter of taking the time to do it. There are certain types of exercises, such as tai chi, that contribute to both physical and mental health. If you find you can't do it alone, don't hesitate to seek professional counseling.

### Diabetes

Diabetes is a risk factor for heart disease, but it can be controlled through medication. If diabetes is well controlled, the acceleration of atherosclerosis is not as rapid as it is in patients whose diabetes is poorly controlled. Diabetic patients should have regular checkups for signs of heart disease.

### Nutrition for a Healthy Heart

by Morrison C. Bethea, M.D., F.A.C.S.
Clinical Professor of Surgery
Tulane University School of Medicine
Chief of Thoracic Surgery
Memorial Medical Center-Baptist Campus
New Orleans, Louisiana

Also coauthor of the best-selling *Sugar Busters!*

Nutrition is often overlooked when discussion turns to the prevention or treatment of health problems today. Obesity, for instance, has become an underappreciated epidemic in the United States, especially among children and young adults. The incidence of diabetes has also increased threefold. According to *Scientific American* (August 1996), the U.S. nutritional industry has become a $33 billion business, and healthcare costs related to obesity exceed $45.8 billion annually. In addition, another $23 billion per year is lost in wages and other forms of compensation because people are absent from work for obesity-related problems. Simply stated, fat has become a $100 billion a year problem for Americans.

Most people diet for one of two reasons: either to improve their appearance or to improve their cardiovascular systems. Although proper nutrition cannot reverse atherosclerosis, it can slow its progression. Therefore, good nutrition is an important factor in the prevention and treatment of many heart-related complications like heart attacks and strokes. That brings up an interesting question — how successful have the traditional "healthy heart" diets been, and are they based on acceptable medical fact or just created for consumer appeal?

Most of these diets have concentrated on removing fat, especially saturated fat, from the diet. The American Heart Association recommends a diet with less than 30 percent total fat and less than 10 percent saturated fat. Some experts have even advocated removing all fat from your diet. However, some fats are necessary for the proper functioning of your body. These include polyunsaturated fats, such as linoleic acid and alpha-linoleic acid, and the monounsaturated fats. Many studies have shown that diets too low in fat are actually harmful. They lower total cholesterol levels but often cause a substantial increase in LDL cholesterol, the bad cholesterol.

Keeping this in mind, the guidelines set by the American Heart Association regarding fat consumption are reasonable and healthy. No one should avoid eating lean and trimmed meats, even red meats, to lower fat intake. However, meats should be baked, broiled, or grilled — not deep fried in oil. When cooking with an oil, always choose one that is high in polyunsaturated and monounsaturated fats and low in saturated fats, such as canola oil or olive oil. All fat need not be eliminated, but fat should be consumed carefully and with moderation.

Unfortunately, the low-fat revolution is having a reverse effect as Americans actually get fatter and cholesterol levels still remain too high in many individuals. Obviously, a low-fat diet is a start, but it is not the complete answer. There must be another culprit.

Most body fat comes from sugar, not fat. The body does not store sugar in

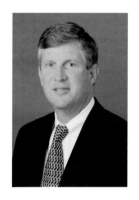

Morrison C. Bethea,
M.D., F.A.C.S.

**Insulin:**
A hormone produced in the pancreas that promotes the use of glucose by the cells and protein formation. Glucose is a simple sugar derived from digested starches, more complex sugars, and other foods. Insulin is also responsible for the formation and storage of fats (lipids).

any appreciable amount, only a few hundred grams as glycogen in the liver and muscles. Most consumed carbohydrates (sugars) are converted under the influence of **insulin** into fat and are stored throughout the body, often in aesthetically undesirable places. In fact, sugar is directly responsible for most cholesterol. Only 40 percent of ingested cholesterol is absorbed from the gastrointestinal tract. Most cholesterol is actually manufactured by the liver under the influence of insulin. The higher the insulin level, the more cholesterol is manufactured. What makes insulin levels rise? Sugar!

Many healthy-heart diets and foods have a reduced fat content but, in most instances, have replaced fat with sugar and, even worse, refined sugar. As fat intake has decreased, refined sugar and processed grain intake has skyrocketed. The average American consumes more than 150 pounds of "added" refined sugar every year.

A healthy diet must address everything — fats (triglycerides); carbohydrates (sugars); protein (amino acids); and fiber. Many people are aware of the harmful effects of too much fat and have taken appropriate steps. Now, people must look carefully at carbohydrate consumption. Attention to correct carbohydrates will involve not only sugar, but also fiber, which has been shown to have a beneficial effect on the cardiovascular system. Only through careful assessment of all foods eaten can anyone make a nutritional difference in their appearance and health. Attention to fat is not enough.

### The Insulin Connection

Until recently, carbohydrates were ignored as a health issue. They are at least as important, and probably more so, than fats in determining weight and cardiovascular fitness. The key to carbohydrates' influence is insulin. Insulin is a hormone secreted by the pancreas in response to a carbohydrate-heavy meal. It is impossible to live without it, but it is possible to live much better without too much insulin. Insulin has many actions, but some of the most important affect body fat, cholesterol levels, and cardiovascular health. Insulin

- ♥ facilitates the transport of sugar across cell membranes
- ♥ promotes conversion of glucose to glycogen and free fatty acids in the liver
- ♥ promotes storage of free fatty acids as triglycerides (fat) and fat cells
- ♥ blocks hormone-sensitive lipase (fat-burning enzyme), and
- ♥ stimulates the production of cholesterol in the liver

The bottom line is that insulin, certainly in excessive amounts, causes the body to produce and store fat as well as produce inordinate amounts of cholesterol.

Insulin is now recognized as an important factor in the development of cardiovascular disease. It is known to act directly on the walls of arteries to produce "atheroma" — atherosclerotic plaques — that can narrow the blood vessels, limit blood flow and oxygen delivery, and result in strokes and heart attacks. Insulin can also cause left ventricular hypertrophy (enlargement of the heart).

### Making Better Choices

Because insulin secretion is a direct result of eating carbohydrates, should everyone stop or slash their carbohydrate intake? Of course not!

The body is primarily fueled by carbohydrates — diets too restrictive in all carbohydrates are unhealthy. However, people should learn to make better carbohydrate choices. This involves avoiding carbohydrates that are highly insulin producing or high-glycemic.

Good carbohydrate choices include high-fiber vegetables, most fruits, and whole grains.

Certain carbohydrates, such as white potatoes, white rice, white bread, corn, and beets, should be avoided or used sparingly. Foods containing more than five grams of added sugar are generally unhealthy. Check the labels of foods for unnecessarily added refined sugar; these foods — even though they may be low in fat — will result in a high insulin response, causing the body to convert and store this sugar as fat.

Eating for a healthy heart and vascular system, as well as maintaining a good appearance and your waistline, involves many facets of nutrition. Just focusing on fat is not enough. People should choose lean and trimmed meats, with an emphasis on reducing saturated fats, and high fiber vegetables and whole grains, avoiding refined and processed products. Also remember to drink plenty of water, about six to eight glasses, throughout the day. However, limit fluids with meals because they dilute digestive juices, making digestion incomplete. Use moderation in portion sizes; too much of a good thing can be bad.

A good nutritional lifestyle will be physically rewarding as well as healthy. Understanding the foods we eat and making good nutritional choices is good pre-

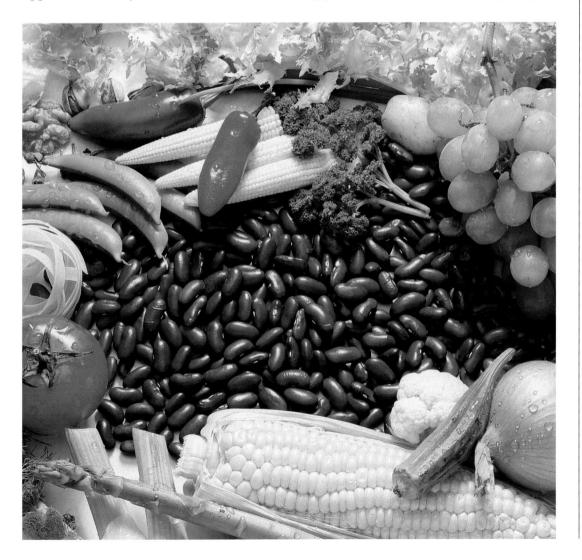

People can learn to make better carbohydrate choices, such as eating high-fiber vegetables, most fruits, and whole grains. Foods that are heavy in refined or simple sugars should be avoided.

ventative medicine. At least in nutrition, the old adage certainly applies: "An ounce of prevention is worth a pound of cure."

## Wine, Alcohol, and the Heart

by R. Curtis Ellison, M.D.
Professor of Medicine and Public Health
Director, Institute of Lifestyle and Health
Boston University School of Medicine
Boston, Massachusetts

Physicians have generally been reluctant to say anything about the health benefits of alcohol. After all, doctors treat patients suffering the effects of alcohol misuse — from drunk driving to spousal abuse to cirrhosis of the liver. They are naturally worried that the public will interpret the message "a little alcohol is good for your health" as an excuse to drink more heavily. Yet there is now a huge amount of scientific data showing that the moderate consumption of alcohol is a powerful preventative factor in heart disease. Likewise, increasing evidence suggests that balanced information on the effects of alcohol consumption may not always lead to increased abuse.

What is the basis for the claim that moderate alcohol consumption may have health benefits?

Epidemiologists have known for many years that people who consume small to moderate amounts of alcohol have less coronary artery disease (CAD) than people who abstain completely. This message was quite a shock to the American public, however, when reporter Morley Safer came on television in November 1991 and talked about the "French Paradox," the name given to the peculiar phenomenon of low rates of CAD in France despite their high-fat diet and cardiovascular risk factors. He attributed it to their regular consumption of red wine.

### Is the French Paradox Real?

For years, we've been seeing large differences in the reported rates of death from CAD among different countries. The rates of premature deaths (before age sixty-five years) among men and women studied at different sites in a study sponsored by the World Health Organization are shown in Table 3-1.

One big surprise is that the French have so few deaths from CAD. This occurs despite the fact that the French consume more fat, and even more saturated or animal fat, than Americans. Furthermore, the French have higher rates than Americans of other risk factors, including elevated blood cholesterol, high blood pressure, and smoking. There are areas in other European countries with rates that are similar to those of the French. The so-called French Paradox (and not the "Spanish Paradox" or "Italian Paradox") lies in the fact that the French consume high levels of animal fat, similar to the intake in Northern Europe, yet have CAD rates similar to those in the Mediterranean countries, where the saturated fat consumption is lower.

There are competing theories to explain this, including a higher intake of fruits and vegetables and a lower percentage of fat intake from red meat, as meat in France is very low in fat and smaller portions are generally served than in the U.S. The theory that has received the most scientific support, however, is that the French

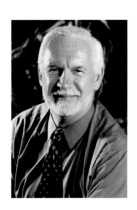

R. Curtis Ellison, M.D.

**Table 3.1:** Premature mortality rates from coronary artery disease (per 100,000 persons aged 35-64)

| Location | Men | Women |
|---|---|---|
| Tokyo, Japan | 37 | 9 |
| Catalonia, Spain | 67 | 10 |
| Toulouse, France | 79 | 11 |
| Area Latina, Italy | 102 | 19 |
| Stanford, California | 189 | 47 |
| Halifax, Nova Scotia | 219 | 53 |
| Belfast, North Ireland | 356 | 88 |
| Glasgow, Scotland | 391 | 133 |
| North Karelia, Finland | 493 | 63 |

consume large amounts of alcohol, on a regular basis, and particularly in the form of wine.

There have been many studies from countries throughout the world connecting the consumption of alcohol to the risk of heart disease. The results have been remarkably consistent: individuals who consume alcohol moderately have fewer heart attacks. In most studies, moderate drinkers experience death rates from CAD that are 20 percent to 50 percent lower than those of people of the same age who are similar in other characteristics except that they do not consume any alcohol. We also see reduced risk of the most common stroke, the **ischemic** or **thrombotic** type, which (like CAD) is related to atherosclerosis.

### How Does Alcohol Reduce the Risk of Heart Disease?

We have identified many of the biologic and physiologic effects of wine and alcohol that relate to protection against CAD. Alcohol affects blood lipids; it increases HDL-cholesterol, the "good cholesterol" that lowers the risk of heart disease. Alcohol also tends to slightly decrease LDL-cholesterol, the "bad cholesterol" that increases atherosclerosis. Thus, individuals who have consumed moderate amounts of alcohol for most of their adult years tend to have less atherosclerosis.

Alcohol also positively affects blood coagulation inside the arteries, which contributes to the second factor in heart

**Ischemia:**
A lack of oxygenated blood flow to a tissue or organ.

**Thrombus:**
Refers to a blood clot, usually in an artery or the heart.

New studies are beginning to show that moderate to light alcohol consumption (one drink a day, six days a week) may have a protective effect on the heart. This explains why some wine-consuming European countries experience relatively lower rates of coronary artery disease despite high-fat diets.

# ATHEROSCLEROSIS: THE GREAT RIDDLE

THE PROGRESS IN HEART SURgery and treatment of general heart disease has been remarkable over the last fifty years. Many conditions that doctors in the 1950s considered fatal are now routinely treatable with a variety of options including drugs (for hypertension, for example), surgery, and less invasive techniques. At the same time these surgical techniques have become accepted, our knowledge of cardiac disease prevention has made incredible leaps forward.

What does the future hold for cardiac therapy? Dr. Michael DeBakey, one of the world's most prominent cardiovascular surgeons, says that atherosclerosis will be the next major medical hurdle. Although the risk factors that contribute to blocked arteries are well known, in about a third of the cases of atherosclerosis, the patients are nonsmokers who eat well and exercise regularly.

"There may even be a viral cause," DeBakey said in a recent interview. "It's the most frustrating problem I've had to deal with, finding the cause of atherosclerosis. Until we know the specific cause of atherosclerosis, we're not going to be able to prevent it. Therefore, until we can do that, we're going to have to deal with the disease. We are educating the public in these risk factors, and there's no doubt they are responding, but the fact remains that the disease is just as prevalent, although we have reduced the mortality of the disease. We will continue to use the methods we have of treating blocked arteries and aneurysms, which are all caused by atherosclerosis."

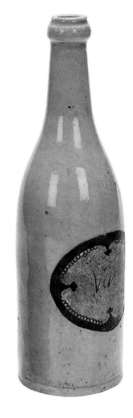

attacks: the formation of blood clots. We now know that alcohol, and especially red wine, decreases the stickiness of the platelets, which form clumps that lead to blood clots.

### The Pattern of Drinking, Not the Amount, Is More Important

Unlike alcohol's effect on atherosclerosis, which develops over many years, the effect of alcohol on thrombosis only lasts for a day or so. For example, after consumption of alcohol, the platelets are less sticky for only a day or two before going back to their usual state or maybe even becoming abnormally sticky.

These results suggest that people who consume alcohol should do so in small amounts on a regular basis, perhaps daily. Unfortunately, most Americans do not have good drinking patterns. They tend to drink nothing all week and then drink heavily — binge drink — on the weekends. This is a very unhealthy way to consume alcohol and is markedly different from the pattern in Europe, where many people have wine with meals every day. Their platelets and other clotting factors are never able to show the rebound effect and become too sticky. The message should be clear: if you drink, consume small amounts regularly. And remember, you cannot "save up" your drinks for the weekend!

Scientific data now suggest that alcohol is best consumed with meals. For any given amount of alcohol, the blood alcohol level rises only about one-half as high when the alcohol is consumed with food as when it is consumed on an empty stomach. Not only does the blood alcohol level remain lower, but combining the fat in a meal with small amounts of alcohol may also have other beneficial effects on the development of atherosclerosis. In a recent study in Italy, the overall mortality for people who consumed wine with their meals was much less than that for those who consumed their wine at other times.

Of all alcoholic beverages, wine is the one that is generally consumed with meals, and some of the benefits attributed to wine (rather than beer or spirits) may actually be related to the pattern of drinking. If one were to select the safest and potentially most beneficial pattern of drinking, it would be regular wine consumption with meals — on most days, but only one or two drinks each day.

### Is Wine the Preferable Beverage for Health?

Many studies cannot show any important differences in heart disease rates on the basis of the type of alcohol usually consumed. On the other hand, we are accumulating new data that suggest that many of the biologically active substances in wine, particularly red wine — substances such as tannins, phenols, resveratrol, and quercetin — are powerful antioxidants, tend to reduce blood clotting, and have other effects that should reduce heart disease risk.

A number of studies have shown that wine drinkers do better than beer and spirits drinkers in terms of disease outcomes. For example, in a large study from the Kaiser Permanente Medical Center in California, researchers found less heart disease among wine drinkers, and not just red wine drinkers, than among drinkers of other beverages. Similar results have been reported from studies in Copenhagen and Scotland. However, at least in some countries, wine drinkers may be different in many ways from beer or spirits drinkers. For example, in the United States, wine drinkers tend to be better educated, have higher incomes, smoke less, and exercise more than beer drinkers. It is difficult to be sure that wine drinkers are healthier because they drink wine or because people who have healthier lifestyles tend to drink wine.

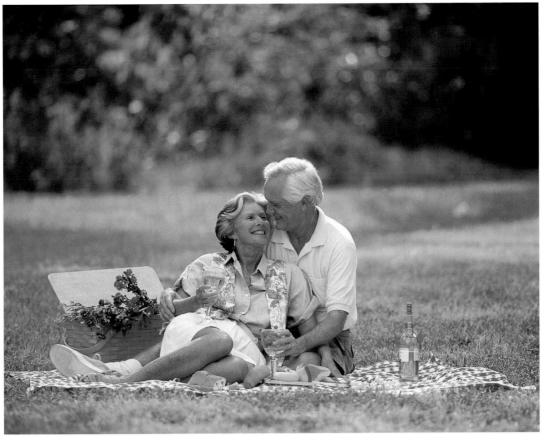

Although all alcohol shows protective benefits, it is perhaps best to drink red wine, which has other health benefits, with meals to aid in absorption and reduce the effect of the alcohol.

I interpret the scientific data as showing that wine probably has additional benefits not found in other beverages. On the other hand, all types of alcohol provide protection against CAD. Patients who don't like wine but are having a cocktail before dinner most nights (and are not having a problem with excessive or inappropriate drinking) can continue to enjoy it.

### Can't We Just Eat a Healthy Diet to Prevent Heart Disease?

Some physicians argue that we do not have to use alcohol to prevent CAD because we know other ways (changes in lifestyle habits) that will prevent heart disease: lose weight and change your diet. But they do not often appreciate how difficult it is for someone to lose 10 to 20 pounds (and keep it off) or how difficult it is for people to permanently adopt a very low-fat and low-cholesterol diet.

Further, our data suggest that the moderate use of alcohol reduces the risk of CAD to a greater extent than would be expected if a healthy lifestyle were adopted sufficient to lower total cholesterol by thirty mg/dl (from 240 to 210 mg/dl) or decrease blood pressure by twenty mmHg (from 140 to 120 mmHg).

### Alcohol and Breast Cancer

Although many studies have shown that breast cancer rates are higher among heavier drinkers, a number of research reports suggest that only a small increase in risk begins to appear among women who normally consume just one or two drinks per day. This is not found consistently in all studies. At our institute at Boston University, we have completed a study of wine, beer, and spirits as they relate to breast cancer by using data from the Framingham Study that has been

# A Few Words About the Dangers of Alcohol

**E**ACH YEAR IN THE UNITED States and around the world, the consumption of alcohol is associated with numerous motor vehicle accidents. In addition, alcohol can be addictive and is the root of many social problems. Alcohol, in excess, is also associated with various health problems, including liver damage and damage to the fetus of women who consumed alcohol during pregnancy. In addition, consumption of large quantities of alcohol over prolonged periods of time can actually cause serious damage to the heart muscle itself.

Recently, however, there has been mounting evidence to indicate that alcohol, and particularly wine, when consumed in moderation, may be beneficial to your heart, particularly in controlling the progression of coronary artery disease.

studying more than five thousand women for twenty-five to forty-five years. We found that the large group of women who never consumed alcohol throughout their lives had the same risk of breast cancer as those who consumed any type of alcohol.

I am not suggesting that all non-drinking women should rush out and start consuming alcohol. Because other studies have shown an increase in risk of breast cancer from even moderate drinking, younger women and women who may be at increased risk for breast cancer should discuss their decision regarding drinking with their own doctors before making changes in their lifestyle. We must keep in mind, however, that a post-menopausal woman in the United States is much more likely to die from heart disease or stroke — diseases for which she would be at a lower risk if she consumed a little alcohol — than she is to die of breast cancer.

### Will Drinking Make One Live Longer?

It depends on how much alcohol is consumed. We know that heavy alcohol consumption or inappropriate alcohol use is very harmful to the individual doing the drinking, those around him or her, and society. But are moderate and responsible drinkers likely to live longer than they would if they did not drink alcoholic beverages? The bottom line for epidemiologists is total mortality. We know that, in most prospective studies, the consumption of one or two drinks a day lowers the death rate. We recently had a report from a very large survey (almost fifty thousand people) done by the American Cancer Society on the risk of dying according to alcohol consumption. Total mortality decreased by 21 percent for men and women who reported that they averaged one or two drinks per day compared with that of nondrinkers.

### What Is the Message?

We know that in the United States and in most other industrialized societies, hospitalization and death rates are somewhat lower for people who drink moderately than for individuals with similar characteristics who do not drink. Thus, from the public health point of view, we should not promote messages or laws directed at preventing alcohol abuse that have little effect on abusers but lead moderate and responsible drinkers to stop drinking. Our health messages should provide scientifically sound and balanced information to permit people to make informed decisions.

In summary, the scientific data are quite clear: light to moderate alcohol consumption is associated with lower risk of heart disease and stroke. We should try to make sure that the medical community, the public, and our policy-makers are kept up-to-date on the scientific findings. And those findings tend to support what St. Thomas Aquinas said more than seven hundred years ago: "If a man abstains from wine to such an extent that he does serious harm to his nature, he will not be free from blame!"

# ANTIBIOTIC PROTECTION FOR DENTAL SURGERY

SOME TYPES OF HEART CONDItions put people at a higher risk to develop infectious endocarditis, or an infection of the heart that can damage heart valves. To protect these patients, cardiologists often recommend antibiotic protection before undergoing surgery, including dental surgery. Your dentist or dental surgeon, in addition to any other doctors, should be made aware if you have one of these conditions before you undergo surgery.

The heart conditions that make a patient susceptible to infectious endocarditis include

♥ People with artificial valves, whether they are artificial or biological

♥ People with most types of congenital heart defects

♥ Patients with mitral valve prolapse with mitral valve regurgitation and/or thickened leaflets

♥ Patients with acquired valvular disease, such as from rheumatic heart disease

♥ Patients with abnormally thickened heart muscle

Patients who have had coronary artery bypass grafting, however, do not generally need antibiotic protection during dental procedures. As always, though, if you have a heart problem, check with your cardiologist and it is recommended to remind your dentist and other doctors about your condition.

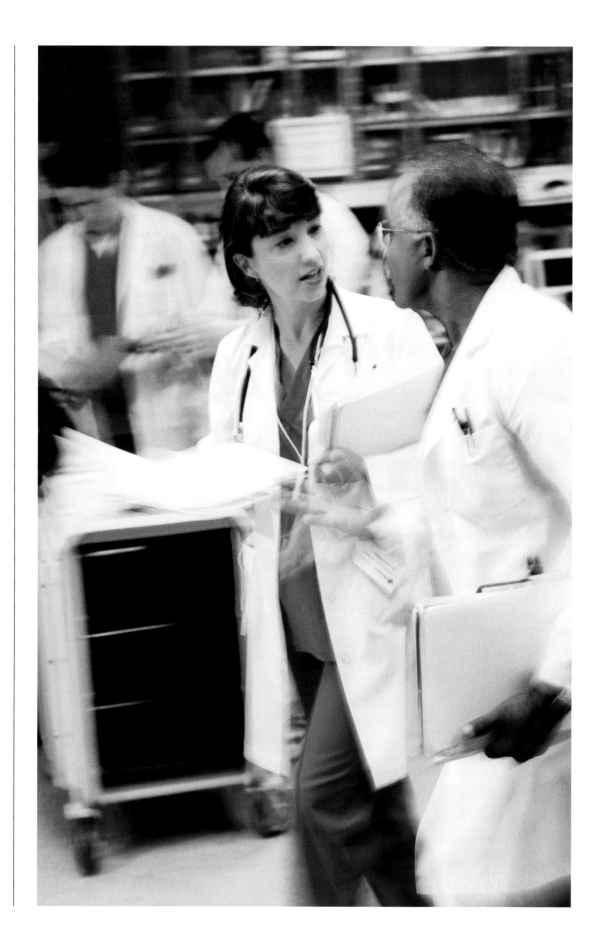

Heart disease can often be identified through signs and symptoms that are detectable before a heart attack or other medical emergency.

## CHAPTER FOUR

# SIGNS AND SYMPTOMS OF HEART PROBLEMS

HEART DISEASE, LIKE MOST DIS-eases, has symptoms and signs that can help you determine if you need to visit your doctor.

A symptom is something like pain or other discomfort. If you were walking barefooted, for instance, and stubbed your toe on a rock, it would hurt. This pain is a symptom. It is subjective and cannot be measured. Your toe may also turn red or black and blue as a result of the injury. This is a sign. You can see the change in the color and so can your doctor.

**History and Physical Exam**

When you visit your doctor's office or go to the emergency room, the first question you will be asked is, "Why are you here?" He is asking you to talk about your symptoms to the best of your ability, such as, "My chest hurts," or "I am short of breath," or "My ankles are swollen," etc.

This information is recorded as the "chief complaint," or the main reason you sought medical help. The doctor will next ask how long you've had this problem and compile what is called a "history of the present illness."

Your general medical history will also be taken: what drugs you are con-suming; if you have had allergic reactions to any medicines; any previous operations. You will be asked about problems related to your head and brain; your eyes, ears, nose, and throat; your lungs and your heart; your abdomen, gall bladder, and intestines; your urinary system and genitalia; your arms and legs; and so forth. That is called a "review of systems."

When the questioning is done, a physical examination will be performed to check the results of the review of systems. Each time you're admitted to the hospital, you will undergo a new history, review of systems, and physical examination.

**Chest Pain**

When people think about heart disease, the first symptom that usually comes to mind is chest pain. However, chest pain can be caused by a number of conditions, only some of which are related to the heart. Following are some common causes of chest pain:

- ♥ gall bladder attack
- ♥ inflammation of the pericardium (pericarditis), which usually hurts more when you breathe

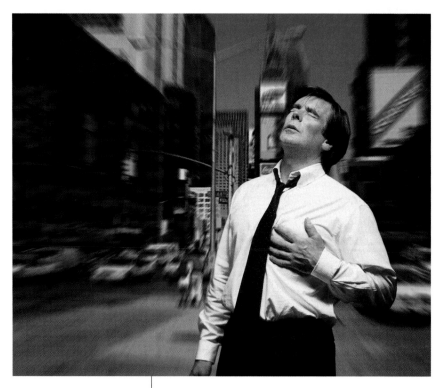

Chest pain, known as angina pectoris, is the classic symptom of coronary artery disease. Chest pain can, however, be caused by other factors.

**Ischemia:**
A condition that occurs when a portion of the body, an organ or tissue, is not getting enough oxygenated blood. It is usually related to a blockage in one of the arteries delivering blood to that area.

♥ back problems
♥ conditions related to the aorta (sometimes the aorta begins to tear apart, called aortic dissection, and this can cause severe pain in the front of the chest or in the back)
♥ conditions in the esophagus and sometimes even a hiatal hernia
♥ inflammation of the lungs
♥ conditions in the upper abdomen

### Angina Pectoris

The most common type of chest pain associated with the heart is a discomfort known as angina pectoris. This condition, related to **ischemia**, is caused when the heart muscle itself does not get enough oxygen through the coronary arteries. Sometimes called simply "angina," the condition is often described not so much as pain but as discomfort. It may be predictable, coming on with exercise and going away with rest, or it may be more unpredictable, coming on at rest and remaining. It can also be brought on by stress or extremely cold

weather. However it presents itself, angina is an important warning mechanism. The body is signaling you to take it easy or a heart attack could develop.

There are several classic symptoms associated with angina, including:

♥ a tightness, heaviness, or pressure
♥ a burning, crushing, or squeezing feeling over a general area in the front portion of the chest
♥ the feeling that somebody has just piled heavy weights on your chest or that your chest is in a vise (it can sometimes almost take your breath away)
♥ a dull, aching pain, usually located just to the left of the breastbone or sternum over the heart
♥ discomfort that radiates from the chest to the back or the neck and even up to the jaw and teeth (sometimes there is only jaw pain that comes and goes with exertion, or sometimes the angina radiates from the chest over the heart, or down one arm or the other, usually the left arm)
♥ in some patients, angina will actually present as a pain or discomfort in the upper abdomen and even cause nausea. When this occurs, it can mimic gall bladder disease, esophageal disease, or stomach ulcers

Angina doesn't always mean pain. Sometimes it just appears as shortness of breath, which doctors refer to as "angina equivalent." In this case, there is usually no pressure or pain.

In fact, some patients experience no symptoms when their heart is not getting enough blood. They may not even have any angina in the midst of a heart attack. This is referred to as a "defective anginal warning system." It is more common in diabetic patients, particularly those who have long-standing diabetes and are being treated with insulin.

Angina that occurs for no particular reason while the patient is resting is referred to as "rest angina." It usually indicates a more severe degree of coronary artery disease. Severe rest angina may even wake up a sleeping person. Usually it can be relieved by putting nitroglycerin tablets under the tongue.

### Heart Attack (Myocardial Infarction)

Although angina doesn't necessarily mean you are about to have a heart attack, any change in your condition should be acted upon quickly. Typical signals of an impending heart attack include angina that is more severe or lasts longer than a few minutes.

The chest discomfort associated with a heart attack, or myocardial infarction, may last for several hours (longer than a usual angina episode) and may not respond to nitroglycerin tablets, or even intravenous nitroglycerin at the hospital. Heart attack victims may require intravenous morphine or other drugs to relieve the pain.

Although heart attack symptoms are usually clear, heart attack victims may not experience any angina and may "just not feel well." In some cases, patients report a sudden onset of heartburn and shortness of breath. These are often explained away as merely indigestion and only later will the actual cause become clear. Sometimes heart attacks are even discovered long after they have occurred, and, in retrospect, patients recall no symptoms at all.

### Difficulty Breathing

The medical term for shortness of breath is **dyspnea**. It is often described as a hunger for air. It can be the symptom of an underlying problem, such as lung disease or anemia, or simply the normal result of exertion, such as vigorous exercise.

There are certain types of dyspnea that occur at night and are usually relat-

ed to heart failure. A person may suddenly wake up very short of breath and have to sit up in bed. A window may have to be opened for fresh air. After sitting upright for a while, the person is finally able to resume a normal breathing pattern. This is called paroxysmal nocturnal dyspnea. Some people must have their head and chest elevated to avoid shortness of breath while sleeping. Some can only sleep sitting up in a chair. This type of dyspnea is called orthopnea.

Dyspnea can be caused by many conditions. In patients with defective heart valves, blood may leak backwards into the lungs. This excess fluid in the lungs causes the lung tissues to swell, resulting in shortness of breath. Other patients may suffer from heart muscle problems, called **cardiomyopathy**. This can cause the blood to back up into the heart and lungs, also resulting in dyspnea.

Shortness of breath associated with heart disease can cause coughing and wheezing, although coughing and wheezing are frequently due to other problems as well, such as lung disease. Smokers often suffer from both heart and lung disease.

Of the most severe forms of heart failure, one type of advanced shortness of breath is called pulmonary edema. In this condition, the lungs literally fill with fluid. Patients are treated with powerful diuretics, which eliminate some excess fluid through the kidneys. They may also be given drugs to help the heart contract more forcefully. In most cases, pulmonary edema can be treated with medicines, but it can be so severe the patient may have to be connected to a mechanical ventilator. If a ventilator is needed, most patients can be removed from it in a day or two. In other patients, depending upon the underlying cause, further intervention may be necessary.

Patients who are short of breath tend to breathe more rapidly. This rapid breathing is known as **tachypnea**. It can be associated with heart failure but isn't always. **Hyperventilation** is a somewhat

**Cardiomyopathy:**
A condition in which the heart muscle is not able to contract or function properly.

**Dyspnea:**
The sensation of being short of breath.

**Tachypnea:**
Abnormal rapid breathing.

**Hyperventilation:**
Breathing fast in such a manner that the carbon dioxide level in the blood falls to an abnormal level.

different type of rapid breathing. If you're hyperventilating, it feels as if you can't catch your breath, and you breathe rapidly. The cause may actually be an anxiety attack unrelated to heart disease. Often a physician is needed to distinguish between tachypnea and hyperventilation.

### Coughing Up Blood (Hemoptysis)

Coughing up blood is occasionally related to heart disease but is more commonly associated with lung disease and other respiratory problems. When it is associated with heart disease, it may occur during acute pulmonary edema, or swelling of the lung tissues. One of the classic causes of pulmonary edema and hemoptysis is a narrowing of the mitral valve, called mitral valve stenosis. This narrowing is a late consequence of rheumatic fever.

### Fatigue

Fatigue, or feeling tired or weak, can be caused by a number of different conditions, including heart failure, depression, a low red-blood-cell count (anemia), or hypothyroidism, meaning your blood is deficient in thyroid hormone. It can also be caused by some drugs used to treat heart disease, like metoprolol, a beta blocker, or verapamil, a calcium blocker. These drugs cause the heart muscle to contract less forcefully. When contracting with less force, the heart muscle does not need as much oxygen and is able to function satisfactorily even when some of the coronary arteries are blocked. On the other hand, because the heart is not pumping as much blood, the patient may feel fatigued, tired, or weak. Sometimes doctors need to adjust drug treatment to reduce fatigue.

Fatigue can also be a symptom of heart failure because the heart is not pumping as much blood.

### Swelling (Edema)

The medical term for swelling, in which tissues become engorged with excess fluid, is referred to as edema. Edema can be caused by a number of

Fatigue is but one of many symptoms that can alert the individual that medical diagnosis and/or treatment is in order.

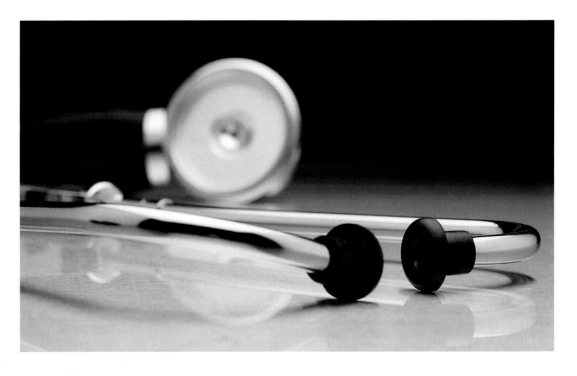

different problems and tends to occur in parts of the body affected by gravity. Swelling may start in the feet and ankles and, as it gets more severe, may involve the entire leg. In certain severe cases it may extend to the abdomen.

Edema can occur in the legs as a result of problems like kidney failure, liver failure, blood clots in the veins in the legs, and local infections in the legs. Sometimes mild swelling in the feet and ankles is related to nothing more than sitting in a chair for a long time, such as in an airline seat during a long flight. It can also be caused by having your legs crossed for extended periods.

If edema involves the lungs, it is usually due to heart failure. The lungs become swollen or edematous, and this is typically what causes the shortness of breath associated with heart failure.

Edema caused by heart failure may first show itself in swollen feet and ankles. The usual treatment is diuretic drugs, which will cause you to eliminate fluid through your kidneys. Heart failure may also be treated with drugs that dilate the vessels, or with a drug like digitalis (also called digoxin or Lanoxin), which has a number of effects but is also believed to cause the heart to contract more vigorously and thereby relieve the heart failure to some degree, thus relieving the swelling also.

A severe form of swelling is called **anasarca**. This swelling extends throughout the body but affects the legs and abdomen more than the chest and the face. It can be caused by severe heart failure. It can also be caused by other problems such as liver failure or kidney failure, and in severe forms of anasarca, one may accumulate extra fluid inside the abdominal cavity, which is called **ascites**.

Edema, anasarca, and ascites, when caused by heart failure, result because the failing heart is no longer able to pump the appropriate amount of blood. As a result, the blood backs up, blood pressure rises in the lungs, and blood is pushed further backwards to the liver and other abdominal organs. This causes the fluid in the blood to leak out through the blood vessels into the tissues.

**Pleural Effusion (Fluid in the Chest)**

Pleura are the thin membranes that line the inner wall of the chest cavity and the surface of the lung. Normally, the pleura of the chest cavity come in contact with the pleura of the lung. Pleural means "related to the pleura," and effusion in this case refers to fluid that has escaped from blood vessels or other small vessels called lymphatics.

Therefore, a pleural effusion is fluid that abnormally collects in the chest cavity between the inside chest wall and the lung. The fluid is not inside the lung. Sometimes, several quarts of fluid can accumulate. When a large volume of fluid accumulates in either the right or left chest cavity, it can interfere with lung function because the lungs cannot fully expand, and this can cause shortness of breath. Pleural fluid usually either is clear or has a slight yellowish straw color. In many cases, it is quite similar to the serum or plasma of the blood, without the red and white blood cells.

There are many causes of pleural effusions. They could develop as a result of heart failure, liver failure, or kidney failure or be related to a tumor in the chest. Sometimes, fluid can accumulate in the chest cavity for other reasons, such as an infection. In this case, the material may be pus. Sometimes the fluid is bloody, and when related to trauma, the fluid may actually be blood.

The treatment of pleural effusion depends on its cause. The simplest and most immediate way to treat a pleural effusion is to do a procedure called a **pleurocentesis**, or "chest tap," in which a small spot of skin on the chest is anesthetized, a needle is inserted through

**Anasarca:**
A generalized swelling of body tissues due to excessive fluid, usually from failure of an organ like the heart, kidney, or liver.

**Ascites:**
An abnormal accumulation of serum-like fluid in the abdomen.

**Pleurocentesis:**
Also referred to as a 'chest tap'. A procedure in which a hollow tube is inserted through the skin into the chest cavity. This is usually done by attaching a needle to a syringe so fluid that is abnormally present in the space between the inner chest wall and lung can be removed.

the chest wall into the chest cavity, and the fluid is drained off. Sometimes, if it recurs or if the pleural fluid is rather thick and won't come through the needle, a small incision is made in the side of the chest and a plastic tube about the diameter of a finger is inserted into the chest cavity to drain this fluid. Rarely, a major surgical procedure is necessary to remove this fluid and treat the underlying cause.

If this fluid is present because of heart failure, it can frequently be treated by medicine that addresses the heart failure. Diuretic drugs cause the patient to excrete excess fluid through the kidneys, and this will help the pleura to reabsorb this excess fluid in the chest cavity.

Small pleural effusions are frequently present after heart operations and usually are reabsorbed naturally during the first few weeks after the surgery. Occasionally, pleurocentesis is necessary to draw off this fluid, and sometimes a second pleurocentesis may be necessary. Sometimes a chest tube has to be placed to remove this fluid. Usually, once it has been treated after heart surgery, pleural effusion does not recur.

### Loss of Consciousness, Fainting, Blackouts (Syncope), and Lightheadedness (Near Syncope)

Losing consciousness, fainting, passing out, or blacking out are medically known as syncope. It is usually caused when the brain does not get enough blood, and it can be related to heart disease and other conditions.

Pilots flying fighter jets like the F-16 can get lightheaded or black out when they make a very tight turn, such as a 9G (nine times the force of gravity) turn, during which blood pools in their legs and not enough of it gets to their head. This problem can be avoided with a special suit that inflates during a tight turn and compresses the legs, abdomen, and chest to keep more blood in the head.

Syncope can be related to disease in the arteries that go from the aorta to the brain. If these become narrow or blocked, the result may be a syncopal episode. In the worst-case scenario, tiny pieces of atherosclerotic material may break off from the artery wall and go to the brain, which can cause a stroke.

A relatively common problem with the aortic valve is aortic stenosis, in which this heart valve becomes blocked and not enough blood gets through. When a person with aortic stenosis is exercising, not enough blood may be getting to the brain. The person may become lightheaded and feel as if they are going to pass out. They may even pass out. It is usually just for a few seconds, but it can be very frightening and even dangerous.

Syncope can also be caused by other heart problems. For example, if your heart beats in an abnormal rhythm called an arrhythmia, your heart rhythm may become very slow, or even miss a few beats or several beats in a row. This causes lightheadedness or even unconsciousness that passes after the heart begins beating again. You may also develop syncope as a result of very fast heart rhythms; so fast, in fact — in the range of 180 to 250 beats per minute — that the heart is no longer able to effectively pump blood. In this case, not enough blood gets to the brain.

### Vasovagal Fainting and Dizziness

Vasovagal fainting (neurocardiogenic syncope) is believed to be the most common type of syncope. It is estimated that 3 percent of emergency room visits in the United States are for this type of fainting. Vasovagal technically refers to the effect the **vagus nerve** has on the blood vessels, but in a broader sense it refers to the effects various nerves have on the heart and blood vessels.

**Vagus Nerve:**
A nerve running from the base of the skull into the abdomen. It gives off branches to various structures, and its main effect on the heart is to slow heart rate.

The two types of nerves that affect the heart and blood vessels are called sympathetic nerves and parasympathetic nerves (like the vagus nerve). If these nerves are too sensitive, they can cause episodes of low blood pressure or slow heart rate or both. This may temporarily starve the brain of blood.

One test used to determine if a vasovagal reaction is the cause of fainting is called the tilt-table test. The patient lies flat on the back on a special table and is connected to an electrocardiogram machine. Under close observation by a physician, the table rotates to an upright position that may cause a vasovagal reaction or other neurologically related type of fainting.

Several medications can effectively treat these types of problems. Occasionally these patients may need a heart pacemaker.

Dizziness is different from lightheadedness in that a person feels uncomfortable, as if the room is spinning, but usually does not feel as if he or she is about to pass out. A good example is the feeling that occurs after getting off a ride such as a roller coaster at an amusement park. Dizzy spells can also be caused by ear disorders or other problems. In many cases, people misinterpret their dizziness as a

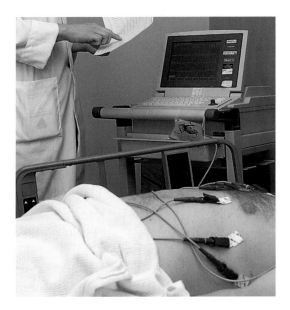

cardiac problem, although it is not related to their heart.

## Palpitations

A palpitation occurs when you can actually feel your heart beating. It may be just one heartbeat that seems stronger than the others or a series of heartbeats — and it can be uncomfortable. Palpitations are sometimes felt when your heart switches into a different rhythm, beats extra beats, or misses beats. Sometimes palpitations are more noticeable at night when you're lying still in bed. They can be felt in your chest, up in your neck, or even in your ear. You may even be able to hear your heart pulsating.

Palpitations can be purely normal, but not always. An abnormal palpitation occurs when you can feel your heart beating very rapidly or skipping beats or there seem to be extra heartbeats. This problem should be brought to your doctor's attention.

Patients who have recently undergone heart surgery frequently complain they can feel their heart beating at night, particularly when they lie on their left side. It's noticed after they are home for a few weeks and have recovered to the point that many of their aches and pains are gone. This type of palpitation is often caused by adhesions or fibrous connective bands forming around the heart due to the heart surgery. One experiences this feeling because the heart pulls on these adhesions as it beats. Usually this is nothing to worry about, and it typically subsides with time.

Your doctor can determine if any palpitation is an abnormal heart rhythm or just the result of one of these other bothersome but less important causes. However, in general, people with heart disease and recent heart surgery also tend to be more sensitive to their symptoms than other people might be. This is understandable.

During an electrocardiogram, or ECG, the heart's electrical rhythm is recorded. This is a useful test for detecting many cardiac abnormalities.

**Skin Color**

Changes in skin color may sometimes be associated with heart disease but can also be due to many other causes. Children's skin may have a bluish tint due to heart abnormalities they were born with in which unoxygenated blood is pumped out to the body. The lips and the fingernails may also be a bluish color. This is referred to as cyanosis.

Adult patients can have cyanosis for other reasons. Lack of oxygen in the blood can be related to heart conditions or other causes such as lung disease.

Interestingly, there is a condition called argyria or argyrosis. *Argenti* is the Latin word for silver. Prior to World War II, there were some antibiotic-type substances that contained silver and were used to treat infection. Over time, the silver accumulated in the skin, turning it a silver blue color. It is a rare condition today. I have seen only one man with this condition and it was very noticeable because his skin was a bright silver blue.

Pale or almost white skin, fingernails and lips are generally not caused by a heart condition but rather by a low red blood cell count, or anemia. In people with darker skin colors, one can look at the color of the tissue beneath the fingernails and toenails to check for cyanosis or anemia.

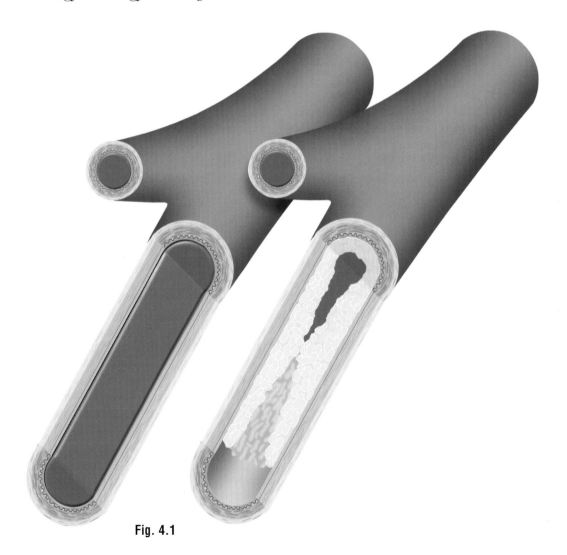

**Fig. 4.1:**
The artery on the left is normal, or open, in contrast with the occluded, or blocked, artery on the right. Blocked arteries can lead to heart attack or stroke by shutting off blood supply to organs like the heart or brain.

Fig. 4.1

66

### Shock

Shock can be caused by a number of different abnormalities and is typically accompanied by very low blood pressure. When shock is related to the heart, we refer to it as **cardiogenic shock**. Cardiogenic shock may be caused by a heart attack in which a large portion of the heart muscle suddenly dies. It may be due to one of the heart valves rupturing, or it may be caused when part of the heart muscle between the left and right ventricles (the septum) ruptures. Another cause may be **cardiac tamponade**, or a buildup of fluid between the heart and the pericardium.

During cardiogenic shock, the amount of blood pumped by the heart cannot keep the blood pressure in a normal range. The pulse is usually very weak and sometimes described as "thready." The skin is usually cool and clammy. Because of the decreased amount of blood getting to the brain, the person's mental condition may be very impaired, even to the point that the person is barely responsive. Breathing may be shallow. Pulmonary edema may be present because the blood is backing up into the lungs, causing the lung tissues to become swollen. Urine output is minimal. If this condition is not treated quickly, the person may die.

### Sudden Changes in Vision, Strength, Coordination, Speech or Sensation

If a person develops sudden changes in vision, strength, coordination, speech, or sensation, this could be due to a stroke. If these signs and symptoms last for only several minutes or less, it is called a transient ischemic attack (TIA). However, if these symptoms persist beyond twenty-four hours, this is called a stroke

or sometimes a CVA, which stands for cerebral vascular accident.

Strokes can result from many different causes. They can be caused by a blood clot breaking loose from the heart or arteries and traveling to the brain. This is called an embolic stroke. An **embolus** is something, usually a blood clot or atherosclerotic material, that breaks loose and travels through the blood vessels. An embolism could occur as the result of an infected heart valve from which a clump of infected tissue breaks off and travels to the brain. Another common type of embolism occurs when a piece of cholesterol breaks off from plaque in an artery and travels elsewhere (Fig. 4.1).

Strokes also occur as a result of a problem in the brain itself, such as blocked blood vessels, the rupture of an aneurysm, or other types of bleeding. Strokes can affect the function of your arms or legs, vision, speech, and swallowing, ability to think, and sometimes other bodily functions. Stroke victims can even go into a coma or die.

### Leg Pain (Claudication)

Leg pain caused by a lack of oxygenated blood getting to the leg muscles is referred to as claudication. This typically results from the same atherosclerotic process that blocks coronary arteries. As you exercise your legs, by walking for example, they feel tired and start to ache. Resting causes the aching and tiredness to go away, and you can get up and walk further. The claudication may occur in various portions of the leg, including the calf, thigh, or buttocks, depending on where the artery is blocked. However, tiredness in the legs or leg pain can also be due to other causes, including disc problems in the lower back.

**Cardiogenic Shock:** A serious condition in which the heart is unable to pump enough oxygenated blood to adequately supply the body's tissues.

**Cardiac Tamponade:** A process in which fluid or blood clots build up between the heart and the pericardium. It interferes with heart function and may cause the heart to fail and even cause death.

**Embolism:** The partial or complete blocking of a blood vessel by an object traveling through the bloodstream (usually a blood clot).

# YOUR VISIT TO THE CARDIOLOGIST

By

## John B. O'Connell, M.D.

Cardiologist
Professor and Chairman
Department of Internal Medicine
Wayne State University School of Medicine
Detroit, Michigan

Physician-in-Chief
Detroit Medical Center

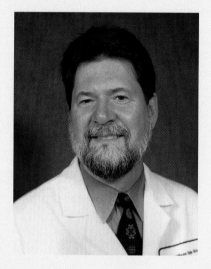

A CARDIOLOGIST IS A PHYsician who has graduated from an accredited medical school and completed three years of internal medicine residency training followed by three or four years of cardiology training. Most cardiologists are part of a larger group, which is sometimes contained within a broader group of medical specialists including primary care physicians. Besides general cardiologists, there are many different subspecialties in cardiology. Those with added knowledge in interpretation of diagnostics are called noninvasive cardiologists. Those with special certification in the use of radioisotopes are called nuclear cardiologists. Cardiologists may also specialize in interventional cardiology, meaning they are experts in the use of angioplasty and stenting. Additionally, cardiologists may specialize in electrophysiology, which is the study of rhythm disturbances or problems with the electrical conduction system of the heart. These cardiologists may prescribe high-

ly specific drugs to treat irregularities in the heart rhythm or use devices (like implantable cardioverter defibrillators and pacemakers) designed to regulate the heart rhythm or trigger the heartbeat. Other cardiologists have specialized in treatment of advanced heart failure and heart transplantation.

## Why See a Cardiologist?

Most people see a cardiologist because of a referral from their primary care physician for chest

pain. In some cases, the cause of the chest pain is known to be coronary artery disease, and the referral is made for more advanced diagnostic testing and treatment; in other cases, the cause of the chest pain is unknown. Other common reasons for referral include shortness of breath, congestive heart failure not responsive to standard medical treatment, irregularities in the heart rhythm, blackout episodes (syncope), or palpitations.

In the past, almost all cardiologists accepted referrals only from physicians. However, a welcomed change is the self-referral, i.e., the patient feels they should see a cardiologist. More cardiologists are welcoming this source of patients.

Sometimes, there is little choice of cardiology referral. This is often the case when your insurance carrier or health maintenance organization (HMO) mandates the specific reason for the referral (requiring extensive documentation by the primary care physician), and the cardiologist is willing to agree to the insurance company's financial arrangements and care plans. This method of referral is the least acceptable to patients and physicians alike.

### How Is a Cardiologist Chosen?

If there is flexibility in referral and the referral is through your primary care physician, that physician will commonly choose a cardiologist with whom they have a close relationship. Communication between the primary care physician and the cardiologist is critical to a successful diagnostic and treatment plan. Your primary care physician knows the most about you and will presumably have a close relationship with you. Consequently, they will be able to interpret the complexities of the visit to a cardiologist. Typically, the cardiologist they choose will be in close proximity and often practice in the same hospital environment and sometimes even in the same professional building or practice group.

Cardiologists are highly visible subspecialists, and, as a result, reputation is another common reason for referral. It is appropriate to ask your physician what other patients may have been referred to this cardiologist or to ask members of your social group or church about that cardiologist.

If you have the option of choosing your own cardiologist, you will probably choose one based on local reputation. However, some standards for academic excellence have been established. Board certification is increasingly a re-

quirement for hospital staff privileges in cardiovascular disease. A cardiologist is certified by the American Board of Internal Medicine in cardiovascular diseases.

Your local medical society has a roster of physicians in your community and their board certification status. Additionally, internet sites such as WebMD's at **www.webmd.com** have a directory of most physicians. The major professional organization for cardiologists is the American College of Cardiology, which also lists cardiologists, including board certification and fellowship (FACC) status, on its website, **www.acc.org**.

Board certification should not be the only criterion because many practicing cardiologists are board certified. Other public databases may list mortality for invasive procedures by each physician.

However, do not be fooled by simple mortality statistics. For example, a cardiologist who is willing to perform highly technical procedures on patients at high risk may have a higher mortality than a physician who routinely selects only the low risk candidates. Physicians who perform high-volume procedures on sick patients are most qualified to care for most problems.

Another major issue relates to the relationship between cardiologists and cardiac surgeons. Many of the diagnostic studies may lead to coronary bypass surgery or valve replacement or repair. The close working relationship between the cardiologist and the cardiac surgeon is part of the equation that should be used in choosing the specialist. Therefore, local reputation,

access, and understanding the quality of the cardiac surgical program should be considered in the decision. Finally, the reputation of the hospital as a cardiovascular medicine and surgical center is also part of the equation because those centers with national reputations for the quality of their cardiovascular medical and surgical teams are highly selective about the physicians on their staff.

### What Will Happen during My First Visit to the Cardiologist?

A typical cardiologist's office has the capability for many diagnostic tests. The cardiologist's staff is familiar with cardiac problems and trained in cardiopulmonary resuscitation.

Before you see the cardiologist, a nurse or staff member will usually review your history, make sure your prior medical records are available, and perform an electrocardiogram (EKG or ECG). This is considered an extension of the cardiac examination. Although many tests provide more specific information, an electrocardiogram remains a major screening tool for rhythm abnormality, evidence of blood vessel disease, and damage to the heart, or heart muscle problems.

However, the ability of an electrocardiogram to give specific diagnoses is very limited. A cardiologist will complete a standard history and physical, and you will be asked to rehash information that you have already given to another physician. This is because of the very specific probing questions to which cardiologists will seek answers in an effort to home in on your problem.

During the initial visit, the cardiologist will probably only obtain tests to help diagnose the problem. Very typically, these will be noninvasive tests (no tubes or instruments inserted into your blood vessels other than perhaps an intravenous line). After these tests, the cardiologist will inform you of the results.

Once the results of the initial tests have been evaluated, further testing may be needed, and an invasive test (in which instruments or tubes are threaded through your blood vessels) may be prescribed. In some cases, you may be referred to a cardiology subspecialist.

During the course of this testing, the cardiologist will communicate directly with your primary care physician. Do not be intimidated if you are self-referred; physicians widely recognize the importance of second opinions, and your self-referral should not place a wedge between you and your primary care physician.

**Typical Diagnostic Tests**

*Noninvasive Testing*
Frequently, noninvasive tests may be used as screening tools before more complicated invasive testing. The most common non-invasive diagnostic tests include those designed to assess the probability of coronary artery disease and review heart muscle function.

The test often used to detect coronary artery disease is the treadmill exercise stress test. In some cases, a simple exercise test is performed in which the patient is monitored by an electrocardiogram during a walk on a treadmill that will increase its speed and slope until either a target heart rate is reached or a symptom or electrocardiographic finding worthy of discontinuation of the test results. In more complicated situations, including an abnormal resting electrocardiogram or poor specificity of treadmill testing in a subgroup population (such as in women, for whom the test is not as accurate), a nuclear or echocardiographic study may be added.

In the case of a nuclear study, a radioisotope, usually either thallium or Sestamibi (Cardiolyte), is injected into your vein during peak exercise, and your heart is imaged. You will be asked to return four to six hours after the initial imaging for a second scan. This image will give the cardiologist a view of what blood flow to your heart is like during rest, and the first image will show coronary blood flow during exercise. If coronary blood flow is abnormal during exercise but normal during rest, coronary artery disease is likely, and the cardiologist may request a catheterization.

In the case of stress testing with ultrasonic techniques, an echocardiogram will be performed at successively harder levels of exercise. If segments of the heart muscle contract less vigorously during exercise than they do at rest, there is evidence for blood vessel disease, and cardiac catheterization in all likelihood will be recommended. In some highly specialized centers, measurements of coronary blood flow may include very sophisticated technology such as magnetic resonance imaging (MRI) or positron emission tomography (PET scanning).

If you are unable to exercise or walk on a treadmill, there are drugs that may be given (dipyridamole, adenosine, or dobutamine) that will enhance abnormalities in coronary blood flow so that they can be imaged with nuclear or echocardiographic techniques.

If your problem relates to congestive heart failure, abnormalities of your heart valves, or increased thickness of your heart muscle, an echocardiogram, or an ultrasound scan of your heart, gives the cardiologist much information. Sometimes the abnormalities in the back of your heart or your chest do not conduct sound waves well. The cardiologist may then suggest a transesophageal echocardiogram (TEE), during which the probe is swallowed and your heart is seen from your esophagus. If you have abnormalities in blood vessels other than in your heart, a Duplex scan utilizing ultrasonic/Doppler techniques to determine flow may be applied.

If your abnormality includes your heart rhythm, a Holter monitor is quite valuable. This is a small device the size of a transistor radio that records your ECG for a day or two while you record any symptoms you may have in a diary. If the palpitations or lightheaded episodes that bring you to the cardiologist occur only once in a while, an event monitor may be utilized. You can take this monitor home and call a station where heart rhythm detection occurs through a telephone monitor.

*Invasive Testing*

If a noninvasive test indicates you have serious problems with your heart rhythm or possible blood vessel disease, an invasive test may be ordered.

Cardiac catheterization with coronary angiography is the most common invasive test. During this test, pressures within the heart are measured, dye may be injected into the left ventricle, and dye is injected into each of the blood vessels that supplies blood to the heart. An x-ray movie of the heart is then made.

If the obstruction to blood flow is localized, it can be repaired by balloon angioplasty and/or stenting (see Chapter Six). That procedure may be done at the same time as the cardiac catheterization. A simple diagnostic catheterization may require only a few hours at the hospital. An interventional procedure may take longer in the hospital, but generally less than one day.

Your cardiologist will discuss the result of your tests. If your problem is not a blood vessel in your heart but one of your other major vessels such as a blood vessel to your legs, the cardiologist may dilate those blood vessels as in coronary angioplasty.

If the problem is a rhythm disturbance, an electrophysiologist can perform an electrophysiologic study, in which your heart is stimulated and the heartbeat measured. Essentially, this is a very sophisticated and highly sensitive electrocardiogram. As a result of this procedure, a recommendation may be made for a pacemaker or for an implantable cardioverter defibrillator. This placement is generally performed by the same electrophysiologist.

## When Does a Cardiologist Refer Patients to a Cardiac Surgeon?

In the event of coronary artery disease, for example, a cardiologist will refer you to a heart surgeon when blood vessel disease affects multiple vessels and angioplasty is not practical. The cardiac surgeon will then review the angiogram and consult with the cardiologist regarding the best surgical approach for coronary artery bypass grafting.

Once the referral to a surgeon is made, your cardiologist will continue to see you immediately before and immediately after surgery. After hospitalization, which is generally less than one week, the cardiologist and surgeon will both see you in follow-up until your surgical wound is healed, at which time the surgeon will typically send you back to the cardiologist for care.

If your postoperative course was not complicated, your cardiologist will typically refer you to the primary care physician but will see you at regularly scheduled intervals: three months, six months, and one year after surgery.

Typically, an exercise stress test will be performed either three or six months after surgery and annually thereafter. Measurement of cholesterol level will occur within six weeks of surgery, and the cardiologist and primary care physician will confer about "secondary prevention," i.e., treatment measures designed to reduce and reverse the blood vessel disease (atherosclerosis) that caused your visit.

Cardiologists work in concert with primary care physicians and cardiac surgeons. They are part of a team of physicians that are directing their efforts toward the well-being of your heart and blood vessels.

However, the ultimate determinant of the success of cardiovascular care is the patient, because you are the fourth member of the team. As a team member, it is your responsibility to ask all the questions you may have.

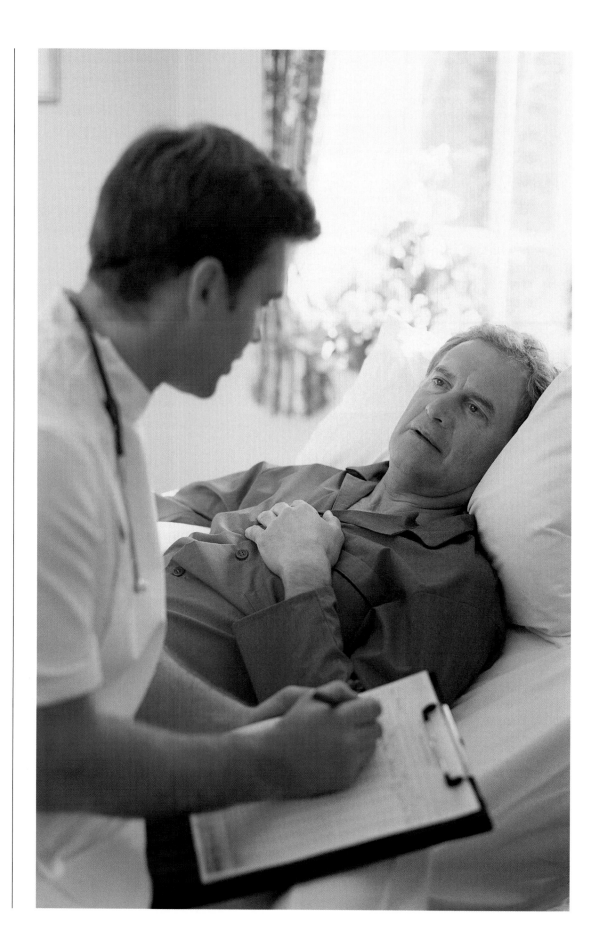

During diagnosis,
a patient's medical
history is obtained.

## CHAPTER FIVE

# DIAGNOSING A PROBLEM

ONCE A PHYSICIAN KNOWS THE symptoms, a series of tests will help determine a diagnosis. "Diagnosis" literally means a determination of the cause of a problem, and diagnostic tests are done to find out what's causing the symptoms. In many ways, doctors are like detectives in that they are presented with a case and have to search out culprits and causes. Diagnosing illness is an art form unto itself, and doctors use some very sophisticated techniques.

### Electrocardiogram

Among the most common tests is the electrocardiogram, which is referred to as either an ECG or an EKG. EKG is short for electrokardiogram, which is a historical spelling that resulted because much of the test's early development was done in Holland. Dr. William Einthoven, professor of physiology at the University of Leiden, received the 1924 Nobel Prize in Physiology or Medicine for his work in developing the electrocardiograph.

An ECG or EKG should not be confused with an EEG, which stands for electroencephalogram and is used to detect brain waves much as the ECG measures electrical activity in the heart.

An ECG is performed by placing electrode patches on the chest and extremities and connecting them to an ECG machine. The sensors pick up electrical activity and send the results to a printer, where they are printed on a piece of paper. Results can also be displayed on something similar to a television screen so they can be constantly monitored in an intensive care unit or other medical facility.

Much information can be obtained from an electrocardiogram, including heart rhythm, heart rate, and estimates of the level of oxygenated blood reaching the heart. If the reading is abnormal, the doctor might be able to determine what is causing the abnormality from that reading alone. The ECG can help determine if a heart attack is occurring and also reveal where in the heart the damage is located. Some forms of congenital heart disease and some forms of valvular heart disease also can be strongly suspected on the basis of an electrocardiogram.

### Exercise (Electrocardiogram) Stress Test

In its simplest form, an ECG exercise stress test is performed to look for coronary artery disease or blocked coronary arteries. Coronary artery disease is not always apparent on a resting electrocardiogram but is often visible on an ECG made while the heart is working and requires more oxygenated blood.

To perform this test, the patient is asked to walk on a treadmill while symptoms, electrocardiogram, and blood pressure are monitored. If the working heart's demand for blood is greater than the amount the coronary arteries can supply, the electrocardiogram may become abnormal, telling the doctor which areas of the heart are not getting enough blood, or are ischemic. Patients might develop angina during the test, which often correlates with changes in the electrocardiogram. Other variables, such as blood pressure and heart rate changes, can occur during the ECG exercise stress test. These might lead a physician to suspect coronary artery disease.

If patients cannot exercise for some reason, the heart is stressed with drugs that dilate the arteries (such as dipyridamole or adenosine). Sometimes drugs are used to make the heart beat faster and harder. Dobutamine is one drug of this type. Atropine is another drug that results in a faster heart rate.

### Ambulatory Electrocardiographic Monitoring

Another form of ECG is ambulatory electrocardiographic monitoring, also referred to as Holter monitoring. In this test, the ECG electrodes are connected from the patient to a portable ECG machine that contains a tape recorder. The patient's ECG is monitored while the patient is performing normal daily activities over a day or two. This is usually done when **arrhythmias** or blackout spells have occurred or are suspected.

Patients are allowed to go home and asked to keep a record of their normal activities during the monitoring period. If a patient has an abnormal event, such as a sensation that the heart rate has sped up or the feeling that an abnormal heart rhythm is occurring, he or she presses a button on the ECG recorder to mark the exact time of the symptoms.

The ECG can also be checked over the telephone. Telephone checks can be helpful in patients with pacemakers because pacemaker activity can be monitored without the need to travel to the doctor's office. To do this, an electronic device with an electrode is attached to the skin and then connected to the telephone. The physician at the other end has to have the necessary equipment so the ECG can be transmitted and printed out.

### Echocardiography

Echocardiography is somewhat like the sonar used to detect a submarine under water. High-frequency sound waves are bounced off the heart to create an image of its structures. This is a relatively simple test using a sound probe placed at various locations on the chest. With this test, a doctor can image the heart while it is actually pumping. These pictures are recorded on video tape for a cardiologist to play back

Usually, echocardiograms are performed in one of two different manners. One type is called a transthoracic echocardiogram. From the patient's standpoint, it is not much different from having an electrocardiogram. The patient lies still while a technician places a probe on the chest and obtains an image, or movie, of the beating heart.

The other type is called a transesophageal echocardiogram (TEE) and is somewhat more involved. The throat is anesthetized, and a sound probe is passed through the mouth, into the throat, and down into the esophagus. The echocardiogram is obtained while the probe is slowly moved back and forth in the esophagus. In the esophagus, the probe is just a half inch from the heart and thus can

**Arrhythmia:**
Any abnormal heart rhythm. Also called dysrhythmia.

74

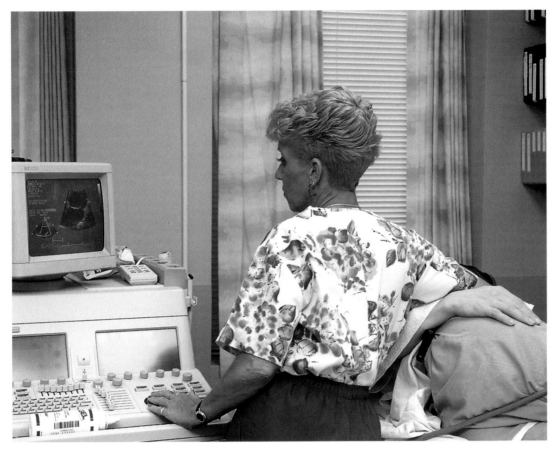

Echocardiograms are very useful for obtaining pictures of the moving heart to diagnose heart disease, valve malfunctions, and other abnormalities. The test, which can be done with probes moved across the chest or inside the esophagus, uses sound waves to obtain an image that can be transferred to a computer screen.

produce highly detailed images of the heart structures.

In most cases, the simpler transthoracic type of echocardiogram is all that is needed. However, a TEE yields a more detailed view of the heart and major blood vessels, which helps if the doctor is assessing the mitral valve or certain other cardiac structures.

With either type of echocardiogram, doctors can see the size of the heart chambers and how well they are functioning. They can see blood clots if present in the heart, fluid around the heart, and problems with valves, such as blockage. Using cardiac Doppler flow studies, they can also see whether heart valves are leaking or if they are narrowed (stenotic). If the patient has an artificial heart valve, doctors can determine whether the valve is functioning properly.

Echocardiograms can also be used to detect problems in the thoracic aorta, which is the part of the aorta in the chest, and to estimate blood pressure in the pulmonary arteries. In certain heart and lung conditions, the pulmonary artery pressure can be abnormally elevated, which is something a physician needs to know.

### Exercise Echocardiogram

The exercise echocardiogram is another type of stress test. This test combines exercise and echocardiogram pictures to show the contraction of the heart. After a resting test is performed, the patient is asked to walk on a treadmill. The results of this test are compared with the resting echocardiogram.

If segments of the heart are no longer contracting well, it can be concluded that these areas are not getting enough oxygenated blood. There may be a coronary artery blockage. If one is unable to exer-

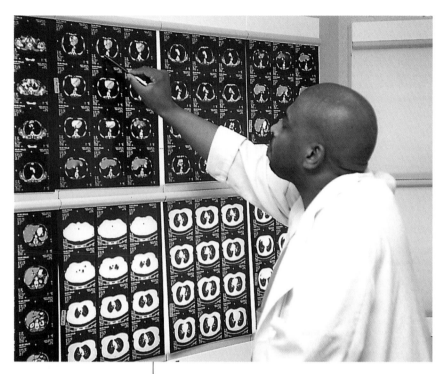

The chest computed tomography scan, or CT scan, is a more sophisticated type of x-ray. This test allows three-dimensional viewing of the heart and is used to help detect abnormalities like aortic aneurysms or aortic dissections.

ray machine to "shoot" the picture from the front.

A chest x-ray is a valuable tool. Doctors use chest x-rays to determine the size and shape of the heart, the shape of the arteries coming out of the heart, and to look at the lungs and other chest structures. They can also tell if the heart or one of its chambers is enlarged. With routine chest x-ray pictures, doctors can frequently tell if calcium has collected on the heart valves or in the aorta or can even see calcium in coronary arteries. Calcium deposits may suggest certain types of disease. If heart failure is present, doctors can determine if the lungs are congested and to what extent. They can also determine how effective a certain treatment is in improving heart failure and decreasing lung congestion.

The ECG and the routine chest x-ray are used as screening tests. They are simple to obtain and very useful. If heart disease is suspected, more sophisticated tests will be obtained.

cise for whatever reason, drugs can be used to induce heart stress. Otherwise, the testing procedure remains the same.

### The Chest X-Ray

Routine chest x-rays are typically taken from two different views. One is called a PA chest x-ray, for "posterior-anterior," which means back to front. The patient stands facing the x-ray film plate with the x-ray machine behind him. The other routine chest x-ray is the lateral view, which is taken either from right to left or from left to right so that the doctor can look at the chest from the patient's side. The PA and lateral views are complementary.

A chest x-ray can also be taken with the patient's back to the x-ray film plate and the x-ray beam aimed from the front through the patient's chest. This is called an AP chest x-ray, for "anterior-posterior." The PA film is usually preferred because radiologists feel it gives a better picture. In an intensive care unit or a patient's room, however, it is more convenient to put the x-ray film plate behind the patient and use a portable x-

### Chest Computed Tomography

The chest computed tomography (CT) is a more sophisticated type of x-ray in which scanning x-ray beams are used to take pictures of the chest from several different angles and provide a two- or three-dimensional view of the heart, lungs, and chest. Chest CTs are very useful for evaluating various abnormalities. In general, the test can be particularly helpful in evaluating conditions like aortic aneurysm, aortic dissection, and fluid around the heart.

There's a form of computed tomography called ultrafast computed tomography that has been used to evaluate the coronary arteries. In this case, as many as seventeen scans are performed per second. These scans are helpful in determining whether a person has clinically significant coronary calcifications. Ultrafast computed tomography is relatively new, and currently the resolution is generally not as good as that of the pictures obtained with a cardiac catheterization, during which radiopaque dye is injected through a catheter directly into the coronary arteries.

### Magnetic Resonance Imaging (MRI)

Magnetic resonance images are produced by the interactions of radio waves and magnetic fields. A computer transforms the signal from these interactions into pictures. There is no exposure to x-rays. The magnet is shaped like a large doughnut within which the patients lie. Unlike CTs, MRI can depict blood vessels and heart chambers without the need for injecting a contrast agent (x-ray "dye") and can picture them in three dimensions or from any angle. Images can also be obtained in movie format to show heart motion and blood flow.

MRI is superior to CTs when differentiating abnormalities next to the heart from abnormalities of the heart itself. Unlike echocardiography, which shares some of these advantages, MRI is not limited by the distance of the organ from the skin or by intervening bone structures and air. In children with complex congenital heart disease, MRI is an important supplement to echocardiography both for diagnosis and for assisting in surgical planning.

For other forms of heart disease, MRI is very helpful in assessing tumors or blood clots in the heart, pericardial disease, and diseases of the aorta such as aneurysms and dissection, and in supplementing echocardiography. MRI can determine cardiac anatomy, how well the heart pumps, and perfusion (blood actually getting to the heart muscle) but cannot adequately picture the coronary arteries. Technological advances should make this possible in the near future, at which time MRI may be able to provide information that is currently obtained from a combination of echocardiography, **radionuclide** studies, and cardiac catheterization.

### Nuclear Perfusion Tests

Another kind of testing uses one of two radioactive agents, thallium or tech-

**Radionuclide:**
A small amount of a nuclear substance that is used during diagnosis of heart disease to help physicians better see the heart and blood vessels.

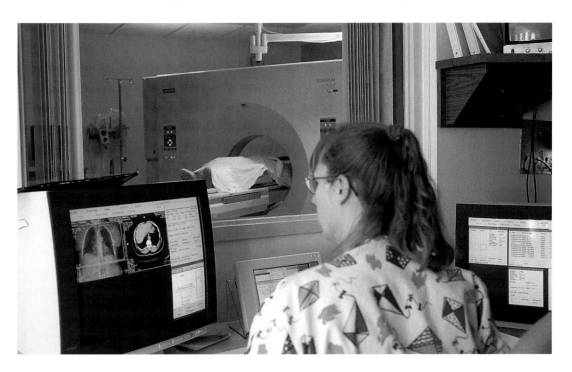

During MRI, or **magnetic resonance imaging**, radio and magnetic waves are used to obtain very detailed images of the heart from any angle. It is especially helpful in diagnosing congenital heart disease in children and problems with arteries and veins.

netium-99m, to study blood flow in patients suspected of having coronary artery disease. Sometimes these tests are used to monitor the progress of disease in patients whose condition has already been diagnosed.

In this test, a tiny amount of radioactive substance, referred to as a radionuclide, is injected into the body, and pictures are produced as the radiation escapes. These substances in the bloodstream are called "tracers" and are detected by a camera similar to a Geiger counter.

Thallium scanning is usually done in conjunction with an exercise stress test. The patient is asked to either walk on a treadmill or pedal a stationary bike. After a vigorous exercise period, radioactive material is injected into the bloodstream, and the patient is asked to exercise for about another minute. Scanning is done with a device that measures ra-

Prior to the actual nuclear scan, patients are often asked to exercise vigorously. During the scan, they lie still while their circulation is watched for signs of abnormality.

dioactivity. The resulting picture will show any areas of the heart that suffer from poor blood flow or no blood flow. With a thallium scan, the patient has a second scan four hours later.

If both tests show adequate blood flow, the heart and coronary arteries are probably normal. If both sets of scans show a "defect," or an area of the heart where there is no uptake of thallium, this indicates that the muscle has probably been replaced by scar tissue from a previous heart attack. If the scan shows faint uptake of thallium during exercise but more normal uptake at rest, it indicates that the heart muscle in that area is probably still alive but the coronary artery may be blocked. In this case, a cardiac catheterization can identify the exact area of blockage.

Technetium-99m is gaining popularity for obtaining similar information because it tends to yield higher quality pictures and more information than thallium. Technetium-99m is commonly used in a form called Sestamibi. With Sestamibi, the resting scan is usually performed before the stress test.

If a patient is unable to exercise on a treadmill, either the thallium or the technetium test can be done by using drugs that cause the heart to mimic its blood flow during exercise.

Nuclear perfusion scans are useful tests and are sometimes used as screening tests to determine whether a person ought to undergo a cardiac catheterization with coronary angiography, which is a more invasive but more accurate test to show coronary artery blockages. Nuclear tests and coronary angiography give somewhat different information and, in many cases, can be complementary. The information taken together may help determine whether a cardiologist will recommend more invasive procedures such as balloon dilatation of the coronary artery, stent placements, or even coronary artery bypass surgery.

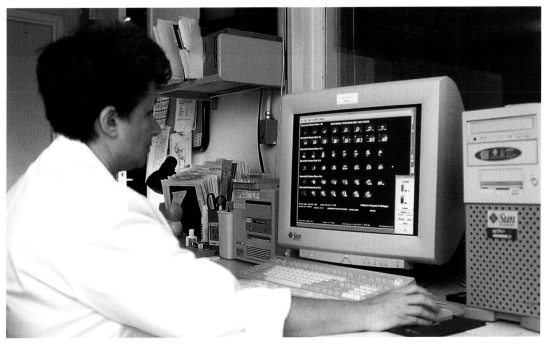

The **positron emission tomography** scan, or PET scan, is a very advanced form of nuclear scanning that reveals circulation of blood through the heart.

### Pyrophosphate Technetium-99m Scanning

The pyrophosphate technetium-99m scan also uses technetium, but a different form than is used in the Sestamibi scan. The pyrophosphate scan is used to determine if a patient has had a heart attack and, if so, how much damage has occurred. Damaged heart muscle will take up this form of technetium within twelve hours after a heart attack. Normally, the propensity for damaged heart muscle to take up pyrophosphate disappears within a week after a heart attack. This test can also be used to determine whether there is ongoing damage from the heart attack and whether the damage is confined to one area. Although this test is useful, it is slowly being replaced with other tests that can each yield some of the same information.

### MUGA Scan (Multigated Acquisition Study)

The MUGA scan is done to determine how well all four chambers of the heart are functioning and how big they are. The results obtained from this test are similar to some of the information obtained from the echocardiogram.

For this test, blood is withdrawn into a syringe containing the radionuclide technetium combined with pertechnetate. The technetium attaches to the red blood cells. About ten minutes later, the blood is reinjected, and a resting scan is taken. If a stress MUGA has been requested, the patient performs stationary exercise, and the heart is scanned at regular intervals.

### Positron Emission Tomography, or PET Scanning

Positron emission tomography, or PET, is currently the gold standard test using radioactive particles and the most accurate noninvasive way to measure blood flow to the heart muscle. In addition to measuring blood flow, it can measure metabolic activity, which means it can determine whether heart muscle cells are alive and functioning. Active heart muscles consume oxygen and glucose, and PET measures this activity.

During a PET test, the patient is injected with a chemical that gives off subatomic particles as it degenerates. The subatomic particles, called positrons, are detected by the PET scanner, and this information is stored in a computer. The computer reconstructs an image of the heart at work, showing which areas are not performing normally. This tells the physician that the coronary artery leading to that area is blocked and may need to be opened with a balloon catheter or surgical bypass grafting.

PET can also tell if an area of the heart is not performing normally because it has been damaged during a heart attack and has now turned to scar tissue. In that case, there would be no need to place a bypass graft to an area that is never going to function normally anyway.

PET is not available at many medical centers because of the cost. Radioactive agents used in this test have a very short lifetime, and therefore a cyclotron, which costs several million dollars, needs to be present at the PET scanning facility to produce these agents. Hospitals without PET scanning use other perfusion tests that also yield adequate information.

### Doppler Ultrasonography

This test is used to measure blood flow through the veins and arteries in the legs or through the carotid arteries that supply blood to the brain. Doppler ultrasound works on the same principle as echocardiography. High-frequency sound waves are bounced off the soft tissue and converted into electrical impulses that are displayed on a screen. In the legs, these tests can be used to determine if there's a blood clot in a vein or blockage of the arteries, which is typically caused by atherosclerotic material.

### Blood Tests

There are scores of different blood tests that can be performed at a hospital, and all of them yield information about various functions of the human body. Some of these are obtained specifically to learn various information about the human heart. If a person is admitted to a hospital emergency room because of chest pain, doctors may draw blood from a vein in the arm to measure what are called cardiac enzymes. The blood is sent to the hospital laboratory for a test to help determine, along with the electrocardiogram, whether the patient is having a heart attack. If heart muscle is damaged, certain enzymes or chemicals

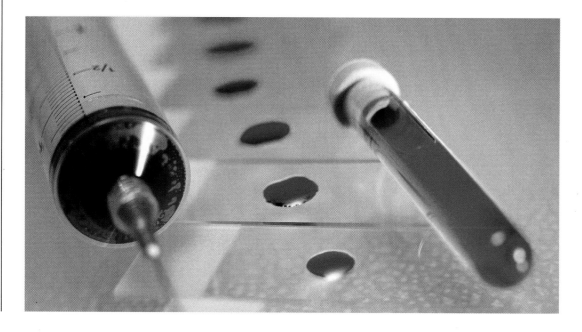

During diagnosis of heart disease, blood samples are often drawn. They can be used to determine whether a heart attack is in progress.

will leak from the damaged or dying heart muscle. Some of these enzymes are very specific to the heart and help determine whether a patient is having a heart attack. One of these is called creatine kinase, or CK. Another is called lactate dehydrogenase, or LDH. Troponin is a type of protein that leaks from the damaged heart muscle and can also help diagnose a heart attack.

If the doctor suspects someone might be having a heart attack, particularly from the symptoms and also from the ECG changes, the patient is usually admitted to the hospital's cardiac care unit for observation. The levels of serum enzymes, such as the CK and the LDH, may not initially be elevated but during the next day or two may become elevated, indicating not only that the heart has been damaged but that portions of it may be dying. The levels of these enzymes suggest how large or how clinically significant the heart attack is. Also, these enzyme levels should start to return to normal levels in a day or two. If they continue to be elevated, the heart attack may be continuing or damage may be occurring over several days. This can be of great concern to the physicians caring for the patient and may indicate that something invasive will have to be done such as obtaining a **coronary arteriogram** in the cardiac catheterization laboratory. It could also mean the patient may need a catheter procedure to open the blocked coronary artery or even require coronary bypass surgery.

**Arterial and Venous Oxygen Levels**

Blood samples are used to determine both arterial and venous oxygen levels. Arterial oxygen content can help determine how well the lungs are working. Blood arterial samples are most frequently obtained from an artery in the wrist or the groin (Fig. 5.1). They can be obtained during cardiac catheterization or in the cardiac care unit.

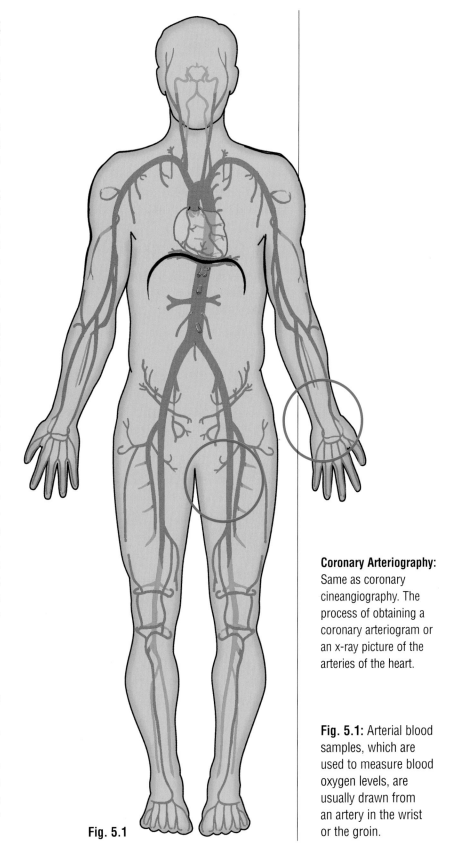

**Fig. 5.1**

**Coronary Arteriography:** Same as coronary cineangiography. The process of obtaining a coronary arteriogram or an x-ray picture of the arteries of the heart.

**Fig. 5.1:** Arterial blood samples, which are used to measure blood oxygen levels, are usually drawn from an artery in the wrist or the groin.

In adults, venous blood oxygen levels are used to determine how well the heart is functioning. A venous oxygen probe can also be part of an indwelling monitoring catheter that's used either during heart surgery or in the intensive care unit (ICU). This monitor provides continuous information that helps physicians determine how well the heart is pumping.

Children who have congenital heart disease have blood samples obtained during the cardiac catheterization procedure. The blood oxygen levels in various cardiac chambers provide clues as to what type of congenital heart defect the child has and even where the defects are located in the heart.

### Cholesterol Level

Cholesterol and triglycerides are substances that can be measured by obtaining a blood sample. Also, the various sub-types of cholesterol such as high-

density lipoprotein (HDL) cholesterol and low-density lipoprotein (LDL) cholesterol can be determined from a blood sample. These important tests reflect how one's body controls the levels of these particular substances, which, if too high or too low, may indicate that one is more prone to develop blockage of the coronary arteries feeding blood to the heart, blood vessels going to the brain, and arteries in other areas of the body. Patients may have to change their diet or take medication to lower the concentration of these substances and thus reduce the chances of a heart attack or stroke.

### Second Opinions

Second opinions are obtained from another doctor, usually one of the same specialty, about a patient's specific medical problem. Obtaining a second opinion is quite common, and, in fact, many insurance companies require a second opinion before important surgery. Sometimes patients feel that they are offending a doctor if they tell a doctor that they would like to get a second opinion. They shouldn't. Most doctors encourage patients to seek a second opinion if they feel the patient is not quite comfortable with the diagnosis.

Obviously, having a cardiac catheterization or a heart operation is a major event in one's life, and patients should feel that they have received informed recommendations about having such a procedure. You should not hesitate to obtain a second opinion unless you are comfortable with the advice you have received. However, sometimes in emergency situations a second opinion is impractical.

In some respects, many patients have actually obtained second or third opinions and may not realize it. For example, the patient's internal medicine doctor or cardiologist may refer the patient to a cardiologist who specializes in cardiac catheterization procedures. After evaluating the pa-

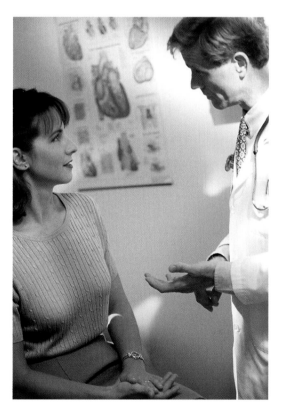

It can be a good idea to obtain a second opinion. Heart surgery and heart catheterizations are major events, and patients should be satisfied with the information about their condition and treatment.

tient and obtaining results from a cardiac catheterization and other studies, the doctors talk with each other and decide whether or not to recommend heart surgery. If the surgery is recommended, the patient is referred to a heart surgeon, who discusses the case with the patient as well as the referring doctor and then makes his or her recommendation for or against heart surgery. From that standpoint, two or three opinions have already been obtained.

How does one go about obtaining an additional opinion or a second opinion from another cardiologist or from another heart surgeon? One way to do it is to simply ask a cardiologist or heart surgeon to recommend another heart surgeon or cardiologist for a second opinion. Usually if you're going to get a second opinion, you would want to get it from somebody other than the doctor's partner because the partner may have a vested interest in agreeing with the first opinion. Also, you would probably feel more comfortable obtaining an opinion from somebody who is perhaps less likely to share exact views with the doctor.

Patients can also ask a family doctor to recommend another specialist. If you are obtaining a second opinion from an-other heart surgeon, you can ask the cardiologist with whom you are dealing to recommend a different heart surgeon. Patients can also check with an insurance company. These companies frequently have a list of specialists whom they will recommend. If you're dealing with a heart surgeon and you want another opinion from a cardiologist, a heart surgeon can also recommend another cardiologist because heart surgeon's deal with many different cardiologists. The local medical societies can also be contacted for advice.

Some people track down second opinions through information on the Internet. Sometimes there are specific doctors listed either in the local area or elsewhere in the country. Sometimes patients obtain their second opinion directly from information available on the Internet or from interfacing with medical people on the Internet.

There are many ways to obtain second opinions, and you should not hesitate to obtain one. Doctors are only human, and sometimes they may interpret a test or other information one way or have opinions on how a certain problem should be treated that may differ from those of another physician of the same specialty.

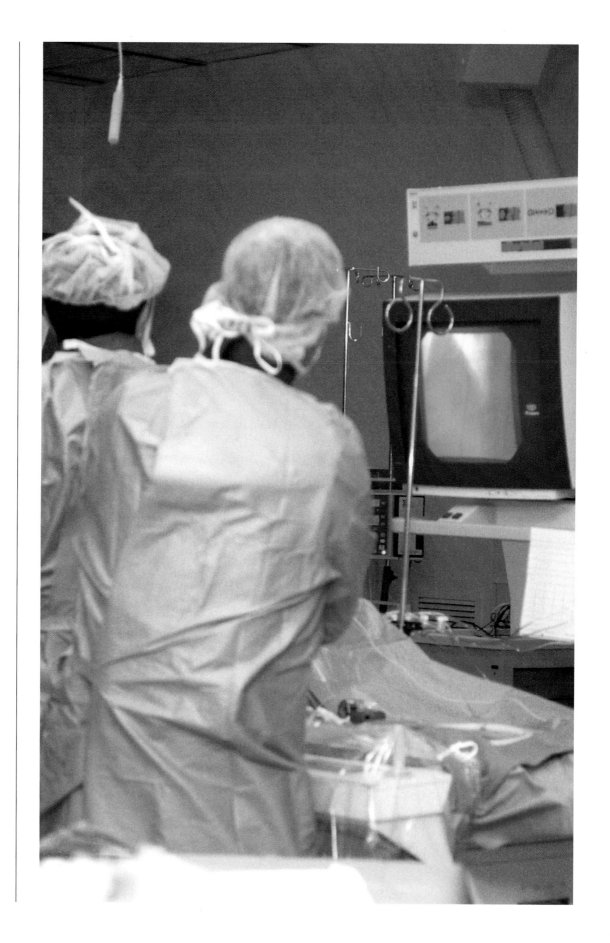

Hospitals have designated cardiac and vascular catheterization labs where specialized procedures are performed by cardiologists and radiologists.

## CHAPTER SIX

# WHAT IS
# CARDIAC CATHETERIZATION?

CATHETERS ARE FLEXIBLE, HOLlow tubes (originally rubber, but now advanced plastic) that are threaded through an artery or vein into the body. They are able to travel from the insertion site in the groin or arm into major arteries and veins, heart chambers, and even the brain. Although cardiac catheterization is not considered heart surgery, it is an invasive procedure that in some cases has replaced open heart surgery. These devices have a wide variety of uses, including

♥ dilating coronary arteries and heart valves using inflatable balloons,
♥ placing stents, or small metal coils, in blood vessels to keep them open,
♥ guiding lasers through the coronary arteries, which are used to open blockages,
♥ introducing devices to close holes in certain types of congenital heart defects such as atrial septal defects, and
♥ enlarging a hole in the atrial septum (the wall between the right and the left atrium).

Today, there are more than one million cardiac catheterization procedures performed in the United States each year.

 **Experimenting on Himself**

The first human heart catheterization is credited to a medical intern from Berlin, Germany, named Dr. Werner Forssmann. Forssmann began his catheter studies on cadavers, passing his rudimentary devices into the right ventricle. He next wanted to conduct an experiment on a living subject but couldn't get approval from his superiors. He decided to use himself. He later wrote about the experience:

*"In a preliminary experiment, I asked a colleague to puncture a vein in my right arm with a large-bore needle. Then I advanced a well-lubricated urethral catheter (used to drain the urinary bladder) ... into the vein. The catheter was easily passed to fourteen inches, but we aborted the experiment, which my colleague considered too risky. I felt perfectly well during the experiment.*

*"One week later, I tried it again without assistance. I proceeded with a venous puncture in my left arm vein and introduced the catheter to its full length of twenty-six inches. I only perceived some sensation of warmth similar to the sensation during intravenous injection of calcium chloride. There was no pain.*

*When I pushed on the catheter, I felt a warm sensation behind the collar bone and near the jawbone."*

Forssmann's 1929 report, which included a photograph of an x-ray showing the catheter in his heart, was received coolly by a medical establishment that was critical of something so outlandish. When he requested permission from his superiors to pursue further studies, he was told his methods were good for a circus but not for a respected hospital.

Nevertheless, Forssmann continued his cardiac catheterization studies on himself and in laboratory animals. He later called himself an outsider with "ideas too crazy to give him a clinical position."

Forssmann was eventually vindicated. In 1956, he shared the Nobel Prize in Physiology or Medicine with two faculty members of Columbia University in New York, Drs. Andre F. Cournand and Dickenson W. Richards, Jr., for work in cardiac catheterization.

**Right:** In 1929, a young German doctor named Werner Forssmann conducted the first heart catheterization on a living human. Forbidden by his superiors to experiment on a patient, he conducted the historic catheterization on himself.

**Angiography:** The process of making a blood vessel visible by injecting a substance that can be seen under x-ray.

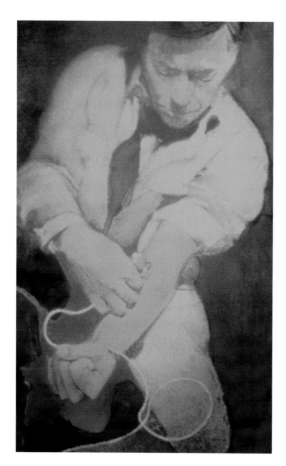

### Catheters Today

Today, catheters are used to both diagnose and treat cardiac disorders. The procedure is usually done on an outpatient basis, and patients who undergo catheterization are often released from the clinic or hospital on the day of the procedure.

Diagnostically, the catheter is an important tool that allows doctors to observe the inside of coronary arteries and actually watch the heart at work. The most popular form of heart catheter procedure is called coronary **angiography**, in which a catheter is used to inject contrast material into the heart's own arteries. It takes anywhere from twenty minutes to an hour to obtain an angiogram.

If it is used in any other artery, such as the pulmonary artery, it is called pulmonary angiography. In the pulmonary artery, angiography is sometimes used

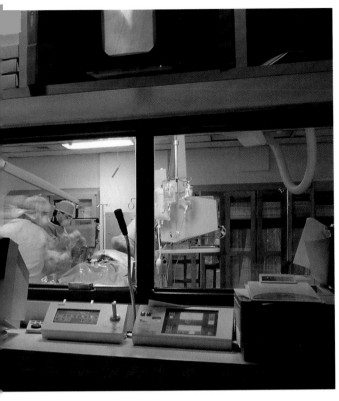

to find blood clots, possibly related to a clot that had broken loose from a vein in the leg or elsewhere and worked its way through the heart and into the arteries in the lung.

### The Coronary Angiogram

Coronary angiograms were first described in 1962 by Dr. Mason Sones at the Cleveland Clinic. Because it allowed doctors to see exactly where the coronary arteries were blocked and what condition they were in beyond the blockage, coronary angiography was a major impetus for the development of the coronary bypass graft operation.

Coronary angiography procedures are done in a special area of the hospital called the cardiac catheterization laboratory. Depending on the size of the hospital's cardiovascular unit, there may be one room or several rooms where catheterization procedures are performed using special x-ray equipment. During the angiography, the patient lies on a special table while the cardiologist performs the catheterization. Heart surgeons typically do not perform coronary angiographies. They are usually performed by an internist who has completed specialty work in cardiology and further specialized in cardiac catheterization.

During the coronary angiogram, the catheter is not in the heart itself. Instead, the dye is injected directly into the coronary arteries where they originate in the aorta. This will determine whether there is atherosclerosis or some other type of blockage in the coronary system. Important information can be gained as to whether blockages are severe enough to require some form of therapy.

Before the catheter is inserted, the skin is cleaned and anesthetized with a local anesthetic. A small needle is used to puncture the vein or the artery, and a wire is threaded through the needle. Next, a larger plastic introducer is placed. The catheter itself, which is a little larger in diameter than a piece of spaghetti, is threaded through the introducer into the blood vessel.

Once inside the body, catheters can be steered through heart valves and into the heart chambers themselves (Fig. 6.1), where catheter-based devices can measure pressure in the various chambers. This is particularly important in diagnosing some types of heart valve disease.

Blood samples also can be taken from the chambers, and the level of oxygen can be measured. This is helpful when looking for possible holes in the heart that are allowing unoxygenated blood to mix with oxygenated blood, or vice versa. It can be an important diagnostic tool in children with some types of congenital heart defects.

Besides coronary angiography, catheters are also used to image the heart itself and other arteries. Radiopaque dyes are injected into the heart's chambers and recorded with x-rays as they course through the heart. This shows how well the heart muscle is contracting and, if

Center:
A cardiac catheterization laboratory. Catheters are used to both diagnose and treat heart disease.

Dr. Mason Sones

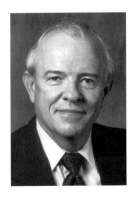

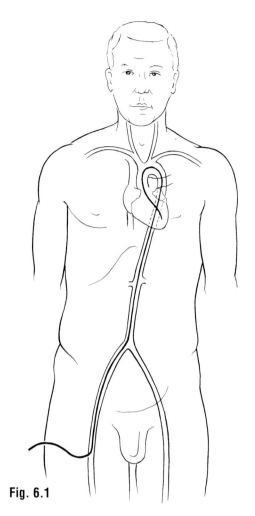

**Fig. 6.1:**
Catheters can be introduced into the heart through a major artery in the groin.

**Fig. 6.1**

**Fig. 6.2:**
Catheters can be used to open blocked arteries (A) in a procedure called PTCA. During PTCA, the balloon-tipped catheter is first guided to the artery segment that is narrowed (B). Next the balloon is inflated and dilates the artery by crushing the plaque against the arterial wall (C and D). When the procedure has been completed, the artery has been reopened (E).

some of the dye flows backwards, it may indicate a leaking heart valve.

After the cardiac catheterization is complete, the devices are removed. If the catheter is inserted through an artery in the arm, the puncture site may have to be stitched closed. If the catheter is introduced through an artery in the leg, pressure held on this artery for a couple of hours will normally allow the puncture to seal over on its own. In this case, the patient will need to lie flat in bed for several hours, and there may be some bleeding after the pressure is relieved.

If the area around the artery becomes swollen because of blood gathering, this is called a hematoma. Occasionally, if the hematoma gets large, a surgeon will have to make an incision and place a few stitches directly into the artery. Currently, how-

ever, there are techniques available to seal the hole as the catheter is removed from the artery, which makes these complications less likely.

Like any invasive procedure, catheterization carries with it other risks. Although it happens rarely, the heart itself can be lacerated by the catheter. This may require emergency heart surgery. Other times, the heart will go into an irregular rhythm. Fortunately, these rhythms usually correct themselves, but they may require some medication. Some patients may become allergic to the dyes that are injected into the arteries. Very rarely, a heart attack or stroke may occur as a result of cardiac catheterization.

**Therapeutic Cardiac Catheterization**

*Percutaneous Transluminal Coronary Angioplasty (PTCA)*

Catheters are also used to treat blocked coronary arteries in a procedure called percutaneous transluminal coronary angioplasty (PTCA). Several hundred thousand of these procedures are performed in the United States each year. The catheter used for PTCA is tipped with a

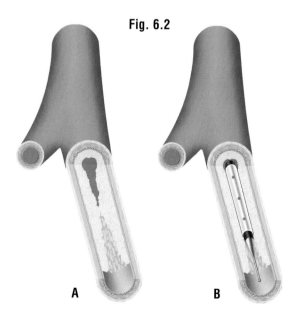

**Fig. 6.2**

A          B

very small, sausage-shaped balloon that is threaded into the coronary artery and into the obstructed part of the vessel. Once it's in place, the balloon is inflated, crushing the plaque and atherosclerotic material against the arterial wall (Fig. 6.2). The balloon may have to be inflated several times.

The PTCA procedure was developed by Dr. Andreas R. Gruentzig at the University of Zurich in Switzerland, although balloon-tipped catheters were already in use to dilate arteries in the leg that were blocked by atherosclerosis. Gruentzig made the existing catheters much smaller so they could be used in the coronary arteries. His first human PTCA was successfully performed in September 1977. Since then, this procedure has rapidly evolved.

Although most PTCA procedures are successful, not all blockages can be relieved with the balloon. Doctors do not usually attempt to use a balloon catheter in the left main coronary artery. There is a risk that the procedure will dislodge atherosclerotic debris that will travel into one or both of the main coronary branches and cause a massive acute heart attack that would likely be fatal. In addition, when any coronary artery is totally blocked, a

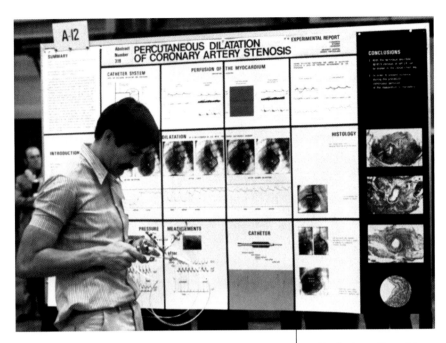

catheter might not be able to get through the blockage. In that case, balloon procedures would not be attempted.

About five percent of the arteries dilated with the balloon catheter will close off before the patient even leaves the hospital. Such an event is usually treated with another PTCA. In a few cases, the patient will have to be taken to the operating room, where a heart surgeon will have to perform a bypass operation.

Dr. Andreas Gruentzig, a physician from Switzerland, performed the first percutaneous transluminal coronary angioplasty (PTCA). During this procedure, a tiny balloon is used to widen a coronary artery that has been partially blocked by plaque. Gruentzig is pictured in the 1970s at a trade show booth sponsored by Boston Scientific, a catheter and medical device company. *(Photo courtesy of Boston Scientific Corporation.)*

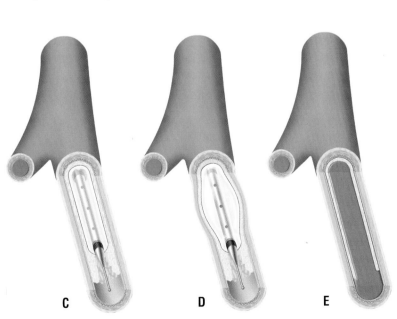

C          D          E

Even after leaving the hospital, about 30 to 50 percent of the four hundred thousand cases of PTCA performed every year restenose, or narrow again to the original level or worse. This often happens within three to twelve months of the procedure, and it is a significant problem.

### Stent Procedures

**Stent:**
A device usually made from metal or other material that is placed in a blood vessel to help keep it open.

**Stenosis:**
An abnormal narrowing of a blood vessel, heart valve or any other orifice or tube-like structure in the body.

In 1993, a new technology called **stenting** came into widespread use as a partial treatment for **restenosis**. Stents were first tested in the coronary artery of a human by Dr. Ulrich Sigwart from Lusanne, Switzerland, in 1987. Stents are small metal coils that are "wrapped" around the PTCA balloon before it is inserted into the coronary artery. Once the balloon catheter is in place, it is inflated, pushing the stent open and lodging it against the arterial wall. The balloon is removed, but the stent stays in place and keeps that area of the coronary artery dilated.

So far, stents seem to perform better than PTCA itself and have improved the safety and efficacy of PTCA. However, a risk of stent stenosis remains when either material forms inside the stent or the blockage occurs just beyond either end of the stent. This is reported in between 10 and 20 percent of cases within six months of stent placement. Nonetheless, the results are promising, and the stenting procedure has become widespread since its introduction.

### Atherectomy

Catheters are also used to treat coronary artery blockage in a technique known as atherectomy. This procedure uses a small device that rotates, much like a miniature drill, to shave off the atherosclerotic blockage. The resulting debris is collected and removed from the artery. The atherectomy procedure is useful in cases with significant blockage, but it is not as widely used as the balloons and the balloons with stents. In a similar procedure, nicknamed the "Roto Rooter," a tiny burr grinds off the hardened blockage material.

### Lasers

Lasers are also used to clear coronary arteries of atherosclerotic plaque. However, the restenosis rate with lasers, including balloon lasers, has not been as good as originally hoped. Nonetheless, research with these procedures continues.

### Transmyocardial Laser Revascularization

Transmyocardial laser revascularization is reserved for patients whose arteries are so diseased both upstream and down that bypasses, balloon angioplasties, or stents are no longer an option. In this case, a laser is used to bore tiny holes in the heart muscle itself, in the hope that new blood channels will develop.

The lasers can be introduced into the left ventricular cavity through the catheter or directly with surgery (See Chapter Eight).

### Catheter Heart Valve Procedures

Besides the coronary arteries, narrowed heart valves can be dilated with balloon catheters (Fig. 6.3). They tend to be quite successful in treating infants and children born with narrowed pulmonary heart valves, and they are also sometimes used to dilate narrowed aortic valves in newborns.

In adults, balloon catheters are used to treat mitral valves abnormally narrowed as a result of rheumatic fever. Although the balloon catheter can be very successful in treating mitral valve stenosis and can spare the patient a heart operation, this procedure is not applicable to every patient.

It is not very effective in treating adult patients with aortic valve stenosis

90

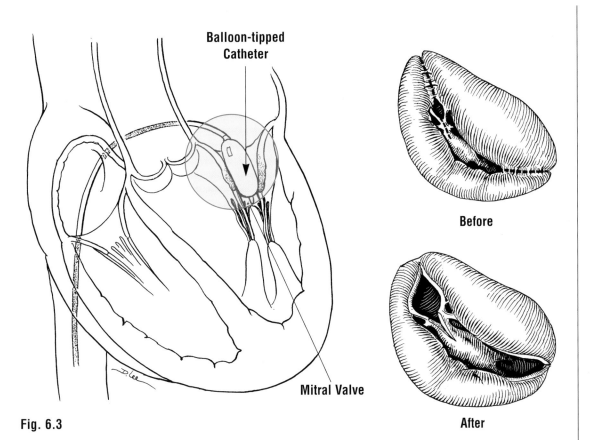

**Balloon-tipped Catheter**

**Mitral Valve**

**Before**

**After**

Fig. 6.3

**Fig. 6.3**:
Balloon-tipped catheters are also used to open blocked heart valves. They can be used in both infants and adults to treat a variety of valvular blockages.

**Coarctation of the Aorta:**
A birth defect in which there is a segment of the aorta that is abnormally narrowed. Typically, this coarcted area is in the descending aorta just after the aortic arch.

**Transposition of the Great Arteries:**
A severe congenital heart defect in which the aorta, which normally comes off the left ventricle, instead originates from the right ventricle, and the pulmonary artery, which normally originates from the right ventricle, originates from the left ventricle.

but is sometimes used in desperate cases, such as when patients have other major medical problems and may not survive a heart operation, or to get critically ill patients in better physical condition for aortic valve surgery.

*Other Heart Catheter Procedures*

Catheters are also used to introduce devices that plug some holes between the two atria, or upper chambers of the heart, called atrial septal defects. This procedure is still undergoing trials under the auspices of the U.S. Food and Drug Administration (FDA).

In some cases, they can plug a patent ductus arteriosus, which is an abnormal vessel connecting the aorta and the pulmonary artery that is present in some children after birth. **Coarctation of the aorta** is another congenital condition and happens when a segment of the descending thoracic aorta is narrowed. This problem is treated surgically, but the narrowing can recur. If that happens, a balloon catheter can sometimes be used to dilate the narrow segment of the blood vessel.

Catheters are often used to make or enlarge a hole in the atrial septum in infants born with a heart defect called **transposition of the great arteries**. Called the Rashkind procedure and Rashkind Balloon Septostomy, it is named after Dr. William Rashkind, a pediatric cardiologist who developed the procedure at the Children's Hospital of Philadelphia. The procedure allows oxygenated and unoxygenated blood from the two sides of the heart to mix, which buys time until surgical correction is done.

Catheters are also used to retrieve foreign bodies such as intravenous lines or other materials that are sometimes mistakenly left in the heart or blood vessels.

# HOW TO CHOOSE A CARDIAC SURGEON

By

## Julie A. Swain, M.D.

Cardiothoracic Surgeon

Professor of Surgery

Gill Heart Institute at the University of Kentucky College of Medicine

Lexington, Kentucky

THE PROSPECT OF UNDERgoing heart surgery terrifies most patients and their family members. Moreover, many cardiac surgery operations, especially coronary bypass procedures, must be done urgently. If it is possible to schedule the operation for a future date, patients will have a greater opportunity to ask questions to guide them in the choice of a surgeon and a hospital. However, if an immediate operation is needed, it should not be delayed.

**When Surgery Is Recommended**

Almost always, a cardiologist will diagnose a condition and, if warranted, will recommend surgery. The cardiologist may then recommend a surgeon or ask the family physician to recommend a surgeon. A personal recommendation by a cardiologist or primary care physician is the most common way a surgeon is chosen. This remains one of the best methods of choosing a surgeon. It is appropriate,

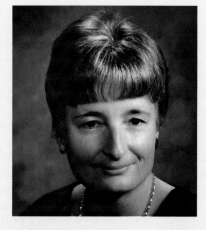

however, to ask questions about the surgeon.

A cardiologist has an obligation to know the "track records" of the surgeons to whom he or she refers. The majority of the referring doctors send patients to the surgeon whom they think will deliver the best care. However, in this era of managed care and other economic factors, referrals might be influenced by other considerations.

**How to Judge Surgical Quality**

The track records of cardiac surgeons have been subjected

to closer scrutiny than those of any other physicians. This is because cardiac surgery is high profile and high cost, and the results are relatively easy to measure and compare. The most common indicator used to judge the quality of a surgeon is the death rate after cardiac surgery.

The average death rate after coronary bypass surgery is three out of every one hundred patients operated upon (3 percent). A patient who is older or has other diseases has a higher risk, whereas younger patients without serious medical conditions are at a lower risk of dying after surgery. To judge the quality of a surgeon or surgery program, one has to know how "sick" their patient population is. Much effort has been made to develop a "risk-adjustment" scale to level the playing field.

**What You Should Know about Cardiac Surgery Databases**

The Society of Thoracic Surgeons, the main professional

92

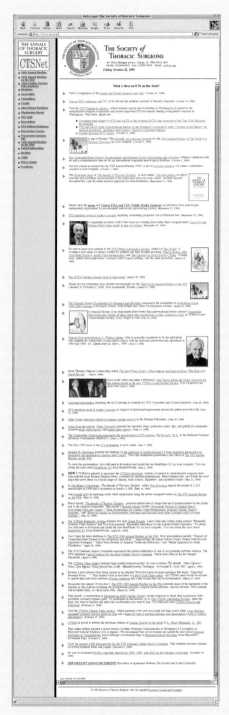

organization for cardiac surgeons, has spent years developing a database for risk adjustment. Although individual surgeon data and hospital data are not available, the national average data can be accessed by the public on the internet at **www.sts.org**. Most of the cardiac surgeons in the country use this database to track their results and to compare themselves with other surgeons.

Other databases exist for regions (such as Northern New England and Cleveland) and for the Veterans Affairs hospitals. New York and Pennsylvania have databases that are available to the public and rate both individual surgeons and hospitals. Surgeons themselves should be enrolled in a database to be able to assess their results. Although many of these databases only rate the quality of results for coronary bypass operations, other operations usually parallel these results.

Still another database at **www.healthgrades.com** contains Medicare data for all heart surgery programs in the United States.

A surgeon may have a very low death rate because he or she is an excellent surgeon. Alternatively, the surgeon may be average or worse and have a low death rate because he or she only operates on the lowest risk patients. Likewise, an excellent surgeon can have a high death rate because he or she operates on the sickest of patients. The databases were developed to help physicians and hospitals sort out these results. For example, a surgeon who operates on very complicated cases may have a death rate of 4 percent (four out of every one hundred patients). If the predicted death rate from the database is 8 percent, then this death rate of 4 percent shows he or she is an excellent surgeon. Conversely, if the predicted death rate is only 2 percent and the actual death rate is 4 percent, the results indicate a worse-than-average track record.

Referring physicians should know the track records of the surgeons to whom they refer and be able to explain these relatively complicated scales to their patients. Likewise, every surgeon should know their results and share them with their referring doctors and prospective patients.

**Is Bigger Necessarily Better?**

There is much controversy about whether the quality of surgery is better at a big hospital where a large number of operations are performed versus at a smaller hospital. Excellent results are obtained by some small programs, whereas lower-quality results may be obtained by some

---

Information on cardiac surgeons can be found on the internet. The Society of Thoracic Surgeons website, left, posts a database at **www.sts.org**. Medicare statistics can be found at **www.healthgrades.com**, below.

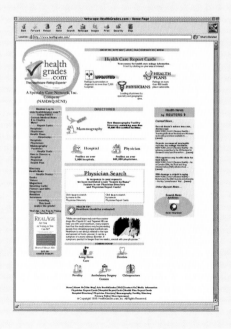

large programs. There seems to be a certain minimum number of operations needed to keep an open heart team trained. This number is about two hundred operations per year.

Almost every state and most large cities have at least one high-quality surgery program. It is advantageous to have medical care close to home for many reasons, including ready access to follow-up care, proximity to family and social support structures, and the ability to be cared for by your own physician.

## Surgeons Perform Operations, Not Hospitals

It may seem obvious, but surgeons perform operations, not hospitals. There may be a wide range between the abilities of different surgeons at the same hospital. However, the quality of a hospital can affect the results of all surgeons.

Surgeons should appreciate the opportunity to have an informed patient and be willing to answer all questions. The rapport patients develop with their surgeon will be important in the postoperative period, and it is important that patients are comfortable talking with the surgeon.

The following questions are suggested to help evaluate the quality of care. Patients may want to give this list to the surgeon to guide the discussion. After talk-

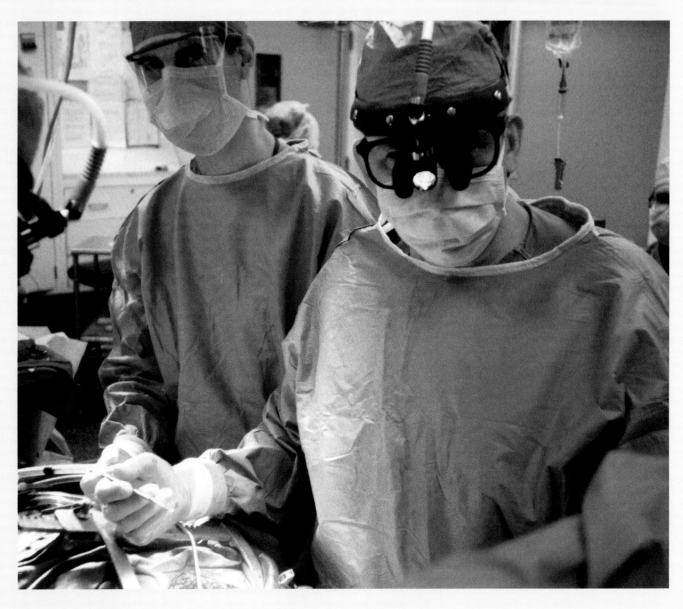

ing with their surgeon, patients may also want to discuss the answers with their cardiologist or primary care physician.

### The Top Ten Things You Need to Ask before Cardiac Surgery

1. How many of these operations has the surgeon personally performed in the past three years? (A prevailing opinion is that a surgeon should perform at least seventy-five open heart surgery operations per year, although more experienced surgeons can obtain excellent results even though they may do fewer operations per year.)

2. What percentage of the surgeon's patients over the last three years have died in the hospital after coronary bypass operations?

3. Does the surgeon use a nationally recognized database to compare his/her results to those of other surgeons? How do the results compare? If a state database exists in your area, how does this surgeon rate?

4. Is the surgeon board certified by the American Board of Thoracic Surgery? (This is the only certifying organization for United States–trained surgeons and requires a rigorous examination process and documented training in a residency approved by the Board.)

5. Is the surgeon a fellow of the American College of Surgeons? (Don't be confused by names such as the "International College of Surgeons." The American College of Surgeons requires a peer evaluation of surgical practice and is the largest professional organization of board-certified American surgeons.)

6. Why did your doctor choose this hospital over any others in which the surgeon operates?

7. How many open heart operations are done per year at this hospital? How long has the hospital had an open heart surgery program?

8. Does the operating room have staff in the hospital twenty-four hours a day for emergencies? (Open heart surgery patients sometimes have to return to the operating room quickly.)

9. Who will assist the surgeon with the operation? (Some states require a second surgeon to be present in the operating room.)

10. Will there be a physician or physician's assistant in the hospital overnight to take care of you if an emergency arises? Are these people trained in cardiac surgical care?

These questions about case volume and quality assessment can also apply to a choice of cardiologist for an angioplasty procedure.

It must be emphasized that the personal recommendation of a trusted physician who is knowledgeable about cardiac surgery is very important and should be used in combination with these guidelines.

Drs. Alfred Blalock (left) and Helen Taussig (right).

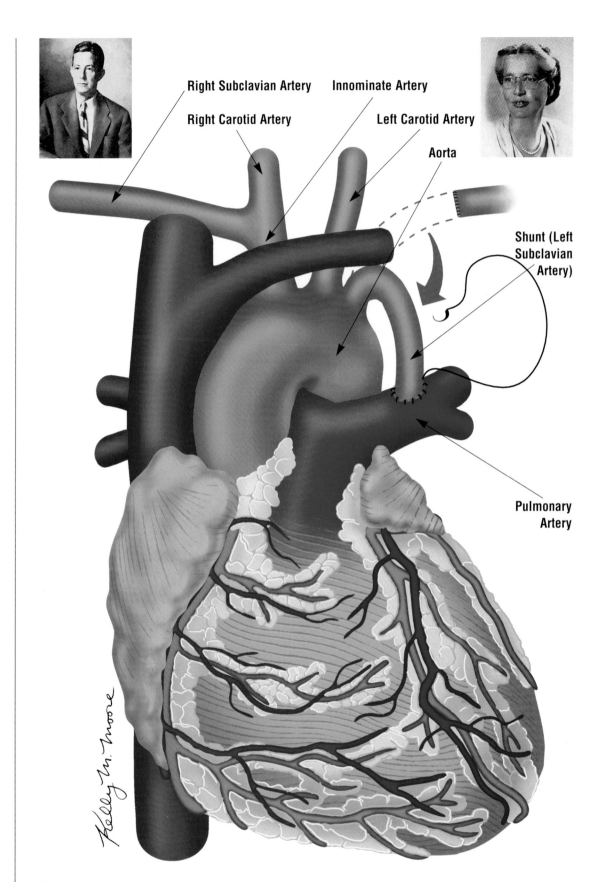

**Right Subclavian Artery**

**Right Carotid Artery**

**Innominate Artery**

**Left Carotid Artery**

**Aorta**

**Shunt (Left Subclavian Artery)**

**Pulmonary Artery**

**Fig. 7.1:**
The famous "blue baby operation," or Blalock-Taussig shunt, was the first surgical procedure developed to treat a congenital heart defect. In this operation, an artery from the arm is connected to the pulmonary artery to help supplement blood flow to the lungs and thus provide more oxygenated blood to the body.

**Fig. 7.1**

# CHAPTER SEVEN

# HEART PROBLEMS OF INFANTS AND CHILDREN

A CONGENITAL HEART DEFECT means an abnormality that is present at birth. Congenital heart surgery started before the heart-lung machine was developed as surgeons started to work on abnormalities of the arteries that came out of the heart. Dr. John Streider at the Massachusetts General Hospital in Boston tied off a patent ductus arteriosus (an abnormal pathway between the aorta and the pulmonary artery) in a child on March 6, 1937. Unfortunately, the patient was quite sick at the time and died four days after the surgery. A year and a half later, in the same city, on August 16, 1938, Dr. Robert Gross at the Boston Children's Hospital operated on a girl seven and a half years old who was short of breath because of the same congenital defect. The patient made a successful recovery. Soon surgeons all over the world were performing this operation.

The next major congenital cardiovascular defect to be overcome was called "coarctation of the aorta." This is a defect in which the aorta narrows and, in some cases, becomes totally blocked, resulting in decreased blood flow to the lower half of the body. Historically, most patients with this defect eventually died of complications by the age of twenty years. In 1944, Dr.

Clarence Crafoord in Stockholm, Sweden, successfully removed this narrow area of the aorta in a twelve-year-old boy.

Only a year later, Gross successfully treated a condition known as vascular ring, which occurs when the aorta and its major arterial branches wrap around the esophagus and trachea in an abnormal manner and compress them. Before this landmark surgical procedure, many infants and children with the condition died of suffocation and/or starvation.

During that same period, doctors announced the famous "blue baby operation" at Johns Hopkins University Hospital in Baltimore. This operation treats congenital heart defects in which the unoxygenated blood returning from the body is shunted through a hole in the heart instead of going through the lungs and is pumped out through the aorta, which causes the child to have a bluish color.

The first patient was a fifteen-month-old girl who had suffered her first cyanotic spell (turning blue) at age eight months. Dr. Helen Taussig, a pediatric cardiologist at Johns Hopkins University Hospital, took her as a patient and consulted with other doctors about trying a new operation. Over the next several months, the baby girl refused most of her

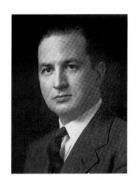

Dr. Robert Gross performed the world's first successful surgical closure of a patent ductus arteriosus, an abnormal pathway between the aorta and pulmonary artery in newborns.

**Table 7-1:** First intracardiac repairs using heart-lung machine or cross circulation

| Congenital Heart Defect | Year | Surgeon | Comment |
|---|---|---|---|
| Atrial septal defect | 1953 | Gibbon | Heart-lung machine (HLM) |
| Ventricular septal defect | 1954 | Lillehei | Cross circulation |
| Complete atrioventricular canal | 1954 | Lillehei | Cross circulation |
| Tetralogy of Fallot | 1954 | Lillehei | Cross circulation |
| Tetralogy of Fallot | 1955 | Kirklin | HLM |
| Total anomalous pulmonary veins | 1956 | Kirklin | |
| Congenital aneurysm, sinus of Valsalva | 1956 | Kirklin | |
| Congenital aortic stenosis | 1956 | Kirklin | First directly viewed correction |
| Aortopulmonary window | 1957 | Cooley | First closure using HLM |
| Double outlet right ventricle | 1957 | Kirklin | Extemporarily devised correction |
| Corrected transposition of great arteries | 1957 | Lillehei | |
| Transposition of great arteries: atrial switch | 1959 | Senning | Physiologic total correction |
| Coronary arterial-venous fistula | 1959 | Swan | |
| Ebstein's anomaly | 1964 | Hardy | Repair of atrialized tricuspid valve |
| Tetralogy with pulmonary atresia | 1966 | Ross | Aortic allograft |
| Truncus arteriosus | 1967 | McGoon | Aortic allograft |
| Tricuspid atresia | 1968 | Fontan | Physiologic correction |
| Single ventricle | 1970 | Horiuchi | |
| Subaortic tunnel stenosis | 1975 | Konno | |
| Transposition of great arteries: atrial switch | 1975 | Jatene | Anatomic correction |
| Hypoplastic left heart syndrome | 1983 | Norwood | Two-stage operation |
| Pediatric heart transplantation | 1985 | Bailey | |

**Table 7-1:**
Within a few years in the mid- to late 1950s, surgeons corrected thirteen types of congenital heart defects. Congenital heart surgery later evolved into its own subspecialty.

**Palliative:**
A treatment that improves a condition but does not cure it.

feedings and lost weight. She weighed only 8.3 pounds at the time the operation was performed by Dr. Alfred Blalock at Johns Hopkins University Hospital on November 29, 1944. During the operation, Blalock sewed an artery that normally supplies blood to the arm to the left pulmonary artery so more blood could get to the lungs and be oxygenated (Fig. 7.1). The successful operation required slightly less than an hour and a half. Although this was not a cure for her heart condition, it improved the patient's symptoms and quality of life substantially.

Thus, within a seven year period, three congenital cardiovascular defects — patent ductus arteriosus, coarctation of the aorta, and vascular ring — were all attacked surgically and treated successfully. However, the introduction of the Blalock-Taussig shunt was probably a much more powerful stimulus to the development of open heart surgery because the operation **palliated** a complex intracardiac defect and focused attention on the abnormal physiology of cardiac disease.

The next major step forward in heart surgery needed to wait for the development of the heart-lung machine, which occurred in the middle 1950s. With the advent of techniques to support the circulation and oxygenate the blood, using either the cross circulation technique of Dr. C. Walton Lillehei or the modified Gibbon-IBM heart-lung machine of Dr. John Kirklin, the cardiac teams of the University of Minnesota and the Mayo Clinic led the way and did many of the first intracardiac repairs for a number of commonly occurring congenital heart defects. Palliative operations, however, continued to be used and developed to improve circulatory physiology without directly addressing the anatomic pathology. The palliative operations somewhat improved the patients' conditions but did not cure them. As the safety of the heart-lung machine steadily improved, surgeons addressed more and more complex congenital abnormalities of the heart in younger and younger patients. Some of the milestones in the development of operations to correct congenital defects using cardiopulmonary bypass appear in Table 7-1.

### Diagnosing a Congenital Heart Defect

The human heart begins to develop at the end of the first month of fetal life and takes about another eight weeks before it resembles an adult heart. During this period, about eight out of every one thousand newborns develop some form of congenital heart defect ranging from very mild to quite severe. The exact cause of congenital heart defects is unknown, but recent information suggests there may be genetic influences. In some cases, they are associated with other medical conditions, such as the mother contracting German measles (rubella) while pregnant. At this point, most doctors don't think congenital heart defects are hereditary in the strict sense of being passed from parent to offspring, but children of parents who were born with such a defect will be somewhat more likely to have a congenital heart defect.

Some congenital heart defects are diagnosed shortly after birth or even while the baby is in the uterus by using ultrasound or echocardiography. They may be diagnosed later when the child is of school age, or in rare circumstances, the congenital cardiac defect remains hidden until adulthood. One indicator of some types of congenital heart defect in a newborn is a faint bluish color in the skin. Some children with heart defects may not thrive, and many suffer from congested lungs, which may be related to heart failure. Heart murmurs can also indicate congenital heart defects, although not necessarily.

If a defect in a newborn is suspected, your child's pediatrician will recommend an electrocardiogram and probably an echocardiogram, which do not require any needle sticks. Other tests used to diagnose congenital heart defects include cardiac catheterization and magnetic resonance imaging. After the heart defect is diagnosed and analyzed, your pediatrician and pediatric cardiologist will develop a treatment plan. This may require nothing more than yearly checkups or perhaps medications. Occasionally, a catheter can be used to dilate a heart valve or to insert a plug to close a hole. Heart surgery may be recommended and, in rare cases, heart transplantation is the best option.

### Specific Defects

There are many types of congenital heart defects. Of the following eleven congenital heart defects, the first nine are relatively common. The last two are much more rare and included for a sense of perspective on the challenges facing a congenital heart surgeon. I also have purely personal reasons for mentioning them. In the 1970s and early 1980s, I was fortunate enough to work with Dr. C. Everett Koop at the Children's Hospital of Philadelphia. It was my privilege to have been involved with the care and surgery of some of these patients. Koop, later to become surgeon general of the United States, was then chief of pediatric surgery and

| Table 7-2: Relative frequency of occurrence of cardiac malformations at birth | |
|---|---|
| **Disease** | **Percentage** |
| Ventricular septal defect | 30.5 |
| Atrial septal defect | 9.8 |
| Patent ductus arteriosus | 9.7 |
| Pulmonary stenosis | 6.9 |
| Coarctation of the aorta | 6.8 |
| Aortic stenosis | 6.1 |
| Tetralogy of Fallot | 5.8 |
| Complete transposition of great arteries | 4.2 |
| Truncus arteriosus | 2.2 |
| Tricuspid atresia | 1.3 |
| All others | 16.5 |

Source: *Heart Disease: A Textbook of Cardiovascular Medicine.*

**Table 7-2:**
This table shows the most common congenital heart and major vessel defects. The ventricular septal defect, comprising almost 30 percent of congenital heart defects, is by far the most common.

had cared for patients with both types of these very rare and difficult defects.

### Ventricular Septal Defect

In this most common congenital defect there is a hole in the septum that separates the right and left ventricles (Fig. 7.2). As a result, blood is short-circuited back into the lungs, putting a burden on both heart and lungs. About 30 percent to 50 percent of these holes, especially the smaller ones, close over time. Patients with large- or moderate-size defects that do not close spontaneously, however, eventually need an operation to close them. Larger defects may have to be closed in the first year of life because they can cause shortness of breath and other symptoms of heart failure. If the defect is not closed, the patient can also develop pulmonary vascular disease, which damages blood vessels in the lungs and can eventually be fatal.

Ventricular septal defects vary in size and location, so naturally some of them are more easily closed surgically than others. While in surgery, the patient's heart and lung function are provided by a heart-lung machine, and the actual hole is closed

**Ductus Arteriosus:**
A tube connecting the pulmonary artery to the aorta. After birth, when the lungs begin to function, this tube normally closes.

**Fig. 7.2: Ventricular Septal Defect:**
In this defect there is a hole in the wall of muscle, or septum, that separates the left and right ventricles. It is usually corrected with a patch.

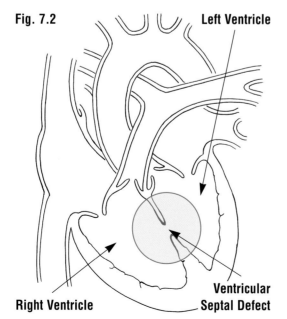

**Fig. 7.2**

Left Ventricle

Right Ventricle

Ventricular Septal Defect

with a patch. The chances of surviving the surgery in childhood and subsequently living a normal life are superb.

### Patent Ductus Arteriosus

While the fetal heart is developing, a tube develops between the aorta and the pulmonary artery. This tube, called the **ductus arteriosus**, is responsible for bypassing the lungs, moving blood from the pulmonary artery to the aorta. Because the fetus receives oxygenated blood from its mother through the placenta, it has no need for functioning lungs. After the child is born, however, the lungs begin to function, and the ductus arteriosus is no longer needed. It normally closes from a couple of hours to a couple of days after birth. However, if it remains open, or patent, it is considered a congenital defect and usually needs treatment (Fig. 7.3).

In some cases, the patent ductus arteriosus is so large that enough blood is shunted back from the aorta into the low-pressure pulmonary artery to actually flood the lungs. Heart failure can develop because the heart is working so hard to pump blood, and much of it is just being short-circuited back to the lungs. In other cases, infections develop in the tube, or over time high blood pressure in the pulmonary arteries can result in what's called pulmonary vascular disease. This disease damages the blood vessels in the lungs where resistance to blood flow increases and, at some point, the blood flow can actually reverse. If this happens, the right ventricle, which should be pumping unoxygenated blood into the lungs, is actually pumping unoxygenated blood through the ductus directly into the aorta. This condition causes blueness, or cyanosis, and is very serious. Fortunately, the open ductus is usually diagnosed well before this condition develops, and the defect can be corrected.

There are three ways to close a patent ductus. In newborn babies, especially

# ♥SIR BARRATT-BOYES: OPENING HEART SURGERY "DOWN UNDER"

WHILE TRAINING TO BECOME a heart surgeon, native New Zealander Sir Brian Barratt-Boyes had the opportunity to spend two years working at the Mayo Clinic.

"I was assigned to various surgeons," he said. "Dr. John Kirklin was one. He had recently begun there, but he was making a name for himself, and in 1955, began doing open heart surgery with the Gibbon-IBM heart-lung machine. It was a staggering responsibility.

"We went through a very rapid learning curve," Barratt-Boyes said. "Some of it was pretty traumatic, but the results were exceptional. I used to be sent as a spy to Minneapolis to see what Dr. C. Walton Lillehei was doing. I reported what was happening so I saw the cross-circulation operations as well, which were very fascinating."

In 1956, he returned to his native New Zealand and entered a kind of creative vacuum. New Zealand was isolated from the medical community. Later, in fact, Barratt-Boyes would be credited with founding modern open heart surgery in the Pacific Rim area.

"If you are working independently and follow your own star and your own ideas, you can sometimes come up with something that wouldn't be the case if you worked in a group, where everybody has their own ideas," Barratt-Boyes said.

It was there that Barratt-Boyes made two contributions to cardiac surgery. In 1962, only a month after Dr. Donald Ross in England, Barratt-Boyes performed the world's second successful aortic valve **homograft** implantation. "It worked extremely well, even in the first patient, who was a young girl of about fifteen with **endocarditis**," Barratt-Boyes said. "She had a successful operation and recovered from her endocarditis. She's now had several children and works outside the home. She is a remarkable person."

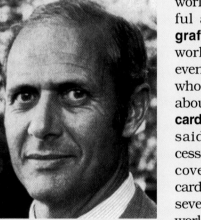

**Brian B. Barratt-Boyes**

After this, Barratt-Boyes, working with surgeons from Japan, helped introduce and popularize open heart surgery in infants by using hypothermia, or lowering the body temperature to protect the brain.

His results with infants, often desperately ill and with complex forms of congenital heart disease, set new world standards. This method was an important stepping stone, and even today most centers use variations of hypothermia techniques in some infants and adult patients.

**Homograft:**
A donor graft, or piece of tissue, taken from a donor and placed into a recipient of the same species.

**Endocarditis:**
An infection involving the heart, caused by bacteria.

**Aorta**

**Patent Ductus Arteriosus**

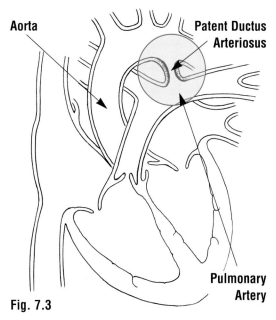

**Pulmonary Artery**

**Fig. 7.3**

Fig. 7.3: **Patent Ductus Arteriosus:** An abnormality in which a tube connects the pulmonary artery to the aorta, mixing unoxygenated and oxygenated blood. This tube is open during fetal development when the lungs are not needed but is supposed to close after birth.

premature newborns, it can frequently be closed by giving a medicine called indomethacin, which causes the ductus to constrict and close. This treatment does not always work, however.

The conventional treatment is surgical closure. This is done by opening the chest on the left side and dividing the ductus and oversewing its ends, or closing it with a tie or a metal clip.

There are also catheters that can be threaded through blood vessels to deliver devices that actually plug the ductus. This avoids a surgical incision in the chest. This procedure has advantages and disadvantages that should be discussed with the pediatrician and the pediatric cardiologist. Trial tests of these devices are being evaluated by the U.S. Food and Drug Administration (FDA).

With all methods, the chances of surviving the closure procedure are better than 99 percent, and in most cases the patient is cured.

**Atrial Septal Defect**

An atrial septal defect (ASD) is a hole in the common wall separating the two atria (Fig. 7.4). There are different types of atrial septal defects. In most cases, they are

well tolerated by children and may not be diagnosed until the child is older — and sometimes not even until adulthood.

Once diagnosed, however, most of these should be closed. Depending on the size, the hole can be sewn up. Larger holes may require a patch of pericardial tissue or an artificial material such as Dacron.

If the hole is not repaired, heart failure can develop because much of the blood pumped by the heart is being short-circuited through the lungs instead of being pumped out to the body, meaning the heart has to work harder to pump more blood. Occasionally, pulmonary vascular disease may develop, or blood clots dislodged from veins in the legs may travel through the ASD and lodge in the brain, causing a stroke. In most cases, the risk of the surgery to repair the defect in children is low, and the survival rate is greater than 99 percent. Devices to close ASDs with a catheter are under development and are being tested at some centers.

There is another, more complex atrial septal defect that may occur with a ventricular septal defect called atrioventricular canal defect. The risks associated with the surgical repair of this defect

**Superior Vena Cava**

**Atrial Septal Defect**

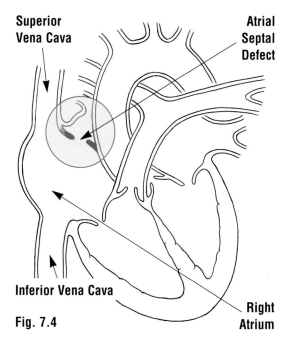

**Inferior Vena Cava**

**Fig. 7.4**

**Right Atrium**

Fig. 7.4: **Atrial Septal Defect:** An abnormal opening in the wall of muscle, or septum, that divides the two filling chambers, or atria, of the heart.

are somewhat higher. Children with Down's syndrome have a higher chance of having atrioventricular canal defect.

Any surgical repair of atrial septal defect requires a heart-lung machine, and afterwards most patients can look forward to a normal life expectancy.

**Coarctation of the Aorta**

In coarctation of the aorta, there is an abnormal narrowing of a short segment of the aorta, usually less than an inch long (Fig. 7.5). The aorta can be narrowed up to 90 percent in this area. Over time, it can become totally occluded. If the aorta is narrowed, blood to the lower body bypasses the narrowing by using collaterals, or tiny channels. In a healthy person, these collaterals are barely functioning, but in patients with coarctation they can become very large.

This defect can be diagnosed at birth or shortly afterwards. Typical signs include high blood pressure in the arms and abnormally low blood pressure in the legs, and strong pulses in the arms and minimal or absent pulses in the legs. Some infants may develop severe heart failure, and an emergency operation may be required. In less severe cases, coarctation of the aorta is not diagnosed until a child is older and sometimes not until he or she is a teenager or an adult.

The life span of people with coarctation of the aorta can be severely shortened if they do not have surgical correction. This is partially because of the high blood pressure in the upper body, which can result in strokes or heart failure. Also, infection is prone to occur at the point of the coarctation, or the aorta can rupture near the coarctation.

In surgery, doctors can remove the narrowed area and suture the normal ends of the aorta back together. Or they can widen the narrowed area with a patch, or replace the narrowed area with a tube made of Dacron. This is a curative

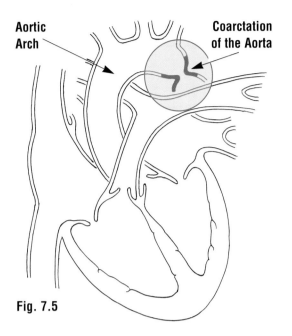

**Aortic Arch**

**Coarctation of the Aorta**

**Fig. 7.5**

Fig. 7.5: **Coarctation of the Aorta:** An abnormal narrowing of the aorta after it leaves the heart.

operation. The chance of surviving repair of isolated coarctation of the aorta is greater than 99 percent. The arteries that supply blood to the spinal cord sometimes originate from the aorta in the area of the coarctation. Because of this, about one in two hundred patients undergoing surgical repair develops some degree of paralysis of the lower half of the body. Occasionally the defect can recur and has to be reoperated on. If it does recur, the narrowed segment can sometimes be dilated with a balloon catheter.

**Transposition of the Great Arteries**

In transposition of the great arteries, the two main arteries coming out of the heart, the aorta and the pulmonary artery, are switched (Fig. 7.6). As a result, when the unoxygenated blood returns from the veins into the heart, it is pumped directly back into the aorta, making the infant very cyanotic. The oxygenated blood that returns from the lungs is pumped back into the lungs through the pulmonary artery, which branches off the left ventricle. When children have any congenital heart defect in which the child is cyanotic or the skin is a bluish color, they are sometimes referred to as blue babies. In some cases of transposition of the great arteries, there also may be other heart defects, such as ventricular septal defect.

Infants suffering from transposition are usually quite cyanotic, and if it is not corrected, they will probably not survive their first year of life. Before the advent of the heart-lung machine, there were some palliative operations developed, but these procedures were not cures. In fact, even today many infants with transposition undergo a procedure to make or enlarge a hole in the atrial septum shortly after birth. This procedure is done in the cardiac catheterization laboratory with a special catheter threaded up through a blood vessel in the groin. The hole in the atrial septum allows mixing of blood and temporarily improves the infant's condition until a surgical repair can be made.

Currently there are a number of ways this defect can be repaired surgically. One technique involves switching the pulmonary artery back to the right ventricle and the aorta back to the left ventricle. This procedure is technically challenging because the coronary arteries that come

off the aorta are quite small, particularly in infants. These tiny coronary arteries have to be moved and reconnected to the aorta in its new location.

With current surgical techniques, the chances of surviving the surgical procedure, depending on the complexity of the transposition malformation, are between 90 and 95 percent. The long-term survival is good for most patients.

**Tetralogy of Fallot**

This complicated condition is actually four different congenital defects occurring simultaneously in the same heart. Tetralogy, in fact, means "set of four," and Fallot was a French physician who was one of the first to describe the condition.

In this defect (Fig. 7.7), 1) there is a ventricular septal defect; 2) blood flow from the right ventricle to the pulmonary arteries is obstructed (the obstruction can be at the pulmonary valve or in the right ventricular outflow tract leading to the valve and/or in the pulmonary arteries themselves); 3) the aortic valve overrides the ventricular septal defect; and 4) the right ventricle is abnormally thickened.

Fig. 7.6: **Transposition of the Great Arteries:** When the two main arteries arising from the heart, the pulmonary artery and the aorta, are switched, causing unoxygenated blood to be pumped back out through the aorta into the circulation. The normal heart at far right is shown here for comparison.

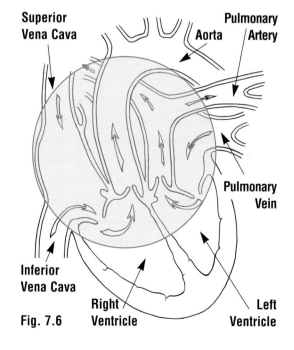

**Superior Vena Cava**    **Aorta**   **Pulmonary Artery**

**Inferior Vena Cava**

**Fig. 7.6**    **Right Ventricle**    **Left Ventricle**

**Pulmonary Vein**

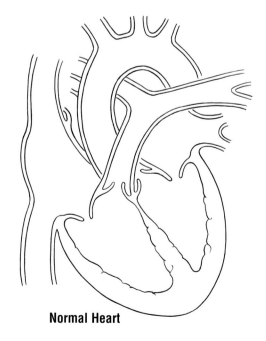

**Normal Heart**

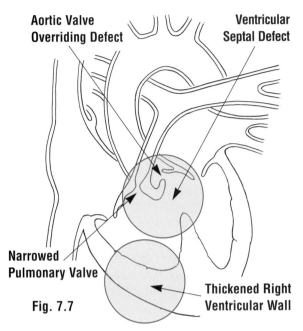

**Aortic Valve Overriding Defect**

**Ventricular Septal Defect**

**Narrowed Pulmonary Valve**

**Fig. 7.7**

**Thickened Right Ventricular Wall**

Because of the location of the ventricular septal defect in relation to the aortic valve and the obstruction of blood flow through the pulmonary arteries to the lungs, unoxygenated blood returning from the body is shunted from the right ventricle to the left ventricle. It mixes with the oxygenated blood returning from the lungs, which results in blueness or cyanosis. In some forms of tetralogy of Fallot, the defects are more severe, particularly in terms of the amount of unoxygenated blood flowing from the right ventricle across to the left ventricle. The more severe the obstruction, the more cyanotic the patient. In some cases, newborns will suffer from severe cyanosis and may have to undergo urgent surgery.

In most cases, doctors recommend that the defect be corrected sooner rather than later, usually within the first six months of life. The surgical repair includes closing the ventricular septal defect and relieving the obstruction of blood flow to the pulmonary arteries. In some special circumstances, however, palliative shunting procedures are recommended before a complete repair is made.

Because of the cyanosis associated with this defect, patients used to be called "blue babies," and the early surgical shunts, like the Blalock-Taussig shunt, that were performed were known as "blue baby operations." These operations would alleviate a good deal of the cyanosis and restore the children to a more normal color.

The chance of surviving a primary surgical repair is greater than 90 percent. Long-term survival in most of the patients whose defect is repaired is good.

If the defect is not repaired, serious complications can develop, including progressive cyanosis, strokes and infections of the brain, pulmonary hemorrhage, and severe hypoxic spells related to a lack of oxygen. Without surgical intervention, most patients with tetralogy of Fallot will not survive until their twentieth birthday.

**Pulmonary Valve Stenosis**

Pulmonary valve stenosis is a narrowing of the heart valve located between the right ventricle and the pulmonary artery (Fig. 7.8). When the valve is very narrow, the patient may have substantial symptoms while still an infant, including a bluish tinge to the skin. This defect can be life threatening. In older children, symp-

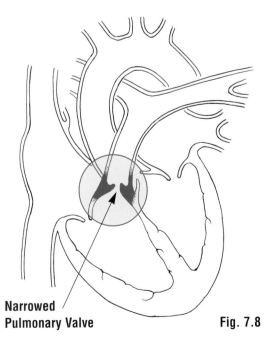

**Narrowed Pulmonary Valve**

**Fig. 7.8**

Fig. 7.7:
**Tetralogy of Fallot:**
A set of four individual defects, including:
1) a ventricular septal defect; 2) an obstruction of blood flow from the right ventricle to the pulmonary arteries;
3) overriding of the aortic valve above the ventricular septal defect;
and 4) an abnormally thickened right ventricle.

Fig. 7.8: **Pulmonary Valve Stenosis:**
An abnormally narrowed pulmonary valve, which is located between the right ventricle and the pulmonary artery.

toms include fatigue or a reduced ability to exercise. The child may stand out because he or she cannot keep up with the other children physically.

The diagnosis is often suspected after hearing a **heart murmur** and obtaining an electrocardiogram. An echocardiogram will likely identify the defect and allow a definitive diagnosis to be made. For simple pulmonary valve stenosis, a balloon catheter is used to dilate the valve, usually with good results. Sometimes surgery using the heart-lung machine is necessary. In some cases, there is also muscular obstruction within the right ventricle, and this tissue needs to be removed. The results, after balloon dilatation or surgery, are usually excellent. The chance of surviving these procedures is greater than 99 percent. The long-term results are usually excellent.

### Congenital Aortic Stenosis

In this defect's simplest form, the aortic valve is abnormally narrowed (Fig. 7.9). Other variations of this defect include narrowing of the aorta immediately above the heart valve or a membrane obstructing blood flow below the aortic valve. In some

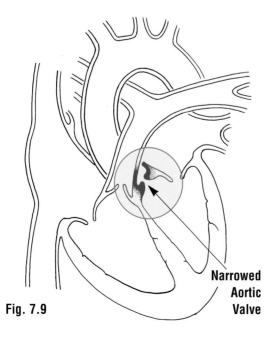

**Fig. 7.9**

**Narrowed Aortic Valve**

cases, an abnormality of the muscle immediately below the heart valve causes obstruction. Children with severe forms of aortic stenosis are likely to have symptoms of heart failure and shortness of breath. This defect may be suspected because of a heart murmur or because of an abnormal ECG. Confirmation of the diagnosis would be made with an echocardiogram. In some instances a cardiac catheterization may be necessary to make the diagnosis.

With the most severe forms, an infant may require emergency heart surgery to open the valve. Some pediatric heart centers use a balloon catheter to open the narrowed heart valve, thus postponing valve surgery until the child is older.

The decision to recommend heart valve surgery depends on how serious the obstruction is. This defect may be so mild that surgical intervention is unnecessary. If surgery is necessary in straightforward and uncomplicated forms of the disease, the chance of surviving the procedure is greater than 98 percent. The chance of surviving the surgery is somewhat lower in more complex forms of the disease, and surgery is higher risk in critically ill **neonates**. With a successful procedure, long-term results are often very good, although in many instances, a second heart valve operation may be needed later.

### Hypoplastic Left Heart Syndrome

Hypoplastic left heart syndrome (HLHS) is one of the most severe and life-threatening malformations of the human heart. "Hypoplastic" means "underdeveloped," left heart refers to the structures that make up the left side of the heart, and syndrome means a group of things that appear together.

The job of the left heart is to receive oxygenated blood from the lungs and distribute it to the body. The left heart includes the left atrium (left filling chamber), the left ventricle (main pumping

**Heart Murmur**:
A noise produced from blood flowing through the heart or other blood vessels or through the lungs.

**Neonate:**
A newborn, or a child within the first several weeks after birth.

Fig. 7.9: **Congenital Aortic Stenosis:** This defect is usually an abnormal narrowing of the aortic valve, which is located between the aorta and the left ventricle. There are, however, several different forms of this defect.

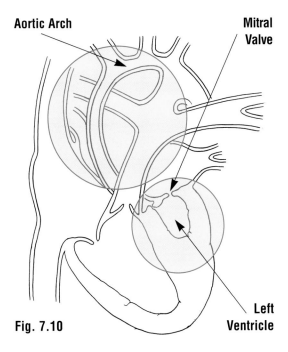

**Aortic Arch**

**Mitral Valve**

**Fig. 7.10**

**Left Ventricle**

chamber), the mitral valve (valve between the left atrium and the left ventricle), the aortic valve (valve between the left ventricle and the aorta), and the aorta. HLHS consists of a wide spectrum of malformations in which one or more of these structures are critically small (Fig. 7.10). Despite the variation that can exist in cases of HLHS, the net result is the same: The left side of the heart cannot do its job properly.

Unfortunately, this is not a rare condition. Data from the New England Regional Infant Cardiac Program found HLHS to be present at a rate of 0.163 per one thousand live births.

Without surgery, 99 percent of patients with HLHS will die shortly after birth. In 1983, Dr. William Norwood at Boston Children's Hospital reported that he had successfully operated on an infant in two separate stages about a year and a half apart. That two-stage operation has greatly improved the chance of survival for infants born with HLHS. Today, Norwood's two-stage repair has evolved into a three-stage repair performed over the first few years of the patient's life.

The goal of these three operations is to bypass the small left side of the heart by making the right ventricle the heart's main pumping chamber. Since the right ventricle will, therefore, no longer be available to perform its usual job of pumping blood to the lungs, the vessels that normally carry the unoxygenated blood (superior and inferior vena cavae) are connected directly to the lung arteries. The flow of unoxygenated blood to the lungs occurs passively without the benefit of an intervening pumping chamber. This type of passive pulmonary blood flow in a heart with only one good pumping chamber is called a Fontan operation — another variation is the Glenn operation. It is applicable not only in HLHS but also in other types of abnormal hearts with a single pumping chamber.

The advantage of the three-stage Norwood procedure is that these operations can almost always be performed; the disadvantage is that it requires three operations and still results in a heart with only one pumping chamber. Furthermore, the long-term results of using the right ventricle (instead of the left ventricle) to pump oxygenated blood to the body are not known.

Dr. Leonard Bailey at Loma Linda University has pioneered the use of newborn heart transplantation for the treatment of HLHS. If a donor heart is available, cardiac transplantation requires only one operation and produces a structurally normal heart with two pumping chambers. Unfortunately, about 25 percent of the newborns who would need a cardiac transplantation die of complications while waiting for a donor heart. After cardiac transplantation, the patient must take antirejection medication for the rest of his or her life. The side effects of these medicines can become serious over time, and rejection of the transplanted heart can occur. Incidentally, Bailey created quite an uproar in the news media in 1984 when a human heart donor was not

Fig. 7.10: **Hypoplastic Left Heart Syndrome:** This literally means underdeveloped left heart. Some or all of the structures on the left side of the heart, including the heart's main pumping chamber, are undersized. It is a very serious congenital defect.

available and he transplanted the heart of a baboon into a desperately ill twelve-day-old premature girl known as "Baby Fay," who was suffering from HLHS.

At this point it is not clear which surgical treatment is better for hypoplastic left heart syndrome. Both, however, are an improvement on previously available treatments. HLHS used to be 100 percent fatal during the first year of life. Although pediatric heart surgeons tend to hold strong opinions, neither the Norwood procedure nor cardiac transplantation is a perfect treatment option for HLHS, and neither approach is clearly superior. In the best centers, roughly 60 percent of patients who undergo either surgery are alive ten years later.

### Ectopia Cordis

This is a rare congenital heart defect. As of 1989, only 219 cases had ever been reported in the medical literature.

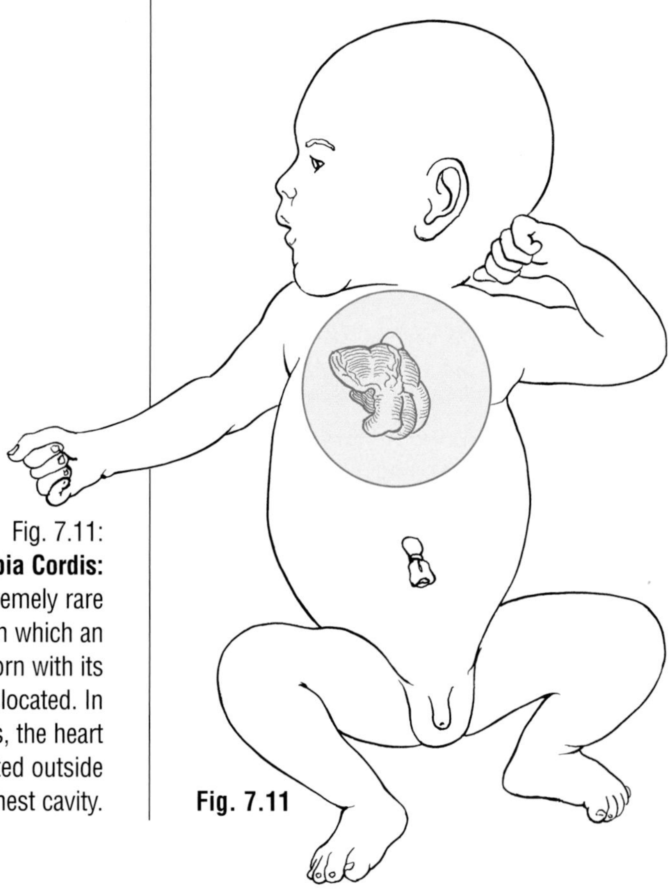

Fig. 7.11:
**Ectopia Cordis:**
An extremely rare condition in which an infant is born with its heart mislocated. In some cases, the heart is even located outside of the chest cavity.

**Fig. 7.11**

Ectopia means displacement, and cordis means heart.

There are four types of this defect: the heart may be located in the neck, either partially or completely in the abdomen, or, almost unbelievably, outside of the body on the chest (Fig. 7.11). Many infants suffering from this defect have other abnormalities inside the heart as well.

When the heart is outside of the body, it is recommended that the infant undergo immediate surgery to put the heart back into the chest. The first successful surgery of this type was performed by Dr. Narish Saxena at the Children's Hospital of Philadelphia in 1975. This case, in which I was involved, was that of a child who had to undergo multiple innovative surgeries and practically lived the first few years of his life in the hospital.

### Thoracopagus Twins

Identical twins occur at an incidence of four per one thousand births. Conjoined twins are identical twins who are joined to each other in some place on their bodies. This form of twin is much rarer and has an incidence of one per fifty thousand to one hundred thousand births. In 1811, in the country of Siam (now Thailand), a Chinese mother gave birth to identical twins joined at the hip. The boys were named Eng and Chang, and they lived unseparated until their death at age sixty-three years. They became famous as a result of being promoted as "freaks" by P.T. Barnum, who called them the "Siamese Twins," and the term has been used since then for all twins who are born attached to each other.

Most Siamese twins are born dead, but there are about four hundred sets known to have lived, ranging in life span from just a few hours to the sixty-three years of Eng and Chang. They can be joined in various places on the body, including the lower back, the abdomen, the hip, the leg, and even the head. About 40

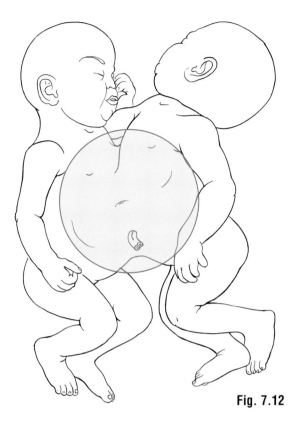

**Fig. 7.12**

racopagus twins." (Thoraco refers to the chest; pagus is a Greek word meaning fixed). Thoracopagus twins may also be joined at the abdomen down to the pubis. They may share a common liver, intestines or even a heart.

For pediatric heart and thoracic surgeons, the division of thoracopagus children ranges from extremely challenging to outright impossible with today's knowledge. My experience in one case with Koop, the chief pediatric surgeon, and Dr. L. Henry Edmunds, Jr., the chief heart surgeon at the University of Pennsylvania, involved a set of Siamese twins with only one heart between them. Before the surgery could be done, the children had to be taken to the operating room and the procedure mapped out ahead of time, position by position, turning them in different ways for each incision. The surgery was considered a success even though we were able to save only one child, but generally success in this very complicated field has been limited. Twin separation remains a challenge for the pediatric surgical community.

percent of the surviving twins are joined at the chest, face to face, looking each other in the eye (Fig. 7.12). They are called "tho-

Fig. 7.12:
**Conjoined Twins:**
Commonly referred to as "Siamese twins," these are a set of twins who are joined at some place on their bodies, including at the chest.

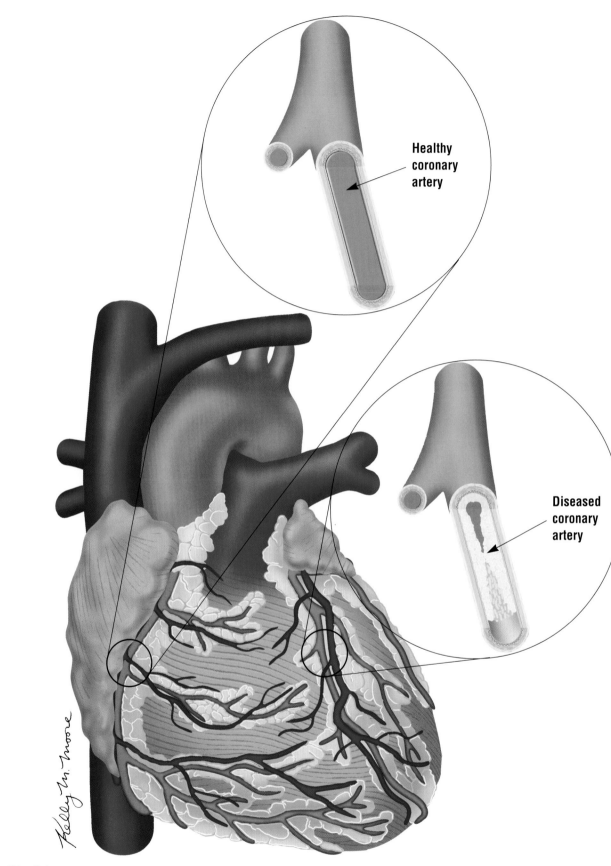

**Healthy coronary artery**

**Diseased coronary artery**

**Fig. 8.1:**
Coronary artery disease is caused by atherosclerosis. During this process, plaque builds up in healthy arteries and gradually clogs them.

**Fig. 8.1**

## CHAPTER EIGHT

# CORONARY ARTERY DISEASE AND TREATMENT OPTIONS

IN THE EARLY PART OF THIS CENtury, Nobel Prize–winning surgeon Dr. Alexis Carrel attempted what may have been the first bypass of a coronary artery. Without a heart-lung machine, however, his animal trial met with limited success.

Little else happened in the dawning field until 1930, when a French surgeon named Dr. Rene Leriche developed a method to attach skeletal muscle to the heart in animals, in hopes that new blood vessels would form. This line of research was pursued by Dr. Claude Beck in Cleveland, who confirmed that new blood vessels did indeed grow into the heart muscle from tissues wrapped around the heart. In his first attempt to treat coronary disease in a human patient, Beck roughened the outer surface of the heart with a burr and sutured a graft of skeletal muscle from the chest to the heart. New vessels formed, and the patient recovered. The patient's angina also disappeared. Beck went on to perform variations of this operation in sixteen patients.

In 1946, a Canadian surgeon named Dr. Arthur Vineberg performed an operation on a patient with a coronary artery blockage. He tunneled the internal mammary artery from the chest wall into the patient's heart muscle but did not directly connect it to one of the heart's arteries. He was hoping new blood vessels would sprout from the mammary artery and connect with the blocked blood vessels in the heart. Over the next several months, new vessels formed, giving the heart a new blood supply. Although the Vineberg operation enjoyed some popularity in the following decades, the chief drawback, as with Beck's operation, was that it took months for new blood vessels to form — if they formed at all.

At about the same time, surgeons began to perform a procedure called **endarterectomy**, which basically meant cleaning out atherosclerotic material from the coronary arteries. Endarterectomies were often quite extensive and sometimes involved almost the entire length of the artery. Although the results were good with larger arteries in the body, the early results with coronary arteries were not good. Some patients survived for years, but in many cases the coronary arteries clotted off soon after the surgery. The high mortality rate was considered unacceptable, and doctors continued searching for new and better ways to treat coronary artery disease. Today, coronary endarterec-

**Endarterectomy:**
A surgical procedure in which atherosclerotic material in an artery is removed and the artery is either sewn back together or a patch is placed over the surgical incision.

**Coronary Artery Bypass Grafting (CABG):**
A surgical technique in which one's own veins or other arteries are used to route blood around a blocked area in a coronary artery.

Dr. Rene Favaloro, below, performed early saphenous vein bypass graft operations to treat coronary artery disease.

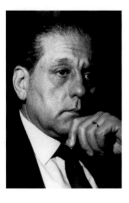

tomy is still used by some surgeons, but it's done in conjunction with **coronary artery bypass grafting**.

 **The Coronary Bypass Evolves**

Even while endarterectomy was being tested on patients, teams of surgeons were approaching the first successful modern coronary artery bypass graft surgery. The story of the bypass begins as early as 1952, when the renowned Soviet surgeon Dr. Vladimir Demikhov was joining the internal mammary artery, which is under the breast bone, to the left coronary artery in dogs. Other surgeons soon began to study coronary artery bypass grafting in experimental animals.

In 1962, the technique received a major boost when Dr. Mason Sones at the Cleveland Clinic reported on a technique called selective **coronary arteriography** (Fig. 8.2). In this procedure, a catheter is threaded up through an artery in either the groin or the arm and used to inject radiopaque contrast material directly into the coronary arteries. This technique supplied the road maps for the surgical treatment of coronary artery disease. For the first time, chest surgeons were able to see the exact location of blockages and plan their surgery.

Meanwhile, the idea of using a piece of the patient's own vein for a bypass graft of a blocked artery was gaining acceptance. During the Korean War, surgeons were more commonly using the saphenous vein from the leg, which is a superficial vein that runs from the groin to the ankle area and is totally expendable (Fig. 8.3), to bypass arteries in the leg that were injured and blocked. As the concept gained widespread acceptance, some doctors began to envision using vein grafts to bypass blocked coronary arteries, and sporadic attempts were made throughout the early part of the decade.

In 1967, at the height of the Cold War, a Soviet surgeon, Dr. V.I. Kolessov from

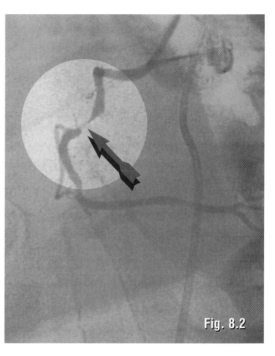
Fig. 8.2

Leningrad, reported in an American surgical journal his experience with internal mammary artery–coronary artery anastomosis for the treatment of coronary artery blockages in six patients. Operations were performed through an incision in the left chest without the heart-lung machine. The following year, Dr. Charles Bailey and Dr. Teruo Hirose from New York published a report on surgery in which the internal mammary artery was used to bypass blockages in the right coronary artery in two patients. In 1968, Dr. George Green, also from New York, used the heart-lung machine to bypass a patient's left anterior descending coronary with the internal mammary artery.

That same year, Dr. Rene Favaloro, a surgeon from the Cleveland Clinic, used the saphenous vein technique to bypass blockages of the coronary arteries in fifteen patients. This group had also had the Vineberg operation, in which a mammary artery was tunneled into the heart to increase blood flow. The saphenous vein bypass graft was inserted between the aorta and the right coronary artery. The bypass was performed by dividing the coronary artery and sewing the vein graft end-to-end beyond the blockage in the right coronary artery. In an addendum to the published paper, fifty-five more cases were added — fifty-two for blockages of the right coronary artery and three others for diseases in the left circumflex coronary artery.

Most surgeons, however, remained extremely skeptical of the coronary bypass operation, especially that in which the saphenous vein was used. This was because, although the saphenous vein bypass grafts worked relatively well for bypassing arterial blockages in the legs, it was not uncommon for these bypasses to clot off and require urgent surgery to save the leg. It was feared that if saphenous veins were used to bypass coronary arteries, particularly those supplying the left ventricle, a blood clot would result in instant death.

By May 1969, all of this was about to change. At the annual meeting of the American Surgical Association, a young surgeon who had recently completed his heart surgery training, Dr. W. Dudley Johnson from Marquette University in Milwaukee, reported on a series of 301 patients who had undergone various operations for coronary disease since February 1967. Many of the techniques he described are still used today. In that report, which was published later that year in a major surgical journal, Johnson stated:

*"The vein graft technique was expanded and used in all major branches (of the coronary arteries). Vein grafts to the left-sided arteries run from the aorta over the pulmonary artery and down to the appropriate coronary (blood) vessel. Right-sided grafts run along the atrial-ventricular groove and also attach directly to the aorta. There is almost no limit to the potential (coronary) arteries to be bypassed. Veins can be sutured into the distal (far end) anterior*

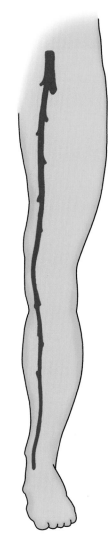

**Fig. 8.3 (above):**
The saphenous vein runs from the groin to the ankle.

**Fig. 8.4 (left):**
The saphenous vein bypass graft, a common bypass technique, using saphenous veins from the legs, is used to bypass blocked portions of the coronary arteries. A double bypass is shown.

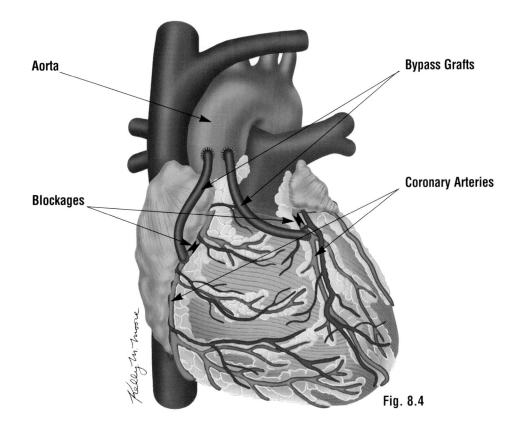

Aorta

Bypass Grafts

Blockages

Coronary Arteries

**Fig. 8.4**

# THE FIRST CORONARY ARTERY BYPASS SURGERY

**D**R. DUDLEY JOHNSON, WHO was one of a handful of doctors who popularized the modern coronary bypass operation, first knew he wanted to practice medicine while in seventh or eighth grade — but he didn't know he wanted to be a surgeon until he got into medical school.

"And then I didn't really have any illusions about being a heart surgeon," Johnson said in a 1999 interview. "But I figured if I had experience in the chest, I could get a little better job in a clinic somewhere, so I also trained to do lung surgery along with general surgery. As it turned out, the doctor in Milwaukee, Dr. Derward Lepley, Jr., who was in charge of the heart surgical realm, which was really in its infancy in the middle sixties, asked me to join him in practice, so I ended up staying in heart surgery."

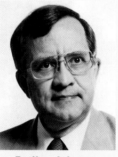

**Dudley Johnson**

It was a fortunate decision for the field of heart surgery. At the time, surgical teams across the country were experimenting with various treatments for arteriosclerosis in the coronary arteries. Endarterectomy, or stripping plaque from the coronary arteries, was an accepted treatment. Bypass grafts, which were being placed into the coronary arteries of animals, remained a controversial procedure that many surgeons thought wouldn't work. Various attempts were made, including one in 1962 by Dr. David Sabiston, who probably performed the first bypass in a human. Unfortunately, his patient died only days later of a stroke.

Meanwhile, a team of doctors in Houston under the leadership of Dr. Michael DeBakey was developing its own bypass program. "If you go back to that period, you will find there was a great deal of work being done in the experimental laboratory on coronary bypass and other types of coronary surgery," DeBakey said. "In 1961, we wrote our last article on our experimental work with animals. We came out with the conclusion that we had about a 50 percent rate at the end of six months with the bypass graft staying open. We said that was very encouraging and we felt that more experimental work ought to be done."

DeBakey's team did continue its animal research — until a historic moment in 1964. The surgical team, having already heard about Sabiston's unsuccessful bypass, was in the midst of an endarterectomy for a patient when an unforeseen opportunity arose. DeBakey recently told the story:

*"This fellow had total blockage of the right coronary, and the only thing he was living on really was his left anterior descending (LAD) coronary artery and a little diagonal branch, and he had a blockage in the left main coronary, right where the LAD began. It was a complicated lesion. When we got in and tried to do the endarterectomy, we kept trying to find the cleavage plane, but we couldn't find it. We knew we couldn't get this fellow off the table unless we restored circula-*

*tion in the one artery that was supplying all the blood to his heart. So we decided right then and there to do what we had been doing in animals. We got a little piece of vein out of his leg and put it in, and it worked."*

This was probably the first successful coronary artery bypass graft surgery. Drs. H. Edward Garrett, Edward W. Dennis, and DeBakey, however, didn't report this success in the medical literature until eight years after the procedure. "In the final analysis, I don't think we deserve all that great a credit for having done the first coronary bypass in a patient," he recently said.

*"It was an accident! I think the most important thing to point out about this was the fact that we were doing experimental work, and if we had not been doing the experiments, we wouldn't have thought of doing it in a patient.... I think that's about as good an example as you can provide for the usefulness of animal laboratory experimental work."*

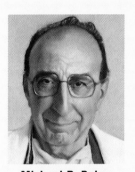

**Michael DeBakey**

**Johnson Shows the World**

While this first successful graft remained pretty much unknown throughout the mid-1960s, other surgeons at various heart centers continued their work. Johnson, by then a heart surgeon himself, remembered visiting the Cleveland Clinic to watch early coronary patch grafts, which only widened the narrow and diseased portion of the artery. After seeing the technique, he went home and "promptly did two such patches."

Johnson, however, did not like sewing a patch onto the most diseased portion of the artery when the disease had obviously spread beyond the patch. "It occurred to me that the diseased area could be avoided completely by opening the artery beyond the disease. A vein could be attached like a patch, and the other end of the vein simply attached to the aorta."

But there was much controversy surrounding a complete bypass procedure, beginning with the technique used to connect the vein graft to the coronary artery and the aorta. Surgeons also debated if more than one vein graft could be placed, or how many "bypasses" were practical.

In 1969, Johnson introduced the modern saphenous vein bypass with the end-to-side sewing technique. He helped settle many of these controversies with his string of successful operations and the multiple-bypass technique he developed, including the double, triple, and quadruple bypass. Since then, he has performed more than ten thousand coronary bypass operations.

"The long-term results of coronary artery bypass graft surgery have been evaluated in several centers. In many subgroups of patients, life expectancy has returned to normal or even better than normal," Johnson said. "Coronary artery bypass graft surgery has stimulated more than nine thousand published reports in the medical literature. It does more to change quality and length of life than what medicine can do for most other major chronic diseases. The coronary artery bypass graft operation does nothing for the basic cause of the disease, however, and prevention is, of course, the ultimate answer."

*descending or even to the posterior margin branches.*

*"Double vein grafts are now used in over 40 percent of patients and can be used to graft any combination of arteries.... This direct approach to coronary flow immediately improves heart function and alleviates most clinical symptoms."*

In discussing Johnson's presentation, a prominent New York surgeon named Dr. Frank Spencer commented: "I would like to congratulate Dr. Johnson very heartily. We may have heard of a milestone in cardiac surgery today.... If the exciting data by Dr. Johnson remains valid and the grafts remain patent [i.e., open] over a long period of time, a total revision of thinking will be required regarding the feasibility of direct arterial surgery for coronary artery disease."

### Coronary Artery Disease Today

Almost fourteen million Americans alive today have a history of heart attack, angina pectoris, or both. In 1999, it was estimated that more than one million Americans will have a new or recurrent heart attack. It will be fatal in about one-third of these cases. At least 250,000 people a year in the United States die of a heart attack within one hour of the onset of symptoms — even before they can reach the hospital. Based on the Framingham Study in Massachusetts, 5 percent of all heart attacks occur in people under age forty years, whereas 45 percent occur in people under age sixty-five years (statistics released by the American Heart Association for 1998).

Since its development, the coronary bypass operation has evolved into the leading surgery to treat clogged heart arteries. Patients who have bypasses are often relieved of angina immediately, and their bypass grafts usually stay open for years to come. Hundreds of thousands of bypass operations are performed every year.

### Coronary Artery Anatomy

Although each person's coronary artery system is somewhat different, most people have two coronary arteries that come off the aorta: the right coronary and the left main coronary. The left main coronary artery is like a short tree trunk, and it usually divides after a half inch or so into two major branches — the left anterior descending coronary and the left circumflex coronary (See Chapter Two).

When physicians talk about coronary arteries, they are usually referring to these three: the right coronary, the left anterior descending, and the left circumflex. Many of my patients wonder how it's possible to have a quadruple or quintuple bypass if there are only three major coronary arteries. As it turns out, the coronary arteries are like branches on a tree. The main trunks split into major branches, which split into smaller branches and on and on until the arterial branches become so small they cannot be seen by the naked eye. Any one of these many, many arterial branches can be blocked, meaning that as many as eight or nine, and perhaps even more, bypasses may be necessary.

### What Causes Coronary Artery Disease?

The most common cause of coronary artery disease is atherosclerosis, sometimes referred to as "hardening of the arteries." In this condition, fatty buildups develop on the arterial lining (Fig. 8.1). These buildups are soft and almost look like cottage cheese. In fact, the word atherosclerosis comes from the Greek "athero" meaning porridge, and "sclerosis" meaning hardening.

As these fatty buildups become larger, they damage the artery wall, and a scar forms. This scar is then infiltrated with calcium, which further hardens the atherosclerotic material. At some point, the arteries become very brittle and calcified, and the buildups gradually narrow the opening until blood has difficulty getting past the blockages.

**Symptoms of Coronary Artery Disease**

When the heart does not get enough oxygen, portions of it may become **ischemic**, which results in a type of pain called angina pectoris. This pain is often described as pressure, and it usually occurs over the breastbone. It can feel like a band tightening around the chest. Some of my patients have described it as a pile of bricks or heavy weights that has been placed on their chest. This could be a pain that goes from the chest to the neck and lower jaw or a numbness down the arm, particularly the left arm. Sometimes it can manifest itself as a discomfort in the upper portion of the abdominal wall. It may be mistaken for heartburn, a gall bladder attack, or even an upset stomach.

Chest pain does not always accompany hardened arteries. Some patients have what is called an angina equivalent. This could be a form of shortness of breath or other symptoms that, after appropriate testing, turn out to be caused by a lack of oxygenated blood getting to the heart muscle.

Diabetic patients, especially those who have been taking insulin for a long time, often lack this angina warning system. These people may have what is called diabetic neuropathies, or diseases related to their nervous system, and may not have the same sensitivity and same warnings that other people would have. This is especially dangerous. People who have a defective warning system could be playing tennis or doing some other strenuous activity with no sign that the heart is not getting enough blood. They could then suffer a heart attack without any warning. Angina alerts people to immediately stop whatever they are doing and rest.

As atherosclerotic material builds up, it may actually starve the heart muscle for blood. Heart attacks occur not only when the plaque on the arterial wall blocks blood flow but also when the artery breaks or ruptures. When this happens, platelets, which are designed to begin blood clotting, attach to the raw surface of the crack and form a growing clump. This further blocks the coronary artery and may result in a heart attack. Even a temporary clumping of platelets can result in a heart attack.

Coronary arteries themselves can also go into spasm and block off. This is believed to be genetically related as some people are more prone to have coronary arteries that will go into spasm. If this happens, the blood flow beyond the spasm is severely compromised, which can cause angina or even a heart attack.

**Heart Attack and Heart Failure**

The medical term for heart attack is **myocardial infarction**. During a heart attack, a portion of the heart muscle dies. Patients usually survive small heart attacks. If the heart attack involves a significant portion of the heart, however, the victim will usually die due to arrhythmias during the beginning of the heart attack.

In the event a patient survives a large heart attack, a considerable portion of heart muscle will turn into scar tissue and no longer contract. This can lead to heart failure. The patient will become short of breath and frequently fatigued because of the reduced amount of blood being pumped by the heart, resulting in a relative lack of oxygen and other nutrients getting to the body's tissues. The patient may develop swelling in the ankles or in the legs or abdomen as the heart fails and fluid backs up into the tissues.

**Ischemia:**
When a portion of the body, an organ or tissue, is not getting enough oxygenated blood. It is usually related to a blockage in one of the arteries delivering blood to that area.

**Myocardial Infarction:**
When a portion of the heart muscle dies. Also referred to as a heart attack.

# Dissolving Blood Clots During Heart Attacks

By

## James Marsh, M.D.

Professor of Medicine and Chief, Division of Cardiology
Wayne State University

IN MOST CASES, HEART ATTACKS are caused by atherosclerosis, which slowly narrows the coronary arteries, and a blood clot that suddenly forms and blocks off the coronary artery completely, thus limiting blood flow to the heart. When a patient comes into a hospital emergency room early in the course of a heart attack, physicians may administer a clot-dissolving drug.

The most common clot-dissolving drug is tPA (tissue plasminogen activator). During the first ninety minutes, this drug will dissolve the clot that is blocking the coronary in about 75 percent of patients, restoring blood flow to the heart and limiting the amount of heart damage.

Because this is a very potent drug that dissolves clots anywhere in the body, bleeding is one possible side effect of tPA. Therefore, patients must be carefully selected to have minimal risk for bleeding. It cannot be used in patients who have had a recent stroke, in patients with severe high blood pressure, or in patients with bleeding stomach ulcers. However, when it is given to carefully selected patients in the first six to twelve hours after the onset of a heart attack, it can definitely improve their outcome.

## Medical Treatment of Coronary Artery Disease

If you develop angina pectoris or what's thought to be an angina equivalent, your physician probably will start with an electrocardiogram. If it's abnormal or in certain cases even if it's normal, your physician may decide to do some form of stress testing. Depending on the results, and sometimes even without testing, your physician may decide to do a type of cardiac catheterization called coronary arteriography, in which catheters are used to inject the coronary arteries with radiopaque dye. This helps doctors see if blockages are present, where they are located, and how severely the artery is blocked.

In most angina cases, the treatment is medication, dietary changes, and exercise. Several medications are popularly prescribed to treat angina:

♥ Nitrates dilate coronary arteries. They do not necessarily dilate the area with the blockage, but they can dilate beyond the blockage and lower the overall resistance to blood flow.

♥ Beta blockers work directly on the heart muscle. Beta blockers cause the heart to contract more slowly and with less vigor, reducing the amount of oxygen demanded by the heart muscle.

♥ Ace inhibitors dilate arteries throughout the body, which lowers the resistance to blood flow. The heart does not have to work as hard to deliver the same amount of blood to the body, allowing the heart itself to get by with less oxygenated blood.

♥ Calcium channel blockers are particularly helpful in patients who have some degree of coronary artery spasm. They prevent the arteries from going into spasm or at least decrease the incidence and severity of the spasm.

**Interventional Therapy**

If a severe blockage is present, more aggressive measures may be needed to get oxygenated blood to the heart. One option is interventional therapy, or the use of catheter-based therapies.

When a coronary artery has a severe degree of blockage — more than 70 percent but usually less than 100 percent — cardiologists may be able to dilate the artery with a balloon catheter (Fig. 8.5). Sometimes even arteries that are totally blocked can be reopened with catheters.

In this procedure, a catheter, which looks like a long piece of spaghetti, is threaded through the arterial system, usually through an artery in the groin or arm. The catheter is tipped with a tiny sausage-shaped balloon that is deflated and guided into the coronary artery and positioned directly opposite the narrowed area. The balloon is inflated, crushing the plaque material against the arterial wall and opening up the artery. It may have to be inflated several times.

A disadvantage to using a balloon is restenosis. Doctors have found that in about 40 percent of patients who undergo this procedure, within a year or less the artery begins to close again, or restenose, which can occur for various reasons. This means another catheter procedure is necessary, or perhaps open heart surgery.

Recently, a device called a stent has been developed to combat restenosis. It is used with the balloon. Stents look like wire or mesh tubes, and they are usually flexible. In this procedure, the stent is placed over the balloon, and both are guided to the obstruction. When the balloon is inflated, the stent expands and is lodged in the artery (Fig. 8.6A). The stent remains in place after the balloon and catheter are withdrawn (Fig. 8.6B). Its major advantage lies in its ability to lessen the chance that the artery will become obstructed again, although it does require placing a foreign object into the coronary artery.

Balloon catheters are not the only interventional option. Another is a tiny drill called a rotablator. This device literally shaves atherosclerotic material off the arterial wall. Under certain conditions, a laser can be used to carve out, or vaporize, some of the atherosclerotic material. These devices are usually not used in a coronary artery that is totally blocked, particularly if that blockage has been present for a long time.

The feasibility of using catheters depends on the severity of the blockage. In some cases, when catheters are forced beyond total blockages, they may perforate the wall of the coronary artery and cause

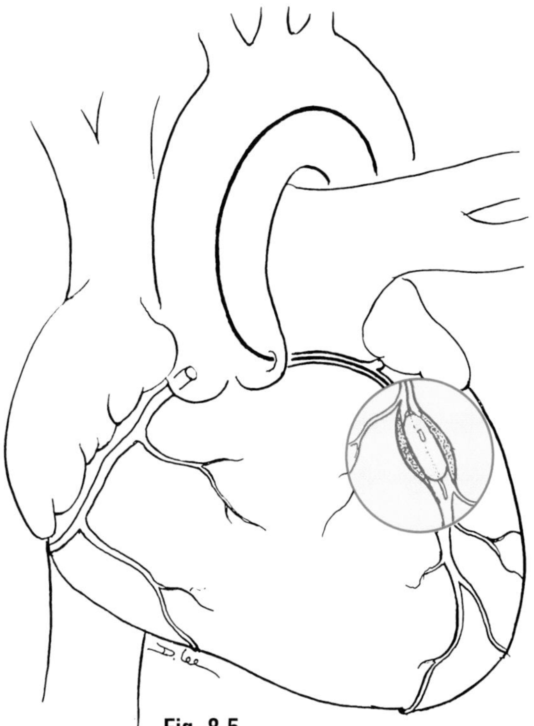

**Fig. 8.5:**
Coronary arteries that are blocked with atherosclerotic material can be opened with a balloon-tipped catheter in a procedure called percutaneous transluminal coronary angioplasty.

**Fig. 8.6:**
Recently, a device called a stent has come into use. This device is placed on the balloon (A) and remains in the artery after the dilatation (B).

**Fig. 8.5**

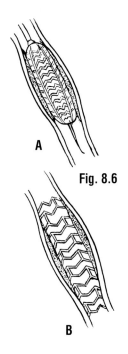

A

**Fig. 8.6**

B

119

**Fig. 8.7:**
These coronary angiography films were taken before and after a stenting procedure. The blocked artery, left, is contrasted with the open artery, right, after a stent was put in place with a balloon-tipped catheter. Introduced in the early 1990s, coronary stents are designed to hold open a blocked coronary artery after a balloon widening.

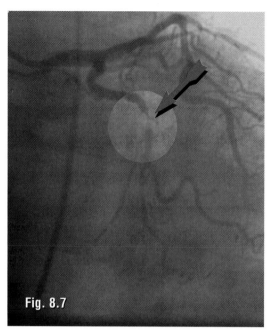
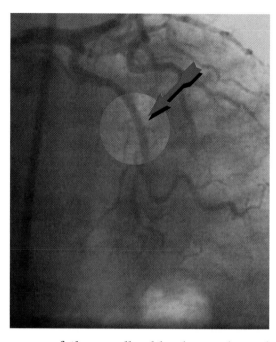

Fig. 8.7

severe complications. In the most important coronary artery, the left main coronary, cardiologists are usually reluctant to dilate blockages or attempt other catheter procedures to open the artery because some of the material could suddenly break off, possibly blocking the blood flow to the left ventricle and causing a fatal heart attack. There are centers, however, where research is being done on using balloons and related techniques in the left main coronary under special conditions.

**Transmyocardial Laser Revascularization**

If interventional catheter techniques aren't viable, doctors usually turn to the coronary bypass graft. There are cases, however, when the coronary artery disease is so severe and so widespread, or diffuse, that there's really nowhere to place the bypass graft.

For these patients, a relatively new procedure called transmyocardial laser revascularization may be considered. In this operation, a laser, used either through a catheter or directly through a surgical incision, is used to burn tiny holes in the heart muscle itself. It is hoped these channels will, over time, connect with some of the smaller blood vessels and form new circulation.

In a September 1999 issue of *The New England Journal of Medicine*, Dr. O. Howard Frazier from the Texas Heart Institute reported on a multicenter study in which ninety-one patients were randomly assigned to undergo transmyocardial laser revascularization and another one hundred one patients were randomly assigned to continued medical treatment.

After twelve months, the study group found that the patients who underwent transmyocardial laser treatment had much better control of their angina than their medicine-treated counterparts. Seventy-two percent were improved compared with only 13 percent of the patients who were receiving continued medical treatment. The group also found that the quality of life was significantly improved in the laser-treated group.

In the group that underwent laser treatment, 3 percent died in the hospital after the surgery. At twelve-month follow-up, 85 percent of the patients who had undergone laser treatment were alive as compared with 79 percent in the medically treated group.

Frazier's report, therefore, indicates that at least up to the first twelve months after the laser procedure, the patients who had the procedure are improved over a similar group treated only with medicines.

### Coronary Bypass Grafting

In patients with substantial left main coronary artery disease, physicians typically choose coronary bypass graft surgery instead of an interventional technique or leaving the disease untreated.

Studies have shown that people who undergo the surgery will, on average, live longer than a similar group who forgo the operation. Patients with triple-vessel coronary disease, in which all three of their major coronary arteries have severe blockages, and particularly those who also have left ventricular dysfunction (perhaps related to a previous heart attack), also benefit from coronary artery bypass grafting and on the average live longer than those who do not have the surgery. Patients with severe double- or single-vessel coronary disease can also be candidates for coronary bypass grafting, depending on the circumstances.

A doctor would often consider recommending bypass surgery if the patient had a substantial blockage of the left anterior descending coronary artery, particularly if the blockage were where it is attached to the left main coronary. Doctors are frequently reluctant to dilate the artery there or put a stent there because it could interfere with the left main coronary.

If the left anterior descending coronary artery is totally blocked upstream but is a good vessel beyond that, as determined by the number of collateral blood vessels feeding it, and the heart muscle is alive beyond this blockage, bypass surgery is often a good choice if angina is bothersome.

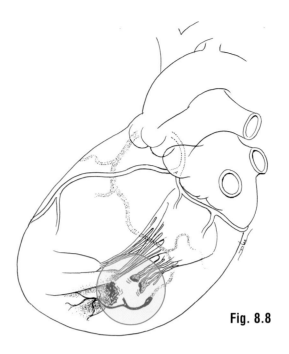

**Fig. 8.8**

**Fig. 8.8:** The papillary muscles, which connect the valve leaflets to the interior wall of the heart, can sometimes rupture during a heart attack. This condition usually results in valve replacement.

### Complications of Heart Attacks Requiring Heart Surgery

If a heart attack has occurred, there are possible complications. These include left ventricular aneurysm, which may require surgery, and post-myocardial infarction ventricular septal defect and papillary muscle rupture, both of which almost always require surgical repair.

### Left Ventricular Aneurysm

When a coronary artery such as the left anterior descending is blocked, a portion of the heart muscle may die and turn into scar tissue. Sometimes, however, as it's turning into scar tissue, the dying or dead tissue stretches and forms a sac (Fig. 8.9A). Later, as the living portions of the heart muscle contracts, some blood may be pushed back into the sac so it actually absorbs part of the heart's pumping energy, thus contributing to heart failure.

These sacs or aneurysms can also be the source of certain types of serious irregular heart rhythms. In addition, blood clots can form in them that can occa-

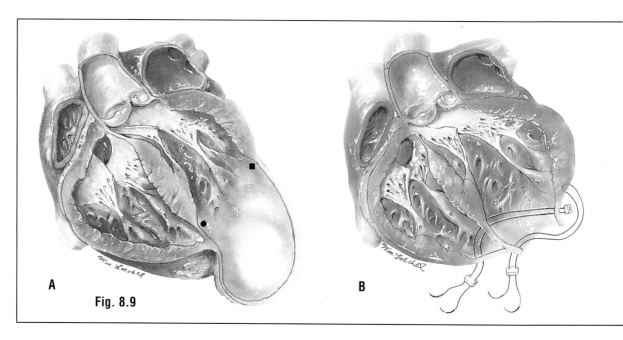

**Fig. 8.9:**
A left ventricular aneurysm occurs when a portion of the left ventricle, the heart's main pumping chamber, balloons out (A), often as a result of a heart attack. It can be corrected surgically by removing the sac-like portion of the ventricle (B) and sewing it back together (C).

Fig. 8.9

sionally break off and travel to the brain and other areas in the body.

Removing a left ventricular aneurysm requires using the heart-lung machine. Much of the scar tissue sac is removed (Fig. 8.9B), and the remaining heart muscle is repaired or sewn back together by using one of several techniques (Fig. 8.9C).

Frequently when performing surgery to remove a left ventricular aneurysm, I will also bypass blocked coronary arteries. A patient who needs coronary bypass surgery may also happen to have a left ventricular aneurysm. In most cases, patients undergoing aneurysm removal, with or without additional coronary bypass grafting, have a good chance of surviving the operation — usually in the range of 90 percent to 95 percent.

### Post–Myocardial Infarction Ventricular Septal Defect

Another complication of coronary artery disease that requires heart surgery is called post–myocardial infarction ventricular septal defect. This happens when the common wall between the right and the left ventricle (the ventricular septum) ruptures after a heart attack.

This is different and a much more serious problem than the congenital type of ventricular septal defect. The postmyocardial infarction ventricular septal defect needs to be repaired relatively soon after it occurs, and the risk of death for this surgery is higher than that for congenital surgery. These patients can be very unstable and sometimes are in cardiogenic shock. This surgery usually requires placement of the intra-aortic balloon pump to assist the heart before the patient is taken to the operating room.

When the surgeon opens the heart to repair the hole, he may find that the heart muscle tissue around the hole is also dying or dead, which makes the hole technically challenging to repair. Nonetheless, the majority of the patients who undergo the repair survive. In some cases, coronary bypass grafting or other heart surgery procedures are done at the same time. Depending on the circumstances, about 70 percent or 80 percent of the patients undergoing this operation survive the procedure and do well.

In many cases, it is a life-saving surgical procedure, and, without the surgery, death may occur within a few days.

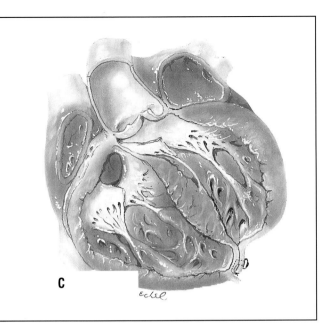

C

**Mitral Valve Replacement for Papillary Muscle Rupture**

Another complication of a heart attack is that one of the papillary muscles, which is inside the left ventricle and helps control the mitral valve, may be involved in the heart attack. The entire muscle may become detached from the ventricular wall (Fig. 8.8). If this happens, the mitral valve will no longer function effectively, blood will flow backwards into the lungs, and they will fill with fluid. The person will suffer from congestion of the lungs and be very short of breath and may go into heart failure or cardiogenic shock.

This is often a surgical emergency that requires the intra-aortic balloon pump to help stabilize the patient's condition while being prepared for mitral valve replacement surgery. This is a high-risk surgical procedure, but it must be done and hopefully will be life saving.

Unfortunately, because this condition is associated with heart attacks, we may be doing several operations at once. We might be placing coronary artery bypass grafts and, in some cases, may even have to remove a left ventricular aneurysm.

The chance of surviving emergency mitral valve replacement for papillary muscle rupture is about 70 percent, and most of the survivors do well providing the left ventricle has not been too badly damaged by the heart attack.

# TRANSMYOCARDIAL LASER REVASCULARIZATION

By

**Lawrence H. Cohn, M.D.** *(pictured)*

Professor of Surgery
Harvard Medical School

Chief, Cardiothoracic Surgery
Brigham and Women's Hospital
Boston, Massachusetts

&

**Sary Aranki, M.D.**

Associate Professor of Surgery
Harvard Medical School
Boston, Massachusetts

IN RECENT YEARS, A TREATment called transmyocardial laser revascularization, or TMLR, has been introduced for coronary artery disease that is so advanced that bypass surgery, balloon catheters, and stents by themselves are not effective. In this new treatment, physicians use a very powerful laser to bore a hole through the surface of the heart into the left ventricular cavity. Until recently, it has been experimental.

Clinical studies under the supervision of the U.S. Food and Drug Administration were performed simultaneously at multiple U.S. centers. Recently, one type of laser (carbon dioxide) was approved as a treatment option for certain patients. Other types of laser are currently in the study phase. Ours was one of the original U.S. sites pursuing carbon dioxide laser treatment.

### The Laser in Medicine

The laser has been used in medicine for more than twenty

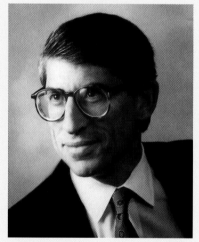

years. Its primary use in medicine is in treating disease. Many eye conditions are successfully treated with a laser, and a laser has been used to dissolve kidney and gall bladder stones. These are but a few of the many applications of lasers in medicine, aside from heart disease, and many more applications are being introduced.

### Who Is a Candidate for TMLR?

Not every person with coronary artery disease is a candidate for TMLR. In many cases, bypass surgery and balloon angioplasty produce good short-term and long-term results. However, in an increasing number of persons, coronary artery disease has progressed to such an advanced and severe form that surgery is no longer possible. These patients typically acquire coronary artery disease at a younger age, are more likely to be diabetic with multiple risk factors, and are more likely to have already had numerous bypass and balloon procedures.

In addition, candidates for TMLR must suffer from severe symptoms, like angina or chest pain, that interfere with their quality of life. Maximal medical therapy must have already failed, and any additional medications must be contraindicated. Also, TMLR treatment is not beneficial for heart failure.

### How Does TMLR Work?

No one has yet determined how the laser treatment improves symptoms and the blood supply to the heart. It was initially thought that the holes created by the laser infuse the heart muscle with a new blood supply directly from the heart cavity (such a system exists in animals such as crocodiles or snakes). However, these channels do not stay open for long, and their role in long-term blood supply is minimal, if any.

Other possibilities include damage to the heart muscle and its nerve supply that eliminates the origin of chest pain. Also, a placebo effect has been postulated, meaning that patients mistakenly believe they should get better because a supposedly very useful treatment was performed. These reasons may explain the improvement of symptoms. Nevertheless, because the symptoms take weeks or sometimes months to improve, the above mechanisms are highly unlikely.

However, it is now believed, although not yet proven, that the laser energy stimulates the heart muscle to sprout new blood vessels that supply blood to deprived parts. This is called angiogenesis and can also be stimulated by certain body proteins.

### The Surgical Procedure

TMLR is performed through an incision in the left side of the chest just underneath the left breast. The heart-lung machine is not required, and the operation is performed on a beating heart. Because the overwhelming majority of these patients have had previous coronary artery bypass operations, it is unsafe to per-form this operation through the sternum, or breastbone. In addition, the back of the heart is more accessible from the left side of the chest without the need to apply too much tension to the heart, which could lower blood pressure during the operation.

Because it takes some time for a new blood supply to the heart muscle to develop after TMLR, the possibility of a reduction in blood supply as a result of the stress of anesthesia and surgery is increased. Therefore, extra vigilance is needed after the procedure to deal with these problems before they become more serious. Aggressive preventative measures include noninvasive monitoring and mechanical and pharmacological support. In addition, all patients are sent to the intensive care unit after surgery for close monitoring.

The operation lasts between one and a half and two hours on an average. Patients can be disconnected from the respirator and their breathing tube removed either in the operating room or as soon as they wake up in the intensive care unit.

### The Results of TMLR

The chance of surviving the operation in the first thirty days after surgery is greater than 95 percent. This risk was initially higher but has improved with more intensive support. The long-term survival after one and two years is comparable to that of those patients who did not undergo surgery.

The major impact of TMLR has been in relief of angina, reduced need for hospital admissions, and an improvement in the quality of life. About three out of four patients have experienced these benefits. The need for hospital admission because of unstable angina was also substantially reduced. Even more encouraging, there has been no deterioration in heart function and no damage to the heart muscle resulting in heart failure symptoms.

### In Summary

We continue to offer TMLR to patients with severe and advanced coronary artery disease in whom conventional treatment either has failed or is no longer possible. It is only offered for symptomatic angina and not for heart failure. The operation is performed through the left side of the chest without the need for the heart-lung machine. The risk of dying from the operation is comparable to that of coronary bypass surgery because of the potential for complications under stressful conditions. Despite this early risk, the survival after one or two years is similar to that of patients who did not undergo surgery. The majority of patients (75 percent) responded with a marked improvement in symptoms and quality of life and less need for hospital admissions. Intensive research on the exact reason for these results continues.

# Women, Race, and Coronary Artery Surgery

By

Reneé S. Hartz, M.D.

Cardiothoracic Surgeon
Professor of Surgery
Tulane University
Tulane Xavier Women's Center of Excellence
New Orleans, Louisiana

CORONARY ARTERY BYPASS grafting (CABG) is the most commonly performed surgical procedure in the United States. There are approximately 325,000 CABG procedures performed every year, and patients who receive this surgery benefit from more than thirty years of experience and published medical data on its relative safety.

Just as CABG is the most commonly performed surgery, more health care dollars are spent treating arteriosclerotic conditions (such as coronary artery disease and stroke) than any other illness in America. These expenditures will dramatically increase as the life expectancy of the U.S. population continues to rise. Currently, men live on average to age seventy-two years and women to age eighty years.

At the same time, the number of female patients undergoing treatment for coronary artery disease is increasing much more rapidly than the number of male patients. In less than fifty years, it is expected,

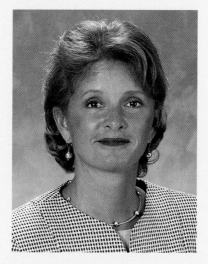

more cardiovascular health care dollars will be spent on women than on men.

Likewise, the medical community has begun to look at the impact of race on CABG, and this is a topic that deserves attention.

When studying the outcome of CABG in large populations, including mortality and incidence of complications, we have found that females and non-Caucasians fare less good. Moreover, women and non-Caucasian patients stand a greater chance of having several

other conditions, each of which on its own increases risk.

**Applications of CABG**

In the early 1980s, the number of women undergoing CABG almost doubled before beginning to level off. Today, about 25 percent of patients undergoing CABG are women. In surgical centers that accept high-risk referrals (such as those that regularly admit 80-year-olds), the percentage of women having CABG may approach 50 percent.

The Society of Thoracic Surgeons (STS) Database is one of the most authoritative sources for statistics on who is having CABG surgery. The largest database for coronary bypass surgery in existence, the STS Database contains records of almost five hundred thousand CABG operations. This study found that between 1994 and 1996, 8.5 percent of CABG-only operations (not including other types of heart operations) were performed on non-Caucasian patients, and 28.2 percent were performed on women.

Medicare statistics also shed light on CABG surgery. In the United States, these figures show that in 1986, the overall national rate of CABG was 25.6 per one hundred thousand people. For Caucasians, the number was 27.1 per one hundred thousand, in contrast to a rate of 7.6 per one hundred thousand for African Americans.

### Risk Factors for CABG in Women

When comparing men and women, several factors have been examined to determine the outcome after surgery. These include age; the presence of risk factors like diabetes, hypertension, and renal failure; body size as it relates to the size of the blood vessels (especially the coronary arteries); and race (Caucasian or non-Caucasian).

*Age*: Because women develop coronary artery disease later than men, women undergoing CABG are often older than men undergoing CABG. For example, although the average age of all patients enrolled in the STS Database remained remarkably constant from 1991 to 1995 (64.5 years), the age of the women in 1995 averaged 66.9 years and that of the men, 63.6 years.

*Contributing Factors*: When undergoing CABG, women are more likely than men to be diabetic or hypertensive or to have pre-existing kidney failure or be experiencing congestive heart failure. They are also statistically more likely to have advanced symptoms of coronary artery disease like severe angina,

unstable or changing angina, or angina at rest.

These factors increase the risk of any type of treatment, especially coronary artery bypass surgery. Furthermore, women are more likely to have their operation on an urgent or emergency basis. All of these factors increase the chance of having a poor outcome after CABG.

On the other hand, women undergoing surgery typically have had fewer previous heart attacks and have fewer diseased arteries than do men.

*Body Size and Diameter of Coronary Arteries*: It has often been said that women have worse outcomes after coronary intervention because they are smaller and their arteries are harder to work with. However, there has been no proven relation between size of the arteries and success in surgery.

### Risk Factors for CABG in Non-Caucasians

Although the risk profiles for Caucasians and non-Caucasians have not been examined as thoroughly as those of men and women, the STS Database shows clear differences between the two racial groups.

*Age*: We found that non-Caucasian patients having CABG are somewhat younger (age sixty-two years) than Caucasian patients (almost age sixty-five years).

*Severity of Cardiac Disease*: Fewer non-Caucasian patients have had previous cardiac operations, although statistically significantly more have severe symptoms that result in urgent or emergency operations. There are no differences in the number and type of diseased arteries in Caucasian and non-Caucasian patients.

*Contributing Factors*: Non-Caucasian patients have a greater chance of having diabetes and kidney failure than Caucasian patients. However, they are much less likely to have emphysema.

### The Operation

*Preparing for Surgery*
For all patients, every attempt should be made to stabilize symptoms and decrease the work load on the heart. In women and non-Caucasians, who are more likely to have severe and unstable symptoms, this may mean early hospital admission or even time in an intensive care unit.

In women, a class of drugs called calcium channel blockers may also be useful because they

**Table 8.1:** Characteristics of women and non-caucasian patients undergoing CABG*

| Preoperative | Postoperative | Procedural |
|---|---|---|
| More renal (kidney) failure | More strokes | Less elective surgery |
| More diabetes | Longer time on ventilator | Less use of LIMA |
| More hypertension | More kidney failure | |
| More serious symptoms | More dialysis | |
| | Higher 30-day mortality | |

*All differences are statistically significant.

have been shown to decrease arterial spasm, a condition that occurs more commonly in female patients.

It is crucial that patients in high-risk categories attempt to lower their operative risk. The lowest priority is an elective operation for which the patient is admitted on the same day of their surgery. An urgent operation is one that is performed on an inpatient basis and within twenty-four hours of a heart catheterization.

The highest-risk operation, and that of the highest priority, is an emergency operation — the patient must go immediately from the catheterization laboratory to the operating room. Caucasian men are more likely to have elective CABG than any other patients.

### Choice of Grafts
### for the Bypasses

It is more often a problem to find good conduits (arteries and veins used as bypass grafts) in women needing CABG because they are more often obese and diabetic and more likely to have varicose veins (or even to already have had their leg veins removed or stripped), and more often have serious arterial blockages in their legs (poor circulation).

Despite this, fewer women have the left internal mammary artery (LIMA) used as a bypass graft during their surgery. Since the LIMA has profound influence on long-term health and has been associated with lower mortality in some studies, attempts should be made to use this vessel as a bypass graft when feasible.

In the past, it was often said that using the LIMA is technically difficult and takes longer, so women and elderly patients (who more often have an emergency operation) usually receive leg vein grafts. These issues are less relevant today because all competent surgeons can rapidly harvest the LIMA (remove it from the chest wall) and because anesthetic techniques have been improved to the degree that almost all patients can be stabilized.

Use of the LIMA has increased dramatically over the previous decade, and the LIMA is currently used in more than 80 percent of CABG operations. Still, a substantial difference persists in its use in men and women and in Caucasian and non-Caucasian patients.

### Results of CABG

*Operative Mortality*

Because of all the involved issues, it is not surprising that overall risks of death in women are somewhat higher than in men. In studies published in the late 1970s and early 1980s, this difference became evident. More recent reports have noted similar results.

In the Coronary Artery Surgery Study of more than eight thousand patients, mortality was 5.3 percent for women, compared with 2.5 percent for men. Moreover, even though mortality has fallen in both genders because of improvements in equipment and techniques, for the almost five hundred thousand patients in the STS Database, the mortality was 4.5

# WOMEN AND CORONARY DISEASE

THE MOST IMPORTANT thing to know about women and coronary artery disease (CAD) is that CAD is the number one killer of women in the United States.

About half of the patients who suffer from heart attacks each year are women. Thus, one should be just as suspicious of coronary artery disease in a woman as in a man. About five hundred thousand women in the United States die each year from all forms of cardiovascular disease.

Almost twice as many women die in the United States from cardiovascular disease as from all forms of cancer.

The incidence of CAD increases after menopause. It's felt this is because patients are not only older, but also because of a lack of estrogen (a female hormone) that gives some protection against atherosclerotic disease.

With estrogen replacement therapy, atherosclerotic disease probably increases at a slower rate.

percent for women and 2.76 percent for men. At the same time, the mortality was 3.9 percent for non-Caucasian patients and 3.3 percent for Caucasian patients.

*Complications of CABG*

Both female and non-Caucasian patients have a significantly greater likelihood of having a stroke or kidney failure after surgery. Women have a greater chance of being treated with a respirator longer than men, despite having a lower incidence of emphysema before surgery. There are almost no differences in the rate of bleeding complications and serious chest infections between the gender and racial groups.

**Postoperative Estrogen in Women Patients**

Women undergoing CABG are likely to be postmenopausal because coronary artery disease is more prevalent in post-menopausal women (young diabetic women are the exception). Many studies suggest that women at high risk for coronary artery disease or those who already have the disease will benefit from estrogen therapy. This group includes women who have undergone CABG or angioplasty.

Hormone therapy is a secondary intervention (as opposed to a primary intervention, in which hormones are used to prevent coronary artery disease). There are seven published studies showing that hormone therapy results in a lower rate of death or complications in women who already have coronary artery disease. One study of 1,091 women, 92 of whom took estrogen after surgery, showed that survival at five and ten years was statistically significantly better in the group who took the hormones.

Another large study is currently testing these results, but, in the meantime, physicians should strongly consider treating all of their postmenopausal CABG patients with estrogen unless they are at very high risk for breast or uterine cancer.

**Conclusions**

Even though the risk may be higher for women and non-Caucasian patients, their long-term benefit from CABG is excellent, and they are likely to experience years of event-free survival (no heart attacks, death, angioplasty, or repeated hospitalization). Women with known or suspected coronary artery disease should discuss CABG with their physicians because the benefit of this powerful intervention outweighs the risk of the surgery for many.

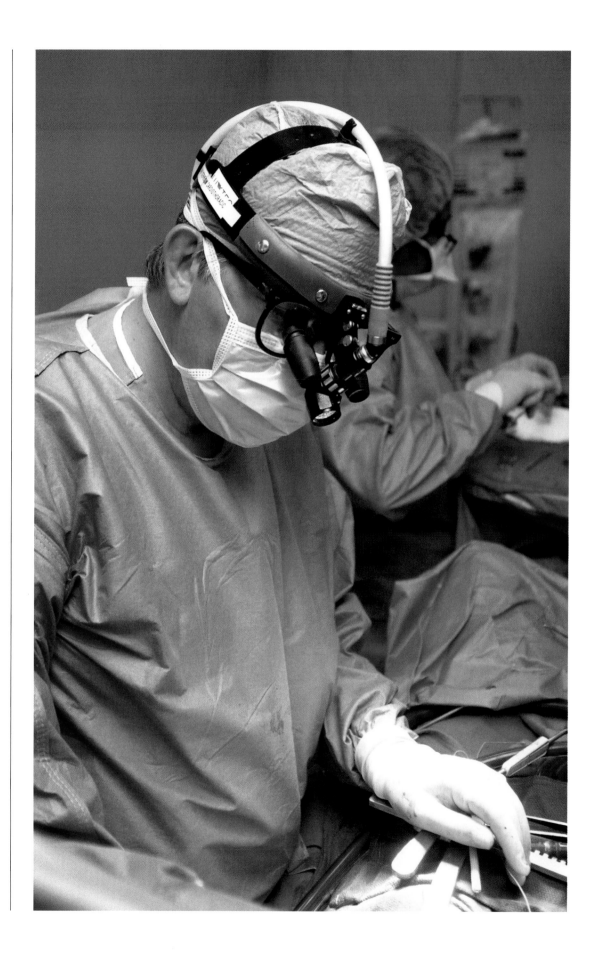

Bypass surgery typically takes about three to five hours. After surgery, most patients remain in the hospital for four to seven days.

## CHAPTER NINE

# THE CORONARY BYPASS: OPERATION AND RECOVERY

THE CORONARY ARTERY BYPASS graft procedure is still the gold standard for patients suffering from left main or multiple coronary artery disease. The final determination that a coronary artery bypass graft operation is necessary is usually obtained from cardiac catheterization using coronary angiography. If the degree of blockage warrants surgery, a standard **battery of tests** is performed before surgery. These tests can be done on an outpatient basis and typically include an electrocardiogram, routine blood work studies, chest x-rays, and urinalysis.

In addition, the blood is typed (found to be type A, B, AB, or O, for example) and cross-matched with donor blood. In some centers, the patient's blood type is determined, but it is not cross-matched against a donor unit of blood in the hospital blood bank because there is about an 80 percent chance that a blood transfusion won't be needed. By avoiding the cross-match, a certain amount of work and expense is avoided. If blood is needed, it can be cross-matched relatively quickly. In other centers, blood for transfusion is actually cross-matched and available. The cross-matching issue depends on the preference of the surgeon and surgical team.

When I first became involved with heart surgery as a medical student more than thirty years ago, patients were routinely admitted for elective heart surgery about a week before the operation, and many, many tests were performed. By the time I became a faculty member at the Hospital of the University of Pennsylvania in 1978, patients were routinely admitted to the hospital one and a half days before heart surgery. Over the next several years, that policy gradually changed; patients were brought in the afternoon of the day before their heart surgery. In the past five years, this has changed further, and now more than two-thirds of the patients undergoing elective heart surgery in the United States are admitted to the hospital on the morning of their heart operation.

Although I would not have believed this was possible twenty years ago, it seems to work well, and there doesn't appear to be any adverse effect from the "admit the morning of the surgery" policy. As a matter of fact, I think if I were to undergo an elective heart operation, I would rather sleep at home in my own bed the night before the operation.

**Battery of Tests**: Includes blood pressure measurement, which is a common and important tool for diagnosing cardiovascular disease.

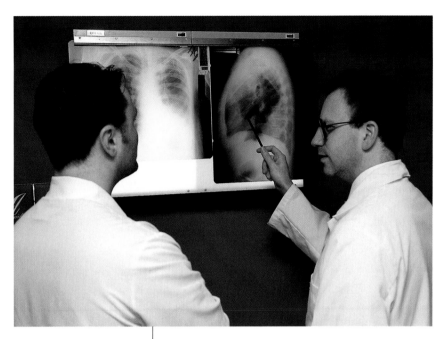

Surgeons viewing a patient's x-ray. The PA, or frontal view, is on the left, and the lateral, or side view of the patient's chest, is on the right.

However, not everyone comes in during the morning of their heart surgery. Some patients are already in the hospital for conditions related to their heart disease or have to be admitted a day or two before their heart surgery because of various pre-existing medical conditions that may need some special attention or "fine tuning" before the heart surgery.

### The Choice of Conduits for
### Coronary Artery Bypass Grafting

During a bypass operation, the surgical team will need to "harvest" a vein or artery from elsewhere in the body to use as a graft. The most commonly used vein is the saphenous vein, which is taken from the leg. This is a superficial vein that runs from the groin to the ankle area and can be seen under the skin in many people when they stand up. It is one of the veins in the leg that may dilate over time and become varicose. In fact, not only is it a vein you can do without, but it can be a nuisance vein.

Although the saphenous vein is generally a good-quality blood vessel and can reach any coronary arteries, there is about a 3 percent to 4 percent

chance per year that it will become narrow or totally blocked. Thus, the long-term patency rate (or chance of the vein staying open) is not as good as that of some other conduits.

Another very commonly used vessel is the left internal mammary artery, which is also called the internal thoracic artery (Fig. 9.1). Using an internal mammary artery is a slightly different approach because one end of it is usually left connected to a branch of the aorta. There are two internal mammary arteries: One runs under the breastbone on the right side; the other runs on the left side. The left one can usually reach the left anterior descending coronary, which generally is the most important coronary artery for bypass. It also has an excellent patency rate — there is about a 90 percent chance it will be open twenty years later.

Sometimes its size is a disadvantage. It may only be a millimeter or less in diameter (there are about twenty-five millimeters in an inch), which is smaller than the coronary artery being bypassed, and sometimes the blood flow through it is inadequate. Occasionally, the internal mammary artery will not reach the point on the coronary that it needs to access. That obstacle can frequently be overcome by disconnecting the "upstream" end and sewing one end to the coronary and one to the aorta or another artery.

The right internal mammary is also frequently used to bypass blockages in the coronary arteries. This artery usually reaches the right coronary, the left anterior descending and some branches of the circumflex. If it does not, the approach is generally the same. The upstream end of the artery is disconnected, and one end is sewn on the coronary artery and the other is attached to the aorta or to another bypass graft.

Another artery used for a bypass operation is the radial artery, which is located in the arm. Although some surgeons were using this artery for coronary bypass twenty-five years ago, recently it has become popular again. There is a single main artery in the upper arm called the brachial artery, which divides into two main branches near the elbow. One branch, the radial artery, runs along the inner forearm toward the thumb. The other branch, the ulnar artery, runs along the outer edge heading toward the little finger. These two arteries reconnect in the hand through an artery called the palmar arch artery. If the palmar arch is intact, it is possible to take a portion of the radial artery for a bypass graft. The reported results with radial arteries so far indicate that the vessel graft has a greater chance of staying open longer than saphenous vein grafts but not quite as long as the left internal mammary artery.

Doctors sometimes use an abdominal vessel called the gastroepiploic artery as the bypass graft. To use this artery, the ab-

domen must be opened. When using this artery, one end of it can be left attached to the stomach while the other end is threaded through a hole in the diaphragm, or breathing muscle, and joined to the appropriate coronary artery. The gastroepiploic artery can also be used as a free graft when both ends are disconnected. In this case, the other end is sewn to the aorta or another coronary bypass graft. The gastroepiploic artery graft seems to have a better patency rate than the saphenous vein graft but a somewhat poorer patency rate than the left internal mammary artery. The disadvantage of using this artery is that the surgeon has to make a second major incision to open the abdomen and devascularize (take part of the blood supply of) a portion of the stomach.

Over the years, doctors have found that using veins from the arms for coronary bypass grafting generally results in

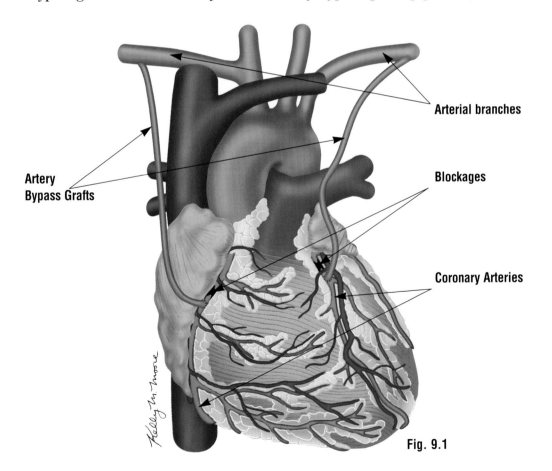

**Artery Bypass Grafts**

**Arterial branches**

**Blockages**

**Coronary Arteries**

**Fig. 9.1**

**Fig. 9.1:** In a coronary bypass operation using the internal mammary arteries, one end of the vessel is left connected to a branch of the aorta, or it can be reconnected to another artery. The other end is sewn into the coronary artery beyond the blockage. This graft vessel has excellent long-term results.

poor patency rates; therefore, in most cases, they are not used unless there is no other choice. In certain other cases, veins from a human cadaver have been used, but, again, the patency rates are not very good. This may be because of a rejection process that occurs from using tissue from another human. Synthetic arteries made of Dacron or other material have also been used. These grafts generally work quite well in other areas of the body, particularly in the larger arteries and the aorta, but the patency rates for coronary artery grafting have not been very good, and these synthetic arteries are not routinely used.

### The Heart Operation

We usually instruct our patients not to eat or drink anything after midnight the night before surgery. When they arrive at the hospital for surgery, patients generally report to the preoperative holding area, which is near the operating rooms. Some intravenous catheters are inserted through the skin, and a sedative is administered. At many heart centers, a local anesthetic is injected into the skin of the neck, and a larger catheter is introduced into the jugular vein and threaded through the right side of the heart into the pulmonary artery.

This catheter, called a **Swan-Ganz catheter**, can be used not only to give medicines but also to measure cardiac and pulmonary-arterial pressure and the amount of blood that the heart is pumping. Although many heart surgical teams routinely use the Swan-Ganz catheter, not all of them do. It depends on the preference of the surgeon, the anesthesiologist, and the heart surgery team.

While the patient is still in preoperative holding, another catheter is placed in one of the arteries so that the arterial blood pressure can be monitored and blood samples can be drawn to check the arterial blood's oxygenation level. This catheter is usually placed in one of the wrist arteries, often the radial artery. If a radial artery will be used for one of the bypasses, the other wrist can be used, or the catheter can be placed in the femoral artery by inserting it through the groin.

The patient is next moved into the operating room, and general anesthesia is induced.

Next, we place a plastic tube about as big as the index finger into the trachea (wind pipe). At some point, usually after the patient is anesthetized, a catheter is placed into the patient's bladder. The patient's chest and legs are swabbed with antiseptic soap solutions, and sterile operating drapes are placed on and around the patient. Now the team is ready to make the first incisions. Usually one surgical team will make one or more shallow incisions in the leg and harvest the vein for the bypass while the other team opens the chest.

To open the chest, an incision is made in the skin. The subcutaneous tissue is divided — this is a layer of fat usually a quarter- to a half-inch thick. In more obese people, however, it can be quite thick. Beneath that, a layer of muscle that is attached to the breastbone is cut through to expose the sternal bone. A saw is used to open the entire length of the sternum. Then a metal retractor is used to separate the sternal edges and hold the chest open.

With the chest open, I free up one or both internal mammary arteries and open the sac around the heart, or pericardium. A powerful anticoagulant, or blood thinner, called heparin is administered directly into the bloodstream to prevent the blood from clotting while the circulation is supported by the **heart-lung machine**. To hook a patient up to a heart-lung machine, stitches are placed so plastic tubes can connect the patient's circulation to the machine. A tube about the size of the index finger is placed into the ascending aorta about three inches above where the

**Swan-Ganz Catheter:** A catheter that is guided into the heart and the pulmonary artery, where it can be used to measure pressures in the heart and pulmonary artery, as well as take blood samples, administer intravenous drugs, and measure cardiac output.

**Heart-Lung Machine:** A machine used to bypass the function of the heart and lungs.

aorta comes out of the heart. This tube delivers oxygenated blood from the heart-lung machine to the patient.

Another catheter is placed through the right atrium. Some doctors use a two-stage **cannula**, with one part going through the right atrium into the inferior vena cava and a second drainage system remaining in the right atrium. In other patients, two separate venous catheters are inserted into these same areas. This depends on whether additional heart surgical procedures might be done and also on the preference of the surgeon. The tube or tubes in the right atrium return unoxygenated blood from the patient's venous system to the heart-lung machine.

Frequently, an additional catheter is placed through the right atrium and manipulated into the coronary sinus. The coronary sinus is a vein that returns blood to the right atrium from the heart itself. This catheter is called a **retrograde coronary perfusion catheter** and is used to give part or all of the solution that will "turn off" the heart during the procedure.

After these catheters are in place, I will begin cardiopulmonary bypass by telling my technician or perfusionist running the heart-lung machine to turn on the machine with a command such as "on bypass." The heart-lung machine then takes over the function of the heart and lungs. After it is activated, most surgeons will cool the patient's body temperature to some level, but not all surgeons do this. There are advantages and disadvantages to cooling. The major advantage is that it adds an additional level of safety to the heart and the brain if some problem were to temporarily develop with the heart-lung machine.

**Retrograde Coronary Perfusion Catheter**:
A catheter that is inserted through the right atrium into the coronary sinus, a vein that drains the heart itself. This catheter is usually used to administer cardioplegia solution, which stops the heart from beating during surgery.

**Cannula**:
A hollow tube that is inserted into a blood vessel, the heart or other body cavity.

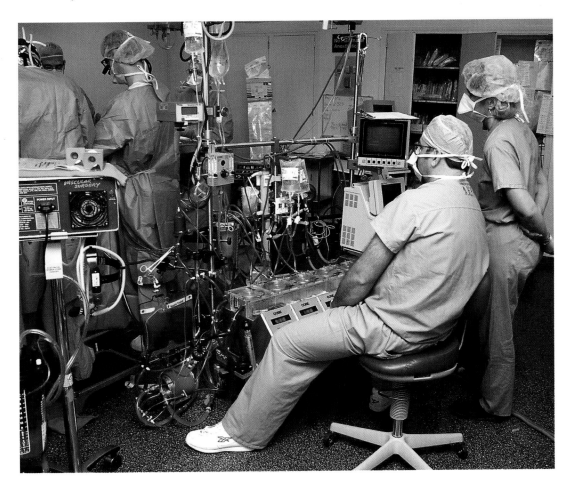

The heart-lung machine is a complex-looking machine that includes pumps with a blood oxygenator to simulate the action of the heart and lungs.

muscle, as does the cooling of the heart. Once again, not all surgeons use these techniques, but the vast majority do.

With the heart stopped and the body supported by the heart-lung machine, the coronary arteries that are to be bypassed are identified. I usually have a mental picture of exactly where I want to put the bypasses and know where the blockages are. Frequently, the last thing I do before scrubbing in, gowning up, and putting on sterile gloves is look again at the movies of the patient's coronary arteries. The images are individual frames from x-rays, which, when shown sequentially at high speed, look like a movie of blood flowing through these arteries. During surgery, most surgeons wear powerful magnifying glasses that increase the size of the relatively small coronary arteries at least two to four times. Some surgeons use a special type of microscope that magnifies the arteries even more.

I next isolate the obstructed coronaries, which tend to be on the surface of the heart. Sometimes they are hidden in a layer of fat on the heart and have to be located. Other times they're in the heart muscle. The coronary arteries are opened beyond the obstruction and measured. The internal diameters tend to be in the range of from one millimeter to two millimeters, which is about the size of a straw from a broom.

### Placing the Graft

With the coronary opened beyond the area of obstruction, I am ready to place the bypass graft. To do this, I join one end of the vessel conduit to the coronary artery with small stitches usually made out of polypropylene. The needle itself is joined to the stitch, and if you hold the needle and suture in your hand, you may have to squint to see them because they are so small.

After all the bypasses, which can range from one up to eight or nine grafts (but

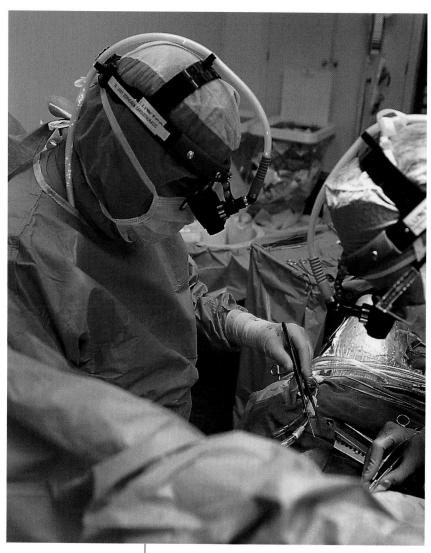

During surgery, heart surgeons wear full operating gowns and 2x or 4x magnifying glasses to help them see the very small coronary arteries and the bypass grafts.

**Cardioplegia Solution:** A solution that stops the heart from beating and reduces its oxygen consumption, thus allowing surgery to take place.

After the patient's circulation is supported by the heart-lung machine, most surgeons will "cross-clamp" the aorta by placing a clamp on the aorta between the heart and the catheter bringing oxygenated blood back from the heart-lung machine. This isolates the heart from the body's main artery. At this point, most surgeons administer a solution called a **cardioplegia solution**, which stops the heart from beating. This is frequently injected into the coronaries through the aorta and also through the retrograde coronary sinus catheter into the veins of the heart.

This stops the heart and cuts down on the oxygen consumption of the heart typically three or four), are sewn to the coronaries, the other ends are joined to the aorta or, in some cases, to other veins or arteries. If I've decided to use an internal mammary artery, one end is already connected to the arterial system.

The bypasses are now complete, and any air that might have gotten into the heart is removed, and the patient's body is rewarmed. The heart usually restarts on its own but sometimes needs the help of a temporary pacemaker or an electrical shock. It might have to be paced a while with a temporary pacemaker until its natural rhythm kicks in. Temporary pacing wires are usually connected to the heart and can be removed a few days after the surgery by pulling them out. Some surgeons choose to leave them in, cut them off at the skin level, and let them retract.

After the heart has started, our patient is weaned from the heart-lung machine by slowly turning the heart-lung machine off as the patient's own heart and lungs take over. In some cases, the heart is too weak to take over for whatever reason, and another attempt or two will be made at letting the heart take over. If these are unsuccessful, I may use an **intra-aortic balloon pump**, which is a pump that is threaded through an artery, usually through the groin, and connected to an external power source. There is a balloon on the tip of a long, thin tube that inflates and deflates in synchrony with the heart, helping the heart to pump blood as the patient gets through the early postoperative period.

In more severe cases when the heart does not take over, some form of ventricular assist device may have to be used. This is relatively uncommon. Most patients are weaned from bypass without the use of any type of mechanical support on the first attempt.

After I check the operative field to make sure that all bleeding has stopped, drainage tubes will be placed, and the sternum will be closed, usually with stain-

less steel wires that are left in permanently. The layers of the tissue are sewn together, and the skin on both the chest and the leg wound may be closed with sutures or metal staples. When stainless steel staples are used to close the skin, they are usually removed a week or two later, although the timing of the removal is the surgeon's preference and may depend on other pre-existing medical conditions.

### The Postoperative Intensive Care Unit

Patients are not yet awake when they leave the operating room and are transferred to an intensive care unit. A portable monitoring system usually accompanies patients so the surgical team, while in transit, can continually read the electrocardiogram and the arterial blood pressure. After the patient arrives in the intensive care unit, various monitoring lines including an **ECG** are connected, and the patient slowly wakes up over the next hour or so. Today, we tend to remove the breathing tube from most patients

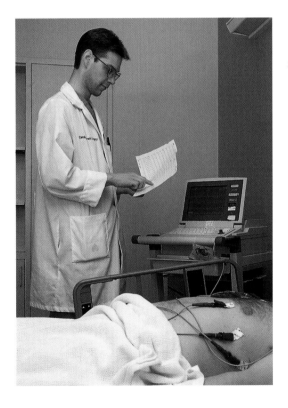

**Electrocardiogram (ECG or EKG):**
A recording of your heart's electrical activity. At left, a patient is shown undergoing an ECG test.

**Intra-Aortic Balloon Pump:**
A pump that is threaded into the aorta, usually through an artery in the groin, and connected to an external power source. There is a balloon on the tip of a catheter that inflates and deflates in synchrony with the heart, helping the heart to pump blood through the early postoperative period.

within the first several hours after the heart surgery. Sometimes, if the patient's breathing has not taken over sufficiently, it may be left in a little longer.

Most patients stay in the intensive care unit overnight and are discharged from intensive care to the step-down unit the next day. Being transferred from the intensive care unit to a step-down unit depends on a few factors. The patient must not need the ventilator. It may also depend on how well the heart and lungs are working, and sometimes it is also related to the surgical team's preference.

When the patient gets to the step-down unit (also referred to as the "floor" or "ward"), he is already drinking liquids and sometimes eating semisolid food. Within a day or two, the diet will rapidly progress to regular food. Patients also often walk up and down hallways, with some assistance, after a day or two on the ward. Discharge from the hospital can be as early as three days after the surgery but is usually about four days to a week after heart surgery, although this can be extended for various reasons. Interestingly, although everybody's pain threshold is different, the midline incision through the breastbone is not very painful. Most patients are sent home with only a mild pain medicine.

With routine coronary bypass operations, the chances of surviving the heart operation and walking out of the hospital are better than 99 percent.

Factors that can increase the risk of the surgery include the relative health of the left ventricle. If it's fairly normal, the risk of the surgery can be very low. If it's badly damaged from previous heart attacks, the risk could be greatly increased. Patients who are in the middle of having a major heart attack and/or in cardiogenic shock during the surgery are at increased risk. Other risk factors include lung disease and other important medical conditions, previous strokes, obesity, and additional heart surgery, like valve replacement, during coronary bypass surgery. Risk is also increased in patients who have had previous heart surgery and in the elderly, particularly in those more than eighty years old.

### Minimally Invasive Direct Coronary Artery Bypass (MIDCAB) Surgery

As medicine and surgery advance, newer techniques are constantly being developed. MIDCAB procedures are coronary artery bypass operations done without the aid of a heart-lung machine and that use novel devices and techniques. Coronary bypass surgery has been performed by some surgeons without the use of the heart-lung machine since the beginning, but the vast majority have used, and still use, the heart-lung machine.

New technology, however, has prompted many heart surgeons to take a long, hard look at performing coronary bypass grafts in selected patients without the use of the heart-lung machine.

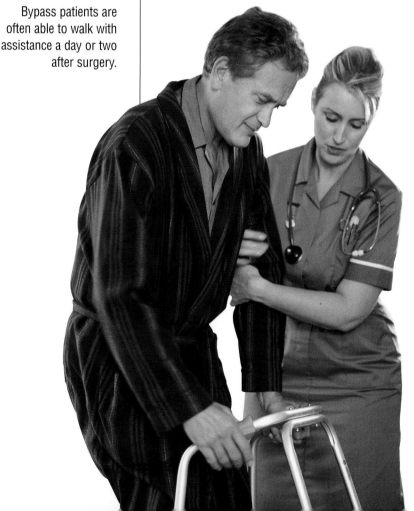

Bypass patients are often able to walk with assistance a day or two after surgery.

Some surgeons now are performing surgery, particularly when only one or two bypasses are needed, through a small incision in either the left or right side of the chest, depending on where the bypass graft is to be placed. This is done without the use of the heart-lung machine. There are certain advantages to performing the surgery without the aid of the heart-lung machine, yet there are many advantages to performing heart surgery with the heart-lung machine. Nonetheless, these techniques are being evaluated at many centers around the world.

If everything goes well and the heart-lung machine is not used, you can have the breathing tube removed sooner after the surgery and may be able to go home a day or two earlier. Some of the surgeons doing the surgery without a heart-lung machine have used videoscopes with remote TV cameras to perform portions of the operation, such as freeing up the internal mammary artery. Some have used videoscopes with special instruments to join the coronary artery to the internal mammary artery. Some surgeons use the routine midline incision through the breastbone but then perform the coronary bypass procedure without the heart-lung machine. Again, there are advantages and disadvantages to doing this.

Not all patients undergoing heart surgery at this time are eligible for these MIDCAB procedures. At one center in California, where the surgeons are prepared to do this in any eligible patient, they have found that over the last three years about 6 percent of the coronary bypass surgeries have been done without the use of the heart-lung machine. In another center in New York that is well known for this type of coronary bypass surgery and has had a lot of self-referrals especially for this type of surgery, the percentage of cases done without the use of the heart-lung machine is about 16 percent of the total number of patients undergoing coronary bypass grafting.

Although the initial results with MIDCAB surgery have been positive, it is probably too early to tell whether the number of MIDCAB operations will continue to grow. After surgeons gain more experience, some may decide to go back to doing most or all of their cases with the aid of the heart-lung machine. Time will tell whether these efforts are worthwhile.

### Complications from Coronary Bypass Surgery

There are complications that can occur during even "routine" coronary bypass surgery. A patient can have a heart attack during or shortly after the heart operation. It may be related to one of the bypass grafts clotting up or possibly to other events related to the heart surgery. The heart may fail even without a heart attack, requiring an intra-aortic balloon pump or mechanical assist device to be placed.

A patient may develop **respiratory insufficiency** or pneumonia and require prolonged stays including treatment with a respirator. Kidney failure may develop. This is more likely in people who have some degree of pre-existing kidney failure and in those with low cardiac output for prolonged periods. Wound infections are another risk with any major surgery. Fortunately, most patients undergoing coronary bypass surgery are at a very small risk, only a few percent, for any serious complications.

Less serious side effects are not so rare, however, and can range from the annoying to something that needs to be fixed with surgery. One of these is excessive blood loss from the chest drainage tubes, which can happen for a variety of reasons. To stop the blood loss, the patient has to be taken back to the operating room. This happens about 2 percent to 4 percent of the time.

Heart arrhythmias, or irregular heartbeats, are fairly common after heart surgery. Most are not serious and are more

**Respiratory Insufficiency:**
When the lungs are not functioning normally.

of a nuisance than anything else. About 20 percent to 30 percent of my patients develop **atrial arrhythmias**, sometimes **atrial fibrillation** or atrial flutter. Also, the ventricles may beat faster than normal. Again, these are usually not serious conditions but may require treatment with medicines. Sometimes, the heart even has to be shocked electrically back into a normal rhythm. The likelihood of these irregular rhythms decreases in the first few days after the surgery, and, by about a month after the surgery, most additional medicines prescribed to treat these abnormal heart rhythms can be discontinued.

### Strokes during or after
### Coronary Artery Bypass Surgery

Patients may suffer a stroke during or shortly after heart surgery. The chances are about 1 percent in a person who has never

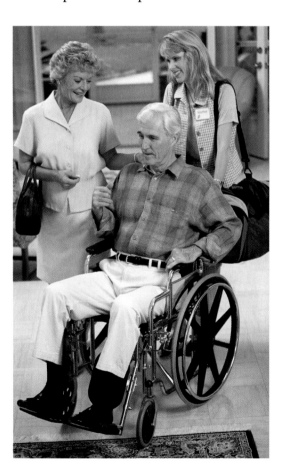

had a stroke before but can be as high as 5 percent or 10 percent in patients who have had a previous stroke. Sometimes strokes can be very severe. The patient may be in a coma and never wake up after the surgery. Fortunately, most strokes are much less severe, and most patients who have a problem with their speech or a weakness in an arm or a leg either totally recover or recover to some degree.

One of the causes of strokes is related to blockages in the arteries that deliver the oxygenated blood to the brain. The two major arteries are called the carotid arteries, and they can develop atherosclerotic disease just as the coronaries can.

When both the coronary artery and the carotid artery blockages are severe, the surgeon will most likely treat both problems at the same time. On the other hand, if one of the two problems is less severe, surgeons tend to first operate on whichever problem is more severe. The preference for which operation to do first or whether to do both at the same time varies with surgeons, and there is a certain amount of information to support one approach versus the other in specific situations.

### Discharge

When the patient is discharged from the hospital, depending on the circumstances, he may have a visiting nurse come to his house for a week or two. This depends on the surgical team's preference and the patient's condition.

If the patient goes home between three and five days after the surgery, he may need to come back to the hospital to get staples removed from the skin of the leg and chest, or a visiting nurse can remove the staples at home.

In most cases, the patient's cardiologist, who has referred the patient to the heart surgical team, will see the patient within the first few weeks or so after heart surgery and may readjust prescription medications. The heart surgeon will

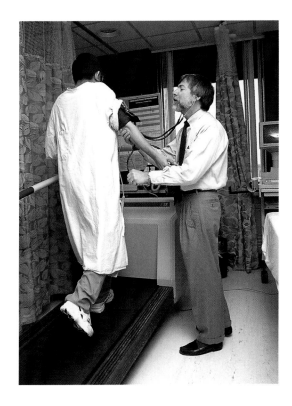

after heart surgery, however, you must first clear it with your cardiologist.

Although patients gain confidence while walking around the hospital ward, once they return home, my patients often realize they're weaker than they think they are. However, they are usually still able to go outside for brief walks. Within a month, most patients are able to walk a mile or two. If the weather is bad or unusually cold, patients often choose to walk inside a shopping mall. Some cardiologists prefer to enroll all of their patients in cardiac rehabilitation programs, whereas others only enroll some, particularly those who get little exercise.

### The Postoperative Exercise Stress Test

Three weeks to two months after the surgery, the cardiologist may prescribe an **exercise stress test.** Some cardiologists order an exercise stress test for all of their patients who have recently undergone coronary artery bypass surgery, whereas other cardiologists are more selective. These cardiologists do stress testing of patients with unusual symptoms, those who are going to do vigorous exercise such as jogging and playing tennis, or people who have jobs that require extra caution, such as commercial airline pilots. If the exercise test result is normal, most cardiologists allow the patient to go back to any type of normal vigorous activity.

### Common Postoperative Complaints

I hear several common complaints when I see patients four or five weeks after coronary bypass surgery. One is poor appetite. In virtually all patients, this improves anywhere from three weeks to two months after the surgery, and in most cases, they will regain weight to their presurgery level. If, on the other hand, they are overweight, they may prefer not to get back to that level, and diet counseling is

usually see the patient three to six weeks after surgery. If the patient is doing well, the patient will usually be transferred back to the care of the cardiologist or internist at that time.

From a surgical standpoint, the only medicine that I routinely recommend is an aspirin a day. Some physicians choose a baby aspirin, and others choose a regular aspirin. Aspirin probably helps keep the coronary bypass grafts open longer, but this has not been proven conclusively. Because aspirin is relatively benign, however, it's worth the effort.

When the patient is discharged from the hospital, the biggest restriction is that the patient should not lift anything heavier than about twenty pounds for the first couple of months while the breastbone is healing. After three months, the patient can generally resume vigorous activity. This could even mean playing professional sports such as ice hockey or other strenuous contact sports. Before attempting any type of vigorous activity

**Exercise Stress Test:**
A test in which patients are connected to an electrocardiogram machine. They are usually asked to walk on a treadmill or possibly pedal a stationary bicycle while their electrocardiogram, blood pressure, and sometimes other vital signs are being monitored.

normally done not only in the hospital but by the patient's own cardiologist. This also applies to special diets recommended by a cardiologist.

Another complaint I frequently hear three to five weeks after the surgery is trouble sleeping. I'm not sure why many of my patients have unusual problems with not being able to sleep. It may be that during heart surgery or time in the intensive care unit, the clock in the patient's brain, or circadian rhythm, gets reset, and it may take awhile to revert to a normal routine. Most patients return to their normal sleep patterns five to seven weeks after surgery.

My patients sometimes complain about night sweats. This problem usually resolves itself, although occasionally night sweats can indicate a serious problem, particularly if they are associated with high fevers. In most patients, however, it is a side effect that seems to be unique to either the heart surgery or a major operation. The condition gets better in a month or two.

Numbness is another complaint, particularly if it is located in the left chest area or left breast in women. It seems to be more common in patients in whom the left internal mammary artery was used for a bypass graft. Some patients notice some numbness along the vein harvest site in the leg, particularly around the ankle area. This can be related to damage to the small branches of the nerve that intertwine with the saphenous vein. These problems usually subside over a couple of months.

Some patients have numbness or tingling in their little finger and the finger or two next to it, either in one or both hands. This common complaint is thought to be related to the fact that when the chest retractor is opened, it stretches the ulnar nerve as it comes out of the spinal cord, loops over the first rib, and goes into the arm. This problem, when it occurs, almost always

subsides, sometimes taking five or six weeks or longer.

Occasionally, patients say their eyeglasses are a bit out of focus. This seems to be a problem that is not specific to heart surgery but occurs following all types of major surgery. I am unclear why this occurs, but ophthalmologists usually say patients should wait a couple of months after a major operation before getting their eyeglass prescriptions changed because their visual acuity tends to return to what it was before the surgery.

Over the years, I have also noticed patients may come in for their heart surgery taking a certain antihypertensive (blood pressure) medication, and go home taking less of that medicine or none. A month later, however, they need that medicine again and don't know why they were not sent home taking it. While patients are in the hospital, particularly while in bed for two to four days, the tone in their blood vessels tends to relax somewhat. When they are up and around again, the tone may not return as quickly, and their blood pressure may be a little lower than it was before the heart surgery. This explains why they may not need the antihypertensive medicines they previously took. However, after about a month or six weeks, when the blood vessel tone returns, they often need to take the same blood pressure medication they took before the surgery.

Patients with diabetes often go home with different insulin requirements than they had before the heart surgery. Sometimes diabetic patients who were not taking insulin go home taking insulin, and sometimes those that are taking insulin, particularly lower doses, will go home and not need insulin. In general, I find that after five to seven weeks, patients tend to require whatever dose of oral antihyperglycemics or insulin they had been taking before the heart surgery.

My patients frequently tell me that when they lie on their side, particularly their left side, they notice their heart beating more than they did preoperatively, and they think perhaps this is dangerous. This is a common complaint and is generally caused by adhesions that have formed around the heart in the healing process. They are feeling the tug of these adhesions as the heart beats. Over time, however, the adhesions stretch, and most patients become used to it and no longer notice it.

Some patients notice a lump at the top of their breastbone that wasn't there before the surgery. If the lump is red and tender, it could signal an infection, but usually the lump appears because there is a layer of fat under the skin that does not hold stitches too well, and the consistency of this fat is somewhat like cottage cheese. To get stitches to hold, we have to place them deeper into the tissue, which tends to wad the tissue up around the stitch. Also, we place deeper stitches because the skin along the middle of the breastbone tends to pull away toward the arms. Over time, the lump will usually even out and return to normal.

Fortunately, over the last ten years, we have seen a decrease in the death rate from coronary artery disease in the United States. This is probably due to a number of factors, including better education of the general public, particularly about diet, cigarette smoking, and, in some cases, changes in life style.

This decrease is probably also due to relentless campaigns by the American Heart Association, the National Institutes of Health, and other groups, including national medical and surgical societies that deal with heart disease. They not only educate the public but also fund research in these areas. We also have better medications, and, certainly, the invasive cardiology field has come a long way, including the use of balloon dilatation and stents to treat various forms of blockages in the coronary arteries. Despite all of this, it appears that coronary artery bypass graft surgery will be around for the foreseeable future and continue to play a major role in the treatment of patients with advanced forms of coronary artery disease.

# STROKES, CAROTID ARTERY DISEASE, AND CORONARY BYPASS SURGERY

By

## Cary W. Akins, M.D.

Clinical Professor of Surgery
Harvard University

Visiting Surgeon
Massachusetts General Hospital

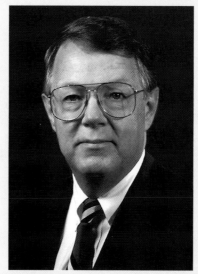

THE MOST DREADED COMplication of coronary artery bypass grafting, other than death, is the occurrence of stroke during the surgery. Unfortunately, as the average age of patients having bypass surgery has risen during the past twenty years, so has the chance of having a stroke. For patients less than age fifty years, the risk of stroke after coronary artery bypass grafting is less than 1 percent; for those patients more than age eighty years, the risk approaches 8 percent to 10 percent.

The causes of a stroke during surgery are many, but they can be grouped under three general headings.

### Problems with Blood Flow to the Brain

Although cardiopulmonary bypass with the heart-lung machine rarely causes poor blood flow to the brain, certain unusual circumstances can occur.

Each time the left ventricle contracts, it ejects blood from the heart and causes a pulse in the arteries throughout the body. The brain, however, is sensitive to the loss of regular pulse, and the heart-lung machine provides a more continuous flow than the normal pulsing flow from the heart. Because there is a lack of pulsation, it is particularly important that an adequate blood pressure be maintained when the patient is receiving assistance from the heart-lung machine to ensure the brain gets enough blood. Partial or complete obstruction of one or both carotid arteries, which supply blood to the brain, can lead to compromised blood flow to the brain while the heart-lung machine is working.

### Bleeding into the Brain

One of the startling and very fortunate findings in heart surgery is that, despite the high doses of very potent blood thinners (anticoagulants) required when the heart-lung machine is used for coronary artery bypass grafting, bleeding into the brain is extremely rare. In fact, it almost never occurs during the operation and thus can be discounted as a cause of stroke during the operation.

### Embolus to the Brain

An abnormal clump of material traveling through the blood vessels is called an embolus. The possible sources of material traveling to the brain include blood clots from inside the heart, debris from plaque in the aorta or the carotid arteries, and particles of material or air from the heart-lung machine.

Surgeons have recently focused their attention on atherosclerosis in the aorta and in the carotid arteries.

Physicians currently have numerous strategies to deal with atherosclerosis when it occurs in the aorta near the heart. This area is of great importance to the surgeon because it is where the blood-return tubes from the heart-lung machine are usually inserted, where coronary bypass grafts may be sewn, and where other clamps and tubes may need to be placed to protect the heart muscle during the operation.

## Atherosclerosis in the Carotid Arteries

In the carotid arteries, the accumulation of atherosclerotic plaque is unfortunately quite common in older patients. When more than half of the carotid artery is obstructed with atherosclerotic material, the risk of stroke begins to climb.

In patients with at least 60 percent obstruction of their carotid artery, a carotid endarterectomy, or surgical clearing of the artery, yields much greater freedom from subsequent strokes than continued medical therapy. A carotid endarterectomy is performed through an incision in the neck. During the procedure, the atherosclerotic accumulation can be removed directly and the artery incision closed.

The subsequent freedom from strokes is obtained not only by patients who have symptoms from their carotid obstructions but also by those who do not have symptoms from them. Thus, the mere presence of a substantial carotid artery blockage can justify a carotid endarterectomy even if the patient does not have symptoms. Unfortunately, the first symptom of advancing carotid artery blockage may be a full stroke.

## Carotid and Coronary Artery Disease

Patients who have substantial carotid artery disease in addition to coronary artery disease are at a much higher risk of stroke during coronary artery bypass grafting if nothing is done to correct the carotid artery disease.

The issue for surgeons in the last several years has been timing the two operations (carotid endarterectomy and coronary artery bypass graft) when a patient has both forms of artery disease. Several approaches have been tried, including performing one of the operations first, followed by the other. In some situations, this may seem to be an acceptable choice, particularly if the disease in one of the arterial systems is very severe and that in the other system is not.

However, recent surgical research has indicated that for the majority of patients with severe disease in both arterial systems, a combined operation is probably the best approach. During such an operation, the blocked coronary arteries are bypassed, and the diseased carotid artery is treated. This approach in our institution and other surgical centers has yielded lower operative death and stroke rates while providing better long-term relief from stroke. One study has demonstrated that doing the two procedures after the same anesthesia induction rather than as separate operations is much more cost effective.

In summary, evidence is accumulating that patients with severe disease in both their coronary and carotid arteries are generally better treated with a combined operation. Continuing studies are being performed that will test whether this combined approach is more effective than the staged approach in all surgical centers. The goal remains lowering the incidence of stroke during surgery, still the most devastating nonfatal complication of coronary artery bypass surgery.

# Minimally Invasive Coronary Artery Revascularization

By

Michael Mack, M.D.

Assistant Clinical Professor of Surgery

University of Texas SW Medical School

Dallas, Texas

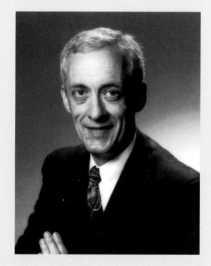

ONE OF THE MAJOR CAUS-es of surgical trauma is the method of entry into the body. Large incisions tend to result in greater trauma, whereas the pain and some complications associated with surgery can possibly be lessened if the physician gains entry through a smaller incision. This approach has led to the concept of "less invasive surgery," a relatively new method of surgery that is accomplished through a few small "keyhole" incisions using a video camera attached to a telescope.

Because of the unique complexities of heart surgery — including the necessity of the heart-lung machine, operating on a moving organ, and the need to sew tiny blood vessels together — cardiac surgery was the last surgical specialty to adopt these new concepts. Starting in 1995, however, a few surgeons began performing coronary artery bypass grafting (CABG) through a three-inch incision between the ribs on the left side of the breast bone. The procedure was performed on a beating heart rather than on a stopped heart, and the minimally invasive direct coronary artery bypass (MIDCAB), or "keyhole" form of cardiac surgery, was born. The "direct" in the acronym means that although the bypass was performed through a small incision, it was done while viewing the heart directly rather than with a scope.

This form of surgery has two benefits for postoperative recovery: Patients do not undergo as much discomfort as a large incision would cause, and the heart-lung machine, which can contribute to the undesirable side effects of heart surgery, is not used.

At first, the MIDCAB operation was basically limited to a single bypass on the front surface of the heart and, because the heart was still moving, the connection of the bypass was technically challenging, and the results of the procedure were appropriately questioned. This issue was largely solved by the introduction of "stabilizers," which are mechanical feet placed against the surface of the heart. This produces a local area of immobilization and allows for precise sewing while the remainder of the heart continues to beat and support the circulation.

In 1995, the Port-Access™ device was introduced by Heartport, Inc., of Redwood, California. This device allows the surgeon access to the heart through a smaller incision while still using the heart-lung machine. It allows not only CABG operations but also surgery on the mitral valve inside the heart. Both are performed through a

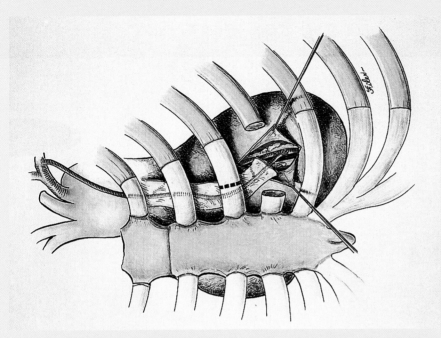

New surgical techniques are allowing surgeons to access the heart through much smaller incisions on the side of the chest. Commonly called "keyhole" surgery, this is possible for a number of different heart operations.

three-inch incision on either the left (CABG) or right (mitral valve) side of the sternum. In addition to the ability to use the heart-lung machine without opening the chest, this procedure offers the ability to safely stop the heart with a balloon catheter placed in the aorta just above the heart.

In 1998, there were about forty-five thousand beating-heart operations performed in the United States (7 percent of all CABGs) and four thousand Port-Access procedures. Findings being published in early 1999 in the medical literature give some early indication that acceptable

results may be obtained by these new approaches.

Currently, most of the focus in the field of minimally invasive cardiac surgery is on the off-pump coronary artery bypass (OPCAB) procedure. In the OPCAB operation, multiple coronary arteries can be bypassed. Although the breastbone is still divided, the heart-lung machine is not utilized, and newer generation stabilizers are used to immobilize each artery to be bypassed in turn while the heart continues to beat. Many experts in the field predict that within five years, more than 50 percent of all CABG surgery will be performed by using this approach.

The field of minimally invasive cardiac surgery is less than four years old, and the early results are promising. However, the results have not yet withstood the test of time. Accurate measurement of its role in managing heart disease will require further comparison, not only with conventional bypass surgery, but also with the "least invasive" form of coronary bypass, percutaneous transluminal coronary angioplasty (PTCA).

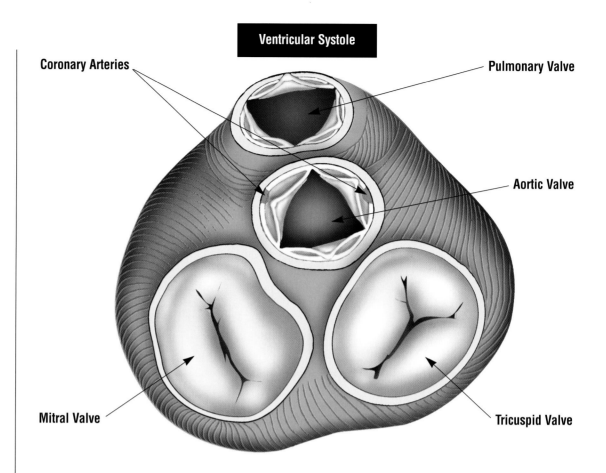

**Ventricular Systole**

Coronary Arteries

Pulmonary Valve

Aortic Valve

Mitral Valve

Tricuspid Valve

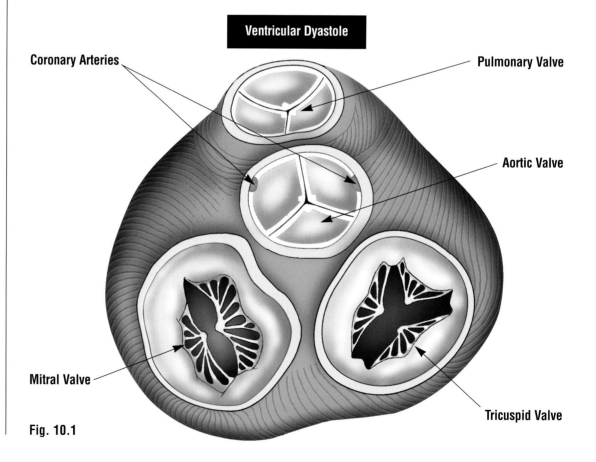

**Ventricular Dyastole**

Coronary Arteries

Pulmonary Valve

Aortic Valve

Mitral Valve

Tricuspid Valve

**Fig. 10.1:**
All four heart valves
are seen from above
here. The pulmonary
valve is seen on top
with the aortic valve
immediately below it.
The two red dots depict
where the coronary ar-
teries originate in the
aorta just above the
aortic valve. The two
lower valves are the
tricuspid, on the right,
and the mitral valve
on the left. The two
illustrations show the
valves during two
stages of the
heart cycle.

**Fig. 10.1**

148

## CHAPTER TEN

# HEART VALVE PROBLEMS

PICTURE A RED BLOOD CELL TRAVeling through the venous system toward the heart. It enters the heart through one of two major veins, either the superior vena cava or the inferior vena cava, and passes into the right atrium. The one-way tricuspid valve opens, and the cell flows into the right ventricle. The tricuspid valve is composed of three leaflets that are connected on their underside (right ventricle side) to string-like structures called **chordae tendineae**, which are connected to muscles called **papillary muscles**. The papillary muscles are outgrowths of the muscular right ventricular wall.

As the right ventricle contracts, the tricuspid valve closes and the pulmonary valve opens, allowing the blood cell to be pumped, or propelled, into the pulmonary artery, which channels unoxygenated blood containing carbon dioxide to the lungs. Like the tricuspid, the pulmonary valve is one-way and composed of three leaflets (also called cusps), although the leaflets differ from those of the tricuspid valve in shape. They look like three small cups. The pulmonary valve does not have chordae tendineae or papillary muscles.

After giving off carbon dioxide and picking up oxygen in the lungs, the newly oxygenated red blood cell returns to the heart through one of the pulmonary veins and into the left atrium. The two-leaflet mitral valve opens, and the cell travels into the left ventricle. Like the tricuspid, the mitral valve has chordae tendineae, which are attached to papillary muscles. When the mitral and tricuspid valves are closed, the valve leaflets look like a parachute, and the chordae tendineae resemble the cords that connect the parachute to the jumper. The papillary muscle is the jumper.

When the left ventricle contracts, the aortic valve opens, allowing the red blood cell to stream out the aorta and into the arterial system that nourishes the body (see Fig. 10.1 for cardiac cycle). The two coronary arteries branch off the base of the aorta (aortic root) just above the aortic valve leaflets.

###  Before the Heart-Lung Machine:

*Opening Narrowed Valves*

The first attempt to open a stenotic (narrowed) heart valve in a human was carried out by Dr. Theodore Tuffier, a French surgeon, on July 13, 1912. After opening the patient's chest, he supposedly pushed the wall of the aorta near the heart through the stenotic aortic valve

**Chordae Tendineae**:
String-like attachments that are part of the mitral and tricuspid valve apparatus that connects the valve leaflets, or flaps, to the papillary muscles on the ventricular wall.

**Papillary Muscles**:
Tiny muscles located in the left and right ventricles that are attached by chordae tendineae to the mitral and tricuspid valves. These muscle structures help control the valve function.

and dilated the valve. The patient survived and was reported to be improved.

About ten years later, Dr. Elliot Cutler, a surgeon at Harvard Medical School, in collaboration with Boston cardiologist Samuel Levine, worked out a procedure to dilate the mitral valve. Their first patient was a desperately ill twelve-year-old girl whose mitral valve had been badly damaged and narrowed from rheumatic fever. She underwent successful mitral valve dilatation on May 20, 1923. Unfortunately, most of Cutler's subsequent patients did not survive the surgery, and he abandoned the procedure.

These sporadic and mostly unsuccessful attempts ceased by 1929, and things remained quiet until 1945, when Dr. Charles Bailey and his team again attempted to treat mitral valve **stenosis**. The first of their five human patients was a thirty-seven-year-old man who was operated on on November 4, 1945. He bled to death in the operating room during the procedure. The second patient was a twenty-nine-year-old woman operated on on June 12, 1946. Her condition improved for the first thirty hours after the

surgery but suddenly deteriorated, and she died forty-eight hours after the surgery. After these two failures, Bailey's home base, Hahnemann Hospital in Philadelphia, refused to allow him to attempt any more mitral valve dilatations. He even became known as the "butcher" of Hahnemann Hospital.

Their third patient, who was treated at a different hospital, was a thirty-eight-year-old man operated on on March 22, 1948. The surgery seemed to go well, but the patient hemorrhaged into the chest cavity on the second postoperative day. He died of complications. Patient four was a thirty-two-year-old man who underwent heart surgery on June 10, 1948. His heart stopped while the incision was being made to start the surgery. He could not be resuscitated and died in the operating room.

The surgical team then immediately regrouped and rushed to Episcopal Hospital, where the fifth operation, this one on a young woman, was started before the bad news from that morning was known and the hospital administration could forbid the procedure. Her mitral valve dilatation was successfully completed. One week later, Bailey brought the patient by train one thousand miles to Chicago, where he presented her to the American College of Chest Physicians annual meeting. She was without symptoms after the surgery and felt better than she had been feeling for years.

On June 16, a few days after Bailey's success, Dr. Dwight Harken in Boston successfully performed his first mitral valve dilatation. Three months later, Sir Russell Brock in England did his first successful similar procedure but did not report it until 1950, when he described six additional successful attempts.

*Targeting the Pulmonary Valve*

On December 4, 1947, Dr. Thomas Holmes Sellers, an English surgeon, completed the first successful surgery on a

**Stenosis**:
An abnormal narrowing of an orifice, blood vessel, or heart valve.

Dr. Elliot Cutler (below) performed the first successful mitral valve dilatation. His patient, a 12-year-old girl (right), had suffered from rheumatic fever. Her surgery was successful.

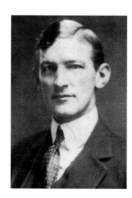

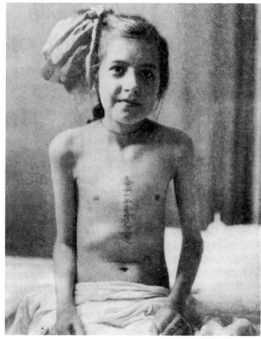

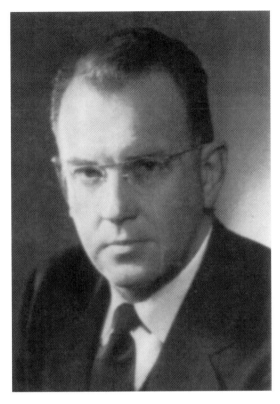

narrowed pulmonary valve. The surgery occurred during an operation for a congenital heart defect called **tetralogy of Fallot**. In this condition, there is an obstruction of blood to the lungs and a hole in the heart. This particular patient also suffered from advanced tuberculosis of both lungs. When Sellers opened the sac around the heart, he could feel the narrowed pulmonary heart valve each time the right ventricle contracted. He passed a special type of knife through the wall of the right ventricle and made slits in the narrowed valve. The patient made a good recovery and was markedly improved.

*The Development of Valve Replacement Surgery*

Like all forms of heart surgery, valvular surgery made great leaps forward as the heart-lung machine came into use. Doctors who had once only imagined the day when diseased valves could be replaced began to actually work to develop implantable valves. Artificial valves were

not a novel idea. The first ones had been developed in the 1950s, when Drs. Charles Hufnagel in Washington, D.C., and J.M. Campbell in Oklahoma independently developed and implanted artificial valves in the descending aortas of dogs. This could be done before the heart-lung machine because the descending aorta is far enough away from the heart. The surgeon merely placed clamps several inches apart on the aorta to interrupt blood flow, opened the aorta, inserted the artificial valve, and then stitched the aorta closed.

These two valves, which were called "cage-ball valves" because of their design, looked similar. After presenting this mechanical heart valve technique in animals at the American College of Surgeons annual meeting in 1949, Hufnagel began to use this procedure in human patients suffering from aortic valve incompetence. The valve implantation did not actually replace the patient's own leaky aortic valve but acted as a supporting or auxiliary valve.

 **The Advent of the Heart-Lung Machine**

Once the heart-lung machine was developed, surgeons began to attempt heart valve replacement with cage-ball valves. The first successful valve replacement was performed by Dr. Dwight Harken and his colleagues at Harvard's Peter Bent Brigham Hospital in Boston. Harken used a cage-ball valve to replace the aortic valve. Many of the techniques described in his 1960 report are similar to those used today for aortic valve replacement.

The same year, Dr. Albert Starr successfully replaced the mitral valve by using a cage-ball valve.

In 1964, Starr and associates reported on thirteen patients who had undergone multiple heart valve replacements. One patient had the aortic, mitral, and tricuspid valves replaced on February 21, 1963.

By 1967, nearly two thousand Starr-Edwards heart valves had been implanted, and the cage-ball prosthesis had gen-

In 1960, Dr. Dwight Harken (left) performed the first successful valve replacement in the normal aortic valve position with an artificial valve. He used a cage-ball valve to replace the aortic valve.

**Tetralogy of Fallot:**
A set of four individual defects, including:
1) a ventricular septal defect; 2) an obstruction of blood flow from the right ventricle to the pulmonary arteries; 3) overriding of the aortic valve above the ventricular septal defect; and 4) an abnormally thickened right ventricle.

# ♥ ALBERT STARR AND THE STARR-EDWARDS HEART VALVE

Dr. Albert Starr (right) was part of the team that developed the Starr-Edwards cage-ball heart valve (facing page). Starr was the first to successfully replace a mitral valve with that valve. The Starr-Edwards valves went on to become the world standard.

AFTER GRADUATING FROM Columbia College of Physicians and Surgeons in 1949, Dr. Albert Starr served a one-year internship at Johns Hopkins Hospital. There, he worked under the world famous surgeon Dr. Alfred Blalock, who had pioneered the Blalock-Taussig operation for children with cyanotic heart disease.

When his internship was completed, Starr returned to New York but was soon drafted into the U.S. Army Medical Corps to serve first as a battalion surgeon in the First Cavalry Division in Korea, then as a surgeon for a Mobile Army Surgical Hospital (MASH) unit. In a single year, he performed more than one thousand major operations.

"Korea was the first war in which you had an almost unlimited backup system to a limited war," Starr said in a recent interview. "It was a war in which there was almost an unlimited supply of human blood available for transfusion on the battlefield. There was also the beginning of antibiotics, and helicopter evacuation so that someone wounded in a firefight in Korea would be back in a MASH within minutes of being wounded, rather than hours or days. The survival rate, if you made it back to the MASH hospital, was about 95 percent."

After his tour of duty, he returned to complete his surgical training at Bellevue and Presbyterian hospitals in New York. By 1957, Starr had finished his thoracic surgery residency and moved to the University of Oregon, Portland, to start

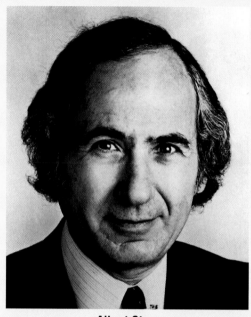

**Albert Starr**

an open heart program. This is where Starr was first exposed to heart valve surgery and the problems surgeons were having repairing diseased valves. After experimenting with all sorts of valve prostheses, Starr became convinced that valve replacement was necessary to save many patients with diseased mitral valves because there was no way to repair badly deformed and diseased mitral valves.

Enter a retired engineer named M. Lowell Edwards. A successful and independently wealthy engineer, Edwards had several important inventions to his credit and originally approached Starr to help him develop an artificial heart.

"I thought he was overreaching, to put it mildly," Starr said. "What I discovered was that he was a very successful engineer, and although he was wearing the typical Oregon golfer's dress, he was very accomplished and had numerous inventions to his credit. One of them was a fuel injection system for rapidly climbing aircraft during World War II. The P-38 and many of our fighter aircraft had his fuel injection system, and a good part of the successful war effort, at least as far as the air war is concerned, is credited to his fuel injection system. In the Battle of Britain, the Spitfires had his fuel injection system, and that enabled them to get up to very high altitudes very rapidly without the system failing."

When Starr pointed out that medicine didn't even have artificial valves yet, much less an artificial heart, the two decided to begin one valve at a time and invent prostheses. They started with the mitral valve and considered every kind of valve known. After drifting from valve to valve, they finally hit upon the ball valve, which showed early promise because it was not as easily occluded by the blood clots that quickly formed around the sutures of more conventional leaflet-type valves.

They quickly learned, however, that blood clots did form in the ball valves — it just took longer before the clot was large enough to block up the free-moving ball. At the time, they were performing their early experimentation in dogs, many of whom were dying from thrombosis months after their valves were implanted. This challenge led Starr and Edwards to the silastic shield, which was basically a retractable diaphragm that covered the sutures and prevented blood clots from forming. This shield created long-term survivors, and soon Starr had a kennel full of active dogs that had undergone mitral valve replacement.

"The chief of cardiology, Dr. Herbert Griswold, knew we had a kennel full of active dogs and came to visit us in August 1960. He looked at all these dogs and said, 'Starr, we have to do this clinically.' That was the first time we began to think about that seriously because I thought it would be a couple years' project at least."

Interestingly, the first valve implanted in a human did not use the silastic shield. Starr, knowing that dog's blood clots very aggressively, figured he wanted the simplest procedure possible and, if the patient's blood clotted, they could always administer anticoagulant medication. This first operation was done in September 1960 on a young woman in her mid-twenties. The Starr-Edwards cage-ball valve prosthesis quickly became established as the gold standard in mechanical heart valve prostheses.

"This generated tremendous excitement and put the Oregon Health Sciences University on the map," Starr said. "We had visitors from all over the world."

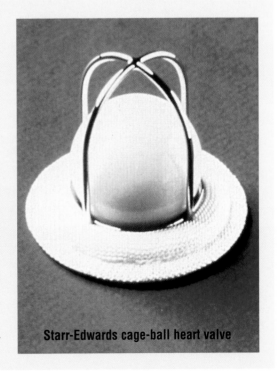

**Starr-Edwards cage-ball heart valve**

153

erated intense excitement and become established as the gold standard for mechanical heart valve prostheses. The valves maintained this status for many years, although today newer, low-profile valves are commonly used. There are, however, still some surgeons implanting the original Starr-Edwards cage-ball valve.

### ♥ Human Valves Used in Other Humans

Not long after the first heart valves were implanted, physicians began searching for better heart valves — including biological valves. Biological valves are valves from animals or human cadavers or valves made from other animal tissue. An aortic **homograft** valve was first used in 1962 to replace a mitral valve in one patient and an aortic valve in another. Survival was short.

That same year, Dr. Donald Ross in England reported the first successful aortic valve homograft implant. He placed the valve in the normal position. A month later, Sir Brian Barratt-Boyes performed the same implantation in New Zealand.

Shortly after his success, Dr. Ross went on to develop another technique. In 1967, he used the patient's own pulmonary valve to replace a malfunctioning aortic valve. An aortic or pulmonary valve homograft was then used to replace the patient's pulmonary valve. This procedure, known as the Ross Procedure, is currently recommended for some younger patients who require aortic valve replacement.

**Homograft**: A donor graft, or portion of tissue, taken from a donor and placed into a recipient of the same species.

Dr. Donald Ross was the first to successfully replace an aortic valve with a tissue valve from another human. He also invented the Ross Procedure, which is still in use today to replace a malfunctioning aortic valve.

## ♥ DONALD ROSS: THE VALVE PIONEER

DR. DONALD ROSS QUALIFIED for his medical degree on the same day as Dr. Christiaan Barnard, a fellow South African. Although the two would take divergent paths — Ross went to England to train and Barnard went to the United States — they remained friends, and both worked to develop heart transplantation. Ross recalled in an interview a conversation he had with Barnard before the first transplantation.

"Barnard came through one day and said, 'I've just been watching Shumway do the transplant of the heart in an animal and I'm going to do that,'" Ross remembered.

Later that same year, a reporter asked Ross when he thought the first heart transplantation would be performed. He predicted sometime within the next five years. Less than a month later, Barnard announced he had performed the first human-to-human transplant. Shortly afterward, Ross himself performed the first heart transplant in the United Kingdom.

Although his work in heart transplantation was cutting edge, Ross became most famous for

**Donald Ross**

Other tissues that have been used for valve implants include the pericardium, fascia lata, or tissue from tendons, and dura mater, which is the tissue that surrounds the brain and spinal cord.

In the 1960s, physicians also began to experiment with valves from other animals, or **xenografts**. This was first done in 1964 by Drs. Carlos Duran and Alfred Gunning in England, who replaced an aortic valve in a human by using a valve from a pig. The early results were good, but these valves often failed after a few years. In France, for instance, Dr. Alain Carpentier and his associates reported on twelve patients with pig valve replacements that all failed by five years. As a result, Carpentier developed a technique to fix the pig valves with a chemical called glutaraldehyde instead of using the accepted formaldehyde. In addition, Carpentier mounted his valves on a stent, which allowed the valves to be used to replace the mitral and tricuspid valves.

Carpentier later wrote:

*"It became obvious that the future of tissue valves would depend on the development of methods of preparation capable of preventing inflammatory cell reaction and penetration into the tissue. My background in chemistry was obviously insufficient. I decided to abandon surgery for two days a week to follow the teaching program in chemistry at the Faculty of Sciences and prepare a Ph.D. (at the University of Paris). It was certainly not easy to become a student in chemistry*

**Xenograft:**
Graft tissue taken from an animal of one species and used in another species. Pig heart valves, which are commonly used to replace heart valves in humans, are one form of xenograft.

his pioneering work with heart valves. This was an area of interest from the beginning of his career. In July 1962, Ross implanted the world's first successful homograft valve (a tissue valve from a human cadaver) only two years after Starr implanted the first artificial valve. Ross recounted this historical implantation:

*"Lord Brock was my mentor and chief and put me onto repeating earlier pioneering work in homograft implantation [in the animal laboratory]. It was a very exciting time. We took human valves and human aortas and stored them by a process of freeze drying so they could keep for months.*

*"One day during surgery while I was scratching away at a calcified valve, the whole thing disintegrated and went down the sucker. We didn't have a valve and there were no valves in England. There were only Starr valves in America. So we took one of those stored human valves,*

*which was freeze dried, reconstituted it and sewed it in."*

Originally, the valve was supposed to be temporary until the surgical team could import a mechanical valve. The patient did well, however, and Ross switched to implanting homograft valves instead of artificial valves.

Over the next several years, he found that an aortic valve homograft worked well in the pulmonary valve position. That discovery led to an important milestone in valve surgery, the Ross Procedure. In this operation, the native pulmonary valve is relocated to the aortic position, and a homograft valve replaces the pulmonary valve.

It is a technically difficult operation that took almost two decades to gain widespread acceptance but it is performed today with excellent results. It has the powerful advantage that the new aortic valve will grow, an especially important quality for small children.

# ♥ ALAIN CARPENTIER

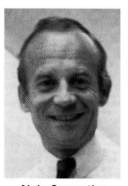

**Alain Carpentier**

Dr. Alain Carpentier (above) was a major figure in the development of pig valves for human hearts. His valves (below) were mounted on cloth rings to help physicians sew them in place.

**Cardiomyoplasty**: A surgical procedure using a muscle, usually the latissimus dorsi muscle in the back, to wrap around a failing heart. The muscle is then electrically stimulated so it will contract in synchrony with the failing heart.

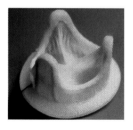

DR. ALAIN CARPENTIER DECIDED to go into medicine after an operation and a month-long stay in a hospital for appendicitis when he was only ten years old. At the time, antibiotics were not widely available, and his recovery was very long and painful, inspiring in the young boy a desire to help the course of healing. Today, he is best known for three major contributions to heart surgery. He developed surgical techniques to repair the mitral valve; he developed a practical method of using heart valves from pigs in humans; and he pioneered a surgical procedure called **cardiomyoplasty**, which is used in patients with failing heart muscle.

Carpentier began his research into heart valve replacement at a time when mechanical heart valves, such as the Starr-Edwards valve, had just recently become commercially available. Physicians were also successfully using heart valve implants from human cadavers, a technique pioneered by Ross and Barratt-Boyes. Inspired by their work, Carpentier began to research biological valve replacements but ran into a snag in French law.

"My surgical master, Dr. Charles Debost, told me if I was interested, I would have to collect homograft valves, just like Barratt-Boyes and Ross did," he remembered in a 1999 interview. "I began to try to collect homograft valves in Paris; however, French law did not permit one to take pieces from cadavers during the forty-eight hours following death to allow the family to make an opposition. Of course, after forty-eight hours, most of the homograft valves I could collect were infected."

After a few months of this, Carpentier began researching the use of valves

*when you are thirty-five years old and an associate professor of surgery.*

*"I began to investigate numerous cross-linking-inducing factors and found that glutaraldehyde was able to almost eliminate inflammatory reaction.... My wife, Sophie, was a tremendous help all these years."*

### Modern Heart Valve Therapy

*Rheumatic Fever*

Today, surgeons are capable of treating a wide range of heart valve defects, which can be caused by a number of conditions. Rheumatic fever is a common cause of heart valve injury requiring surgery in adults. People of any age can contract rheumatic fever, but it's most common in children between the ages of five years and fifteen years. It is caused by bacteria known as streptococcus and is usually related to a severe type of sore throat sometimes called a "strep throat." Most people who have strep throats do not develop rheumatic fever, and appropriate treatment with antibiotics dramatically decreases the risk of developing rheumatic fever. Rheumatic fever usually occurs from two weeks to a month after the strep throat infection.

Symptoms of rheumatic fever include aches and pains in the joints. The pain in the joints tends to migrate from one joint to the next, and it's not always located in the same joint. Rashes can occur. Lumps, called subcutaneous nodules, can develop under the skin. Victims sometimes develop uncontrolled movements of the legs and from other animals, or xenografts. It was this effort that led him to his work with glutaraldehyde and the technique to successfully replace any of the four heart valves with xenografts. He called these tissue heart valves, which were mounted on a cloth sewing ring, "bioprostheses," a term that is still used today.

At the same time, he also developed what he considers his most important contribution to valve surgery: reconstruction of the mitral valve, as opposed to replacement of it. This question of valve replacement versus valve repair used to be answered during surgery. Today, Carpentier credits medical technology like echocardiography with greatly improving valve analysis.

"In the old days, I adopted a policy that I would try to repair the valve for fifteen minutes and if I was not satisfied after fifteen minutes, I would just replace the valve," he said. "Progressively, the number of valves I had to replace diminished. Today, of course, is very different because we see patients at an earlier stage and we have the echocardiography technique, which I call the stethoscope of the next century because it is so useful."

Valve repair was a superior option to replacement, according to Carpentier, because of the drawback of valve prostheses. "The reason I developed these two techniques almost simultaneously is the fact that, in 1966 to 1967, the only existing solution when a patient had a valvular problem was replacement with a mechanical valve," Carpentier said. "I was struck by the fact that one of my patients was a painter and was obliged to stop his artistic activity after the operation. He was a well-known artist, and I found it a real tragedy that although the mechanical valve made it possible to save hundreds of lives, there was this problem of emboli (blood clots breaking away from the valve) and the need for anticoagulation."

arms, called chorea. Patients with rheumatic fever can also develop an inflammation of the heart muscle called carditis, which can result in shortness of breath and fatigue. Fever can also be present.

Although it doesn't always do so, rheumatic fever can cause damage to any or all of the heart valves. The aortic and mitral valves are most commonly affected.

A second episode of rheumatic fever can further damage the heart, particularly the heart valves. Patients with damaged heart valves may need heart surgery relatively soon after their rheumatic fever. However, most people who need heart surgery will require it much later, sometimes late in life, even though they contracted rheumatic fever as a child. About half of all patients who require heart valve surgery as adults because of rheumatic fever damage do not even know that they had rheumatic fever.

*Infectious Endocarditis*

Bacterial and fungal infections are another threat to both the heart and the heart valves (Fig. 10.5). In many cases, the exact reason for the infection is unknown. During a dental procedure, for example, bacteria may gain access to the bloodstream. Antibiotics should be given before a dental procedure to those who have a diseased or artificial heart valve to help prevent infectious **endocarditis**, or infection of the heart muscle. Other causes include surgery and illicit intravenous drug use.

In most cases, infections of the heart and heart valves can be treated with

**Endocarditis**:
An infection inside the heart.

antibiotics. In some cases, however, one or more of the heart valves can be severely damaged by an infection and may require heart surgery to repair or replace the valve.

*Prolapsed Mitral Valve*

**Mitral valve prolapse**, or MVP, is a condition in which the leaflets of the mitral valve do not meet properly, usually because the chordae tendineae are too long (Fig. 10.2). Sometimes one or both valve leaflets are also abnormally enlarged. When the leaflets do not meet correctly, the heart valve may make an abnormal noise when it closes. This can be heard with a stethoscope. If they do not touch each other when they close, blood from the left ventricle can leak back into the left atrium. This can cause a heart murmur.

Some patients may have chest pain related to mitral valve prolapse. They may develop cardiac arrhythmias, or irregular heartbeats, and shortness of breath. Medications may alleviate these symptoms. Fortunately, the great majority of patients with mitral valve prolapse lead a normal life and do not need a surgical procedure. Some people with diagnosed mitral valve prolapse are also encouraged to undertake an antibiotic regime both before and after dental work, even teeth cleaning.

The cause of mitral valve prolapse is unknown. It is more common in women. Occasionally, patients require heart surgery, particularly if the chordae tendineae connecting the prolapsed mitral valve to the heart wall rupture.

**Aortic Valve Disease**

The aortic valve is responsible for regulating the flow of blood from the left ventricle into the aorta. As time goes by and the valve is subjected to stress, calcium may deposit on the leaflets and cause the valve to become stenotic, or constricted (Fig. 10.3). This process is accelerated by rheumatic fever. The leaflets (cusps) become scarred. Over time, the scar tissue increases, and the valve itself becomes calcified.

Aortic valve stenosis is also related to a condition known as a congenital bicuspid valve. In this condition, the aortic valve, which normally has three leaflets, has only two. The bileaflet valve does not usually cause problems in childhood, but after many years it tends to scar. As with rheumatic fever or stenosis, calcium builds up, and the valve orifice becomes very narrow. Bicuspid aortic valves tend to calcify in some people by age twenty years or thirty years. They

Fig. 10.2:
**Mitral valve prolapse**, or MVP, occurs when the valve leaflets do not meet properly. The mitral valve on the near right is healthy. The mitral valve on the far right is prolapsed.

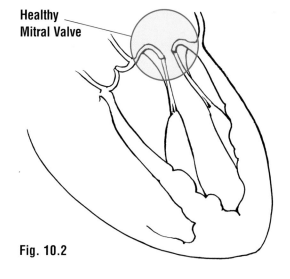

Healthy Mitral Valve

Fig. 10.2

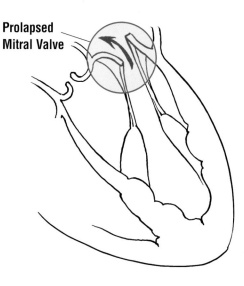

Prolapsed Mitral Valve

usually become symptomatic between ages thirty years and sixty years.

Stenotic aortic valves cause stress on the left ventricle, which is forced to work harder to push blood through the narrowed opening. As a result, the ventricular heart muscle will thicken, or hypertrophy, until it actually outgrows its blood supply. Finally, the left ventricle will no longer be able to force enough blood past the valve.

In this case, the heart itself may begin to fail, and patients usually start to develop symptoms including lightheadedness, or they may even pass out because not enough blood is getting to the brain. Irregular heartbeats and **angina pectoris** are also symptoms. This kind of angina occurs not only because the heart muscle outgrew its blood supply but also because not enough blood is getting past the narrowed aortic valve and into the coronary arteries that supply the heart.

Heart failure, signaled by shortness of breath and fatigue, is also associated with aortic valve stenosis. These symptoms are more commonly brought on by exercise, which increases the body's demand for oxygen. The severity of symptoms of aortic stenosis does not always correlate with the severity of the blockage. Sometimes the first sign of severe aortic stenosis is sudden death.

*Diagnosing Aortic Stenosis*

This condition can be diagnosed by using a number of different techniques. The first clue is frequently obtained with a stethoscope, which reveals a heart murmur that is rather typical of aortic stenosis. Further testing will be performed, including the two definitive tests that reveal aortic stenosis: echocardiography and cardiac catheterization. If the aortic stenosis is severe enough to warrant heart surgery, the patient will frequently undergo both tests.

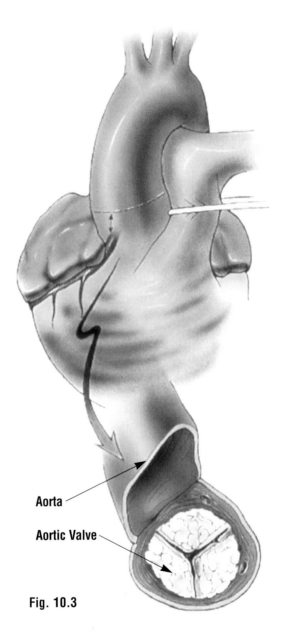

Aorta

Aortic Valve

**Fig. 10.3**

Fig. 10.3:
**Aortic Valve Stenosis:** A condition in which the aortic valve is narrowed, which stresses the left ventricle because it has to work harder to get blood through the valve.

**Angina Pectoris:** Chest pain that occurs when the heart is not getting enough blood. Often described as pressure, like a band tightening around the chest, or a dull, aching pain over the front left side of the chest. It can also be a pain radiating down the left arm or, occasionally, it can radiate into the neck or jaw.

*Aortic Valve Incompetence*

Aortic valve incompetence, also called insufficiency or regurgitation, usually occurs when the three leaflets of the aortic valve do not come in contact with each other when the valve closes. Some of the blood that has just been pumped into the aorta leaks back into the left ventricle. This makes the left ventricle much less efficient because it pumps the same blood twice.

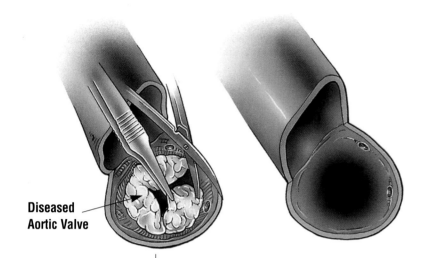

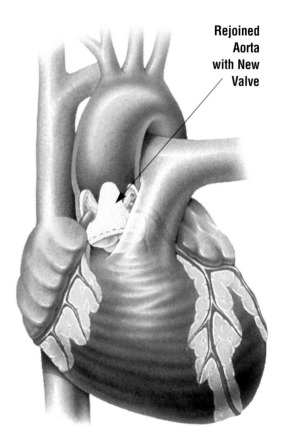

**Rejoined Aorta with New Valve**

**Diseased Aortic Valve**

To correct aortic valve stenosis with a porcine valve, physicians remove the diseased aortic valve (above) and sew in a xenograft (below). The final illustration (above right) shows the aorta incision stitched closed.

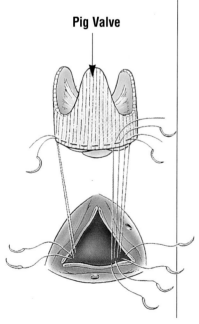

**Pig Valve**

Aortic valve incompetence can be caused by rheumatic fever (Fig. 10.4). It also can result from infective endocarditis or a number of other causes.

Aortic valve incompetence ranges in severity from mild to severe. Mild to moderate aortic valve incompetence is generally well tolerated. Most patients with mild or moderate aortic incompetence can lead a normal life and have a normal life expectancy. If the leakage becomes great, however, the left ventricle will start to dilate and fail. Patients can develop signs and symptoms of congestive heart failure, including shortness of breath and fatigue, and their ankles may become swollen. A definitive diagnosis is made with echocardiography and/or cardiac catheterization.

In some cases, aortic incompetence can appear rather quickly and be severe. This could be related to an infection in which one of the heart valve leaflets is destroyed, or it can happen as a result of trauma sustained in an automobile accident when the chest strikes the steering wheel. There can be other causes. In these situations, emergency heart surgery with heart valve replacement is necessary.

*Aortic Valve Stenosis and Incompetence*

A combination of aortic valve stenosis and incompetence is usually related to rheumatic heart valve disease but can also be due to bicuspid aortic valve or aging. In either case, as the valve becomes deformed, narrowed, and stenotic, the leaflets no longer come together. Not only is the blood obstructed as it tries to leave the left ventricle, but when the left ventricle relaxes, some of the blood leaks back into the chamber. Heart valve surgery may be needed.

**Mitral Valve Disease**

*Mitral Stenosis*

Mitral valve stenosis is usually caused by rheumatic fever, although some babies are born with an abnormally narrowed mitral valve. In this condition, the two leaflets of the mitral valve gradually fuse together, making it difficult for the blood traveling into the left atrium from the lungs to pass through the mitral valve and into the left ventricle.

As this condition becomes more severe, shortness of breath develops because blood backs up into the lungs. Fatigue is also a common symptom.

In some cases, the patient may cough up blood. (However, there are many other causes of coughing up blood [hemoptysis].) Depending on the degree of mitral valve stenosis, some form of intervention may be necessary. This might involve using a balloon catheter to dilate the stenotic mitral valve and could also mean heart surgery.

*Mitral Valve Incompetence*

Mitral valve incompetence, which is also referred to as mitral valve regurgitation or insufficiency, occurs when the two leaflets of the mitral valve no longer meet each other when the valve is closed. Because the leaflets do not meet, some of the blood that should be ejected into the aorta is squeezed through the faulty mitral

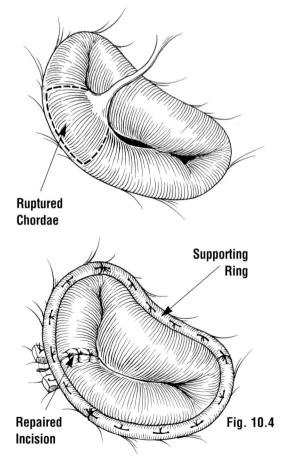

**Ruptured Chordae**

**Repaired Incision**

**Supporting Ring**

Fig. 10.4

valve backwards into the left atrium as the left ventricle contracts. The resulting higher pressure in the left atrium sends blood backwards into the lungs.

This condition can cause shortness of breath and fatigue. The heart also has to work harder because some of the blood that's being pumped is going backwards. As a result, the left ventricle will dilate and begin to fail, adding to the shortness of breath. Patients also have swollen ankles and become fatigued. If this problem becomes severe, heart surgery will most likely be required.

Another condition is called **myxoid degeneration**, in which some of the tissues in the heart are weakened, and the valve is prone to incompetence. This condition can affect varying parts of the mitral valve. For example, the chordae, which attach the valve to the underlying muscles, can rupture (Fig. 10.4). Likewise, the papillary muscles can rupture. Papillary muscle rupture is usually related to a heart attack. This condition requires emergency heart surgery.

*Mitral Valve Stenosis and Incompetence*

As with the aortic valve, the mitral valve may deform so that it obstructs the flow of blood into the left ventricle and prevents it from closing normally because the two mitral leaflets no longer touch each other. In this condition, the valve is narrowed and incompetent, sending some of the blood back through the deformed valve. Depending on the severity of this problem, heart surgery may be required.

**Tricuspid Valve Disease**

*Tricuspid Valve Stenosis*

The tricuspid valve may become stenotic as a result of rheumatic fever, or it may be narrow at birth (Fig. 10.5). Tricuspid valve stenosis from rheumatic fever, particularly that severe enough

**Myxoid Degeneration**: Degeneration of the middle layer of tissue in blood vessels and heart valves.

**Fig. 10.4:** The mitral valve is attached to the ventricular wall by chordae. If these rupture, the mitral valve becomes incompetent. The surgeon removes that portion of the valve where the ruptured chordae is located (above), then sews the valve together and places a supporting ring (below).

to require heart surgery, is relatively uncommon.

If the valve is severely stenotic, blood returning from the veins to the heart will have difficulty getting into the right ventricle. As a result, the liver may become engorged, and fluid can build up in the abdomen. This fluid buildup is known as **ascites**. The legs and ankles may swell. If there's a small hole in the heart between the right and the left atrium, some unoxygenated blood may pass through this hole, and a patient may appear blue (cyanotic). Heart surgery may be required to correct this problem.

*Tricuspid Valve Incompetence*

Tricuspid valve incompetence is relatively common and usually related to dilatation of the tricuspid valve annulus, or the ring around the tricuspid valve that anchors the valve. This is commonly related to either long-standing mitral valve disease or pulmonary arterial and/or pulmonary venous hypertension, meaning the pressure in the pulmonary arteries and veins is elevated, forcing the right ventricle to work harder.

Over time, the right ventricle enlarges and begins to fail. As it does, the annulus may dilate and cause the tricuspid valve to leak blood back into the right atrium, causing similar signs and symptoms as in tricuspid valve stenosis (narrowed valve).

During an episode of endocarditis, bacteria or fungi can destroy the leaflets of the tricuspid valve. Depending on the severity of the condition, heart surgery may be required, and the valve may be repaired or replaced.

**Ascites:**
An abnormal accumulation of serum-like fluid in the abdomen.

**Fig. 10.5:**
This illustration shows four possible valve disorders. The pulmonary valve (top) suffers from congenital stenosis. The aortic valve (middle) suffers from stenosis and incompetence resulting from rheumatic fever. The tricuspid valve (far right) suffers from stenosis and incompetence. The mitral valve (near right) suffers from incompetence due to bacterial infection. The growths on the valve's surface are clumps of bacteria, and a hole has been eaten through the valve leaflet.

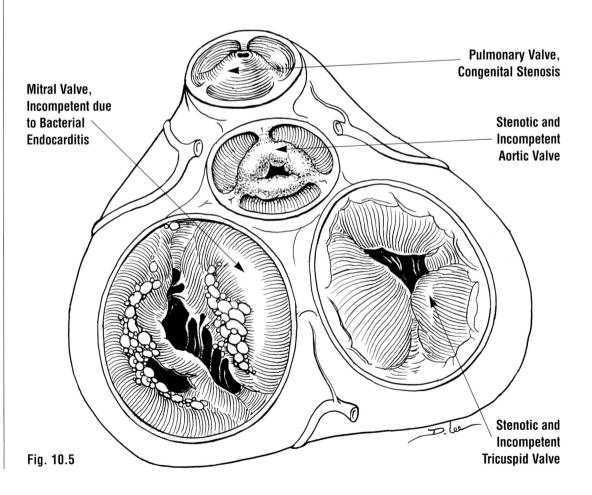

**Mitral Valve, Incompetent due to Bacterial Endocarditis**

**Pulmonary Valve, Congenital Stenosis**

**Stenotic and Incompetent Aortic Valve**

**Stenotic and Incompetent Tricuspid Valve**

Fig. 10.5

Dr. Agustin Arbulu, a heart surgeon at Wayne State University in Detroit, has shown that when a tricuspid valve is severely damaged because of antibiotic-resistant infection and the infection is the result of illicit intravenous drug abuse, a good method of treatment is to remove the infected tricuspid valve and not replace it. This removes the source of the infection. If an artificial valve is put in, it too will likely become infected since the patient frequently resumes the illicit drug use.

### Tricuspid Valve Stenosis and Incompetence

This combination is usually related to rheumatic heart disease, and the problem is similar to mitral and aortic valve incompetence/stenosis in which the valve is both leaky and narrow. Depending on its severity, this condition may require heart surgery.

## Pulmonary Valve Disease

### Pulmonary Valve Stenosis

Pulmonary valve stenosis (narrowing) is most commonly of congenital origin in the United States (Fig. 10.5). Although it may occur as a result of rheumatic fever, this is relatively uncommon in the United States. Pulmonary valve stenosis can be treated with a balloon catheter, which is used to dilate the valve. Sometimes, however, heart valve surgery is needed.

### Pulmonary Valve Incompetence

Pulmonary valve leakage (incompetence) is usually related to abnormally high pressure in the pulmonary arteries or pulmonary veins. This, in turn, may be due to a problem with the pulmonary blood vessels or with the aortic or mitral valves. In this case, the right ventricle may fail, causing the pulmonary valve annulus to dilate and

leak. The pulmonary artery may also dilate and cause the valve to leak. It is uncommon to need heart surgery for this condition.

The pulmonary valve may also become incompetent as a result of bacterial endocarditis. Sometimes, the valve may need to be replaced.

### Heart Valve Balloon Dilatation

When heart valves, including the pulmonary valve, the mitral valve, or even the aortic valve, are narrow (stenotic), they can sometimes be dilated with a balloon. The balloon is attached to a catheter and inserted into the bloodstream through an artery or vein. After the catheter is placed within the narrowed heart valve, the balloon is inflated, which dilates the valve. If the valve is both stenotic and incompetent, however, physicians generally do not try to dilate the valve with the balloon catheter. Although the obstruction may be relieved to some degree, the valve would likely become more incompetent, thus trading one type of heart valve problem for another.

Mitral valves that are narrowed from rheumatic fever can sometimes be opened successfully with balloon catheters, similarly to the treatment of pulmonary valve stenosis. In fact, Dr. Zoltan Turi, a cardiologist at Wayne State University in Detroit, has shown in two randomized studies (published in the journal *Circulation* and *The New England Journal of Medicine*) that in certain patients, balloon catheter treatment for rheumatic mitral valve stenosis yields results that are as good as or better than surgery.

Balloon catheter therapy for congenital aortic valve stenosis can sometimes be life saving. This technique can buy time and delay heart valve surgery in some infants until they are in better condition to undergo elective heart valve surgery.

Balloon catheter therapy can also be used for rheumatic aortic stenosis or bicuspid aortic stenosis. However, the longer-term results tend to be unsatisfactory. Aortic valve balloon catheter therapy is used in some adult patients who are desperately ill, perhaps even being treated with a mechanical ventilator. It is designed to improve their condition and decrease the risk of the aortic valve operation. It is also sometimes used in patients more than eighty years old who have numerous other serious medical problems, in hopes that their symptoms will improve, even though in most cases the improvement is short lived.

### Heart Valve Surgery Repair versus Replacement

Most heart surgeons believe that if a heart valve can be repaired with the likelihood of relatively good long-term results, repair should be attempted rather than valve replacement. Although many excellent artificial heart valves are currently available, the perfect heart valve substitute has yet to be developed. If any one of the four valves is stenotic, physicians may be able to open the closed valve with a scalpel by carefully opening the fused leaflets, or commissures. This is called commissurotomy or **valvotomy** (Fig. 10.6). It is most commonly done in patients who require heart surgery for congenital pulmonary stenosis and those requiring mitral valve surgery for mitral valve stenosis related to rheumatic fever. The short-term and long-term results in both cases are quite good.

For mitral valve incompetence and tricuspid valve incompetence, there are numerous repair techniques that can be used depending on the circumstances.

### Heart Valve Replacement

If the heart valve cannot be repaired, physicians will most likely recommend heart valve replacement with either a mechanical heart valve or a tissue (biological) heart valve.

**Fig. 10.6:**
During a **valvotomy**, a surgeon can treat a narrowed valve by widening the valve with a scalpel (above). The corrected valve (below) will allow blood to move through more freely and therefore place less stress on the heart.

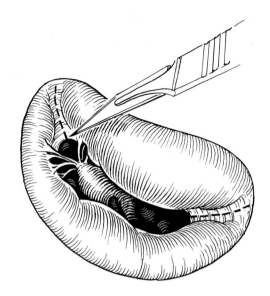

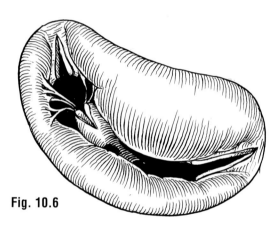

Fig. 10.6

When it comes to mechanical heart valves, some surgeons still use the original cage-ball valves. These valves have a good, long-term track record. Some patients have had the cage-ball valves for more than thirty years.

The newer mechanical heart valves are made from carbon. They tend to be low profile so they take up less space and have better flow characteristics. These types of valves have been put on pulse duplicators with which accelerated wear can be tested. Tests of one hundred simulated years of use show very little actual wear on the valve. These tests indicate that, in most cases, satisfactory function can be expected for many years.

The biggest disadvantage of the mechanical heart valves is that most patients need to take an anticoagulant, also referred to as a "blood thinner," to prevent blood clots from forming on the valve itself. The most common anticoagulant is coumadin, otherwise known as warfarin. Patients who take coumadin need to get their blood tested periodically. When coumadin treatment is first started, the blood is tested every day or two, but after a few weeks, it is usually tested every couple of months to make sure the level of anticoagulation is appropriate. If the anticoagulation is too great, the patient is more prone to develop bleeding problems, which can include bleeding into the stomach, intestines, brain, or kidneys. A person with bleeding ulcers would be prone to bleed more. If you were cut, you would have a problem with abnormal bleeding. The coumadin treatment can be reversed in an emergency situation if necessary.

Another problem related to mechanical heart valves is blood clots that occur even if the anticoagulation level is appropriate. These clots can form on or near the artificial valve and travel to various parts of the body, causing strokes and other problems. Fortunately, the incidence of this is small. It is somewhat more common in patients who have mechanical artificial heart valves than in those with tissue heart valves. The biggest advantage of

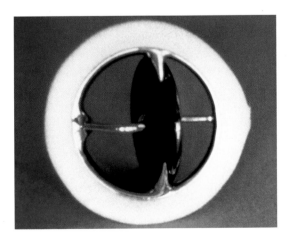

the mechanical valves is that the current models tend not to wear out.

Both mechanical and tissue heart valves are more prone to become infected than your own normal heart valves. Currently, the most commonly used tissue valves come from a pig. The pig valve can be used to replace any of the four human heart valves. Another type of tissue valve is made from the pericardium of a cow. The results with this valve seem comparable to those with the pig valve.

The problem with tissue valves is that they wear out, which occurs more rapidly in children and young adults. The degeneration of these tissue valves is slower in older adults, particularly those more than seventy years of age. In patients less than seventy years old, about 15 percent to 30 percent of the tissue valves wear out within ten years. The rate of valve deterioration increases greatly after the valves have been in place for ten years.

Another type of tissue valve is the aortic homograft valve, which is used to replace the aortic valve and sometimes the pulmonary valve. These valves come from a human donor and are removed right

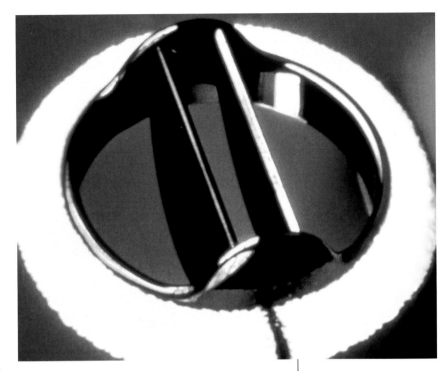

Above: A modern, bi-leaflet, low-profile heart valve made of carbon.

Left: A tilting disc mechanical heart valve made by Medtronic.

after death. Like pig valves, they tend not to last as long in younger people and last longer in patients fifty years of age or older. The incidence of blood clot problems with these tissue valves is generally quite low. Most patients with tissue valves do not need to be anticoagulated.

Some patients who undergo aortic valve replacement have a procedure called the Ross Procedure. During this operation, patients have their own pulmonary valve removed and used to replace the aortic valve. The pulmonary valve is then replaced with a human pulmonary or aortic valve homograft. This seems to be a particularly good operation for children, in whom the valve may grow with the child. Some groups have reported excellent results with this procedure, whereas others are less enthusiastic about it. Centers that have considerable experience with the Ross Procedure tend to have the best results.

### The Heart Valve Operation

Many aspects of heart valve operations are similar to those of other forms of cardiac surgery. The patient is usually admitted to the hospital the morning of the operation. The procedure is performed after general anesthesia is induced. Operations are performed through a midline chest incision (from the base of the neck to the upper abdomen) through the breastbone, although some surgeons prefer to use other incisions depending on the circumstances.

The pericardium is opened, and the patient is connected to the heart-lung machine. The heart or a major blood vessel is opened, and the heart valve is repaired or replaced. After that, the heart or blood vessel is sutured closed, and the patient is disconnected from the heart-lung machine. The chest incisions are closed in layers with stitches, and the skin is closed with stitches or staples.

Afterward, the patient is transferred from the operating room to the intensive care unit (ICU). At this point, a mechanical respirator is breathing for him or her, and will for at least several hours. The patient is typically in the ICU for a day or two. Discharge from the hospital typically occurs from four days to nine days after the surgery.

When the patient returns home, he or she will be able to go out for walks. It will be about a month before driving a car is recommended. By then, many patients are

A pig valve without a stent (inset) can be used to correct various abnormalities of the aortic valve.

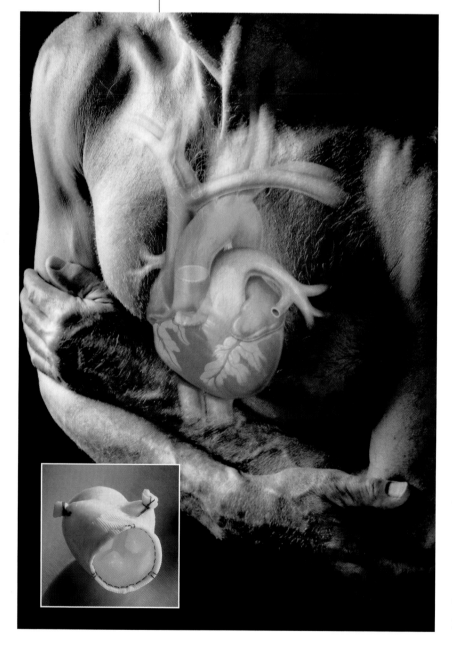

walking a mile or two a day. Some cardiologists feel that all of their patients should be enrolled in a cardiac rehabilitation program, whereas others feel that only more sedentary people need a formal rehabilitation program. Professional athletes might be able to resume normal strenuous activities, depending on a number of variables, about three months after heart surgery. Cardiologists determine when and what level of activity can be resumed and when it can be started after heart surgery.

The midline incision (through the breast bone) that is currently used for most valve replacement surgeries is not very painful for most people. Patients are usually discharged with a prescription for a relatively mild pain medicine.

So how many heart valves can be replaced in the same person? The aortic valve is the most commonly replaced. The second most commonly replaced is the mitral valve. Third is replacement of both the aortic and mitral valves during the same operation. Sometimes the aortic, mitral, and tricuspid valves are all replaced at the same time. More typically, the aortic and mitral valves are replaced, and the tricuspid valve is repaired. This treatment is usually reserved for long-standing aortic and mitral valve disease in which the tricuspid valve has become incompetent as a result of the other two valves causing stress on the right ventricle and tricuspid valve. Occasionally, the mitral and tricuspid valves are both replaced. Rarely, the aortic and tricuspid valves are replaced at the same time.

I am aware of one patient, a young girl, who had stenosis of all four valves related to rheumatic fever. All four valves were opened at surgery with a commissurotomy procedure. She was alive and well one year later. I am also aware of one patient who underwent replacement of all four valves. This was at the Mayo Clinic. The patient survived for about six months and then died of unrelated complications.

# ROBOTIC HEART VALVE SURGERY: IS THIS REALITY OR MYTH?

By

Randolph Chitwood, M.D.

Cardiothoracic Surgeon
Professor and Chairman, Department of Surgery
East Carolina University School of Medicine
Greenville, North Carolina

IN THE LAST SEVERAL years, the public has become entranced by the idea of reducing both the psychological and the physical effects of heart surgery. Minimally invasive techniques have recently emerged as one way to speed patient recovery, reduce discomfort, and reduce the economic impact of these expensive operations. Unfortunately, despite rapid, multiple advances in other surgical specialties and interventional cardiology, heart surgery has lagged behind in the development of less invasive methods.

Cardiac surgeons have been afraid of accepting the added risk of performing major heart operations through tiny incisions and obtaining less-than-excellent results. In fact, our surgical teachers, many of whom are featured in this book, taught that exposure of the entire heart and great vessels was central to performing safe, technically excellent surgery.

In the early 1960s, it was a feat to have patients survive even simple heart valve operations.

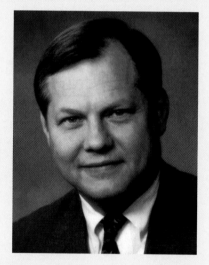

Most patients were at the end stages of their cardiac disease, the heart-lung machines were crude, and heart valve prostheses were in early evolution. Moreover, these were uncharted waters for surgeons regarding technique and postoperative care. In spite of these impediments, pioneers in heart surgery took the necessary first steps.

Years later, minimally invasive cardiac surgery is emerging with no less skepticism and criticism. However, simultaneous near-meteoric advances have been made in both Europe and the United States. After just three years, we are beginning to see improvements in our specialty and what may be a renaissance in cardiac care. Evolving technology has afforded us opportunities to make these changes safely.

Many of us think it is time to make bold steps in cardiac care. Advances in heart-lung perfusion, surgical mini-cameras (endoscopes), "smart" instruments and robotics, and cardiac cellular protection have catapulted us to a better position. Moreover, standard heart operations are safer than ever. For example, both coronary bypass and heart valve operations in uncomplicated cases can be performed with only a 1 percent to 2 percent operative mortality, even in the elderly.

Why should we try to improve on these outstanding results? Technology has allowed some surgeons to envision ways to improve heart operations. Still, most heart surgeons perform operations through large breastbone incisions. Patient recovery is slow because of muscular and skeletal tissue trauma rather than the operation on the heart itself. Thus, surgeons are now asking themselves: Can quality coronary bypass and valve operations be done through tiny access ports using endoscopes and miniaturized instruments, and even robotic assistance?

## Minimally Invasive Valve Surgery — The Beginnings

The trek to a completely closed chest heart operation may be compared to a Mt. Everest ascent. There are multiple levels of accomplishment established before reaching the summit. This surgical trek began at a "base camp" that was the conventional valve operation with a breastbone incision. All new procedures are being compared to this gold standard.

Although widespread adoption has been slow, many cardiac surgeons already have learned to use less invasive techniques to replace and repair valves and place coronary artery grafts. They can do this safely, with demonstrated expertise and improved outcomes.

The first minimally invasive valve operations were done in 1996 through smaller incisions yet under direct vision. Clinical results in the last three years have been excellent. Dr. Delos Cosgrove of the Cleveland Clinic Foundation and Dr. Lawrence Cohn of Brigham and Women's Hospital pioneered much of this early work.

Operative results have been excellent in hundreds of patients who had both aortic and mitral valves repaired and replaced through smaller chest incisions

(four to five inches) with a 1 percent operative mortality.

Others have followed and shown that these results can be reproduced in many local hospitals. Using more expensive aortic balloon occlusion devices, namely the Port-Access™ device (Heartport, Inc., Redwood City, California), the Stanford University and New York University groups have operated through even smaller chest incisions (3 inches to 3.5 inches) to repair and replace mitral valves effectively with a 2 percent mortality.

## Video-Assisted Minimally Invasive Mitral Valve Surgery: Trekking to Robotic Heart Surgery

Once these valve operations, performed under direct vision through a smaller incision, were accomplished, the door was

opened to the use of tiny cameras for secondary vision. This allowed surgeons to operate through even smaller incisions. Ultimately and hopefully, physicians will be able to perform true closed-chest cardiac surgery by using a monitor or head-mounted visual display to see the inside of the chest. The use of computer-assistance and robotic techniques may one day allow a completely endoscopic heart valve operation. These devices continue to evolve at a very rapid pace.

Dr. Alain Carpentier in Paris performed the first video-assisted mitral valve operation in February 1996. Three months later, our group at East Carolina University performed the first videoscopic mitral valve replacement in North America. Since then, more than ninety minimally invasive video-assisted mitral valve replace-

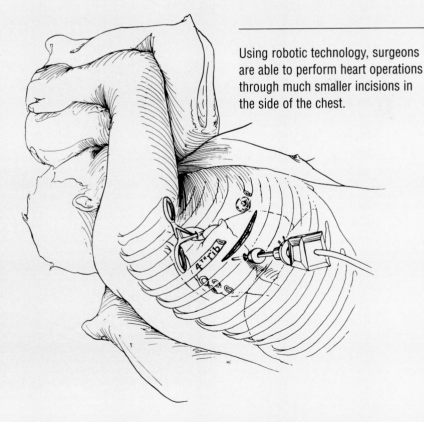

Using robotic technology, surgeons are able to perform heart operations through much smaller incisions in the side of the chest.

ments or repairs have been done at our center. Details of the results in the first thirty-one patients were published, as was the technique.

To perform these operations, an even smaller (2.5-inch) chest incision was used, and intracardiac instrument manipulation was performed using videoscopic vision. There were no operative deaths, and midterm results were excellent. Both transfusion and ICU requirements were markedly less than with the breastbone incision, and the length of stay averaged 3.5 days. There have been few major complications. Each videoscopic operation is now performed with an effort similar to that in a conventional operation. Overseas doctors have also pioneered videoscopic mitral valve surgery, working through tiny, two-inch incisions, and have had excellent results in more than two hundred patients.

### Robotics: The Final Ascent

Surgeons and patients reviewing this emerging area of heart surgery will have to judge whether widespread, truly endoscopic or even robotic (computer-assisted) valve operations are possible. In the past, three-dimensional vision was not possible unless the surgeon viewed the operation with his or her eyes. Recently, however, new video devices have been developed that are very

promising. Using both three-dimensional Zeiss™ and Vista™ systems, doctors in Germany, as well as our group, have performed "video-directed," or completely endoscopic, mitral valve replacements.

Each surgeon worked with either a head-mounted display or a television monitor. Currently, three-dimensional intracardiac cameras are somewhat large (10 to 15 mm); however these are evolving rapidly toward the 5-mm size. These three-dimensional devices give us a look inside the heart as never seen before — the small papillary muscles look like trees, the fine chords to the valve

now appear as ropes, and the valve itself looks like a parachute rather than a small (about 1.5-inch) potato-chip-like structure.

Many of us have worked with evolving robotic methods. Early costs have been great and video-dexterity expertise difficult to develop. However, it is clear that new technology will allow voice-activated camera manipulation, scaling and tremor elimination of instrument motion, camera tracking of the operative field, flexible intracardiac articulation of small instrument tips, and three-dimensional vision.

During computer-assisted or robotic cardiac surgery, the

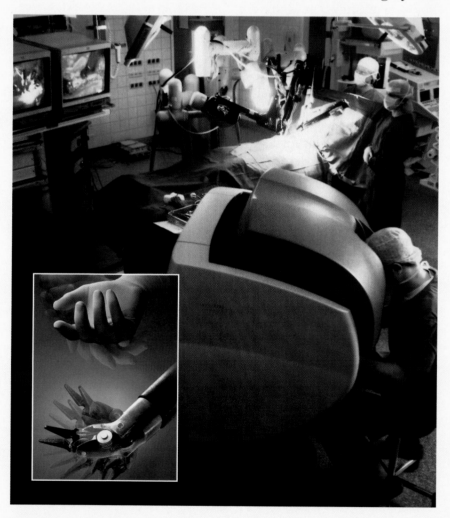

The robotic operating room at the Leipzig Heart Center in Germany. Inset: The wrist-like robotic instrument is capable of intricate movement.

surgeon moves the instrument within the chest by manipulating instrument-like electronic sensors. The robotic unit requires a "master" and a "slave" unit. The surgeon sits at a master console located a distance from the patient, and the slave unit is within the patient's chest. The physician's hand and wrist motions are translated directly to the robotic instruments, which are inserted through the chest wall.

There are two effector components common to all surgical robotic systems. Advanced computer technology has enabled direct translation of electronic data from the master console into fine mechanical motion in the slave unit. The camera tracks the operative site, and instrument tips are controlled by complex sliding internal cables within mechanical arms.

Unfortunately, complex instruments can be made only so small and still function well. Moreover, mechanical limitations and chest anatomic variations have caused intrathoracic instrument conflicts (much like sword fighting). Despite these limitations, massive progress in robotic cardiac surgery has been made in the last two years. To date, we have done thirty mitral operations using the Aesop™ (Computer Motion, Inc., Santa Barbara, California) voice-activated camera-directing robot. This device has made the operation easier for surgeons and reduced operative time but has not decreased costs or improved operative quality. However, it has provided the first step in robotic cardiac surgery.

On May 21, 1998, Carpentier and Dr. Didier Loulmet at Broussais Hospital in Paris successfully performed the world's first truly robotic-assisted heart operations in mitral valve patients. In these cases, intracardiac "wrist" instruments were manipulated from outside the chest. The surgeon, sitting at a master console, "drove" the instrument in the heart using the slave robot. This device provides true telemanipulation of a variety of coronary and valve instruments within the chest.

One week later, Dr. Friedrich-Wilhelm Mohr's group in Leipzig successfully performed five mitral repairs using the same system. This latter group has performed more than twenty mitral repairs totally endoscopically using a DaVinci™ device (Intuitive Surgical, Inc., Mountain View, California).

Recently, I had the opportunity to be the first American to perform a true robotic mitral valve repair while working in Leipzig with Mohr's group. The operative facility and translated hand movements with this device are superb; however, other challenges surely await us. The Leipzig group has brought the field of robotic coronary and valve surgery from fantasy to reality and to the forefront.

Other groups in France, Belgium, and Germany are beginning to apply this device to cardiac operations. To date, both the DaVinci™ and Zeus™ surgical robots await FDA approval in the United States. Early results using these true robots appear to parallel those of both prior videoscopic operations and of conventional mitral valve operations.

Thus, within the last three years, cardiac minimally invasive surgery has developed from a concept to a working application. The current enthusiasm of surgeons worldwide, combined with rapid technological development and communications, appears to be moving us toward even less traumatic and maybe "microinvasive" cardiac operations. Yes, the spirit of innovation for better patient care is in the air! Yet many techniques are evolving so rapidly that large multipatient series have not been done. However, data from series of patients are beginning to be collected, and analysis of these data should be enlightening.

Surgeons always will ask themselves: Is this new method really offering our patients reduced trauma, fewer complications, more rapid recovery, and better long-term results, compared with traditional operations? A healthy mix of scientific skepticism and wisdom must be exercised. The public must ask penetrating questions regarding efficacy and outcomes. Yes — some of us believe that microinvasive reconstructive cardiac surgery will be a reality, and robotic cardiac surgery will probably be a reality rather than a fantasy. But the trek up Mt. Everest is not over — we have just arrived at a new base camp.

# MINIMALLY INVASIVE HEART VALVE SURGERY

By
Delos M. Cosgrove, M.D.
Chief of Cardiothoracic Surgery
and
A. Marc Gillinov, M.D.
Staff Cardiothoracic Surgery

The Cleveland Clinic Foundation
Cleveland, Ohio

THOUSANDS OF PEOPLE benefit from heart valve repair or replacement every year. Heart valves require surgical correction when they become narrowed (stenotic) or when they begin to leak (become regurgitant). Although there are four heart valves, surgery is most often necessary for diseases of the mitral valve and the aortic valve. When these two valves become severely dysfunctional and cause symptoms, valve repair or replacement is indicated; there are no effective non-surgical treatments.

Traditionally, during heart valve surgery with the heart-lung machine, the heart was approached through a long incision down the middle of the chest. The breastbone, or sternum, was split in two, allowing access to the entire heart and the great vessels. This incision is called a median sternotomy. Recently, however, it has become apparent that heart valve surgery can be accomplished through a far smaller incision.

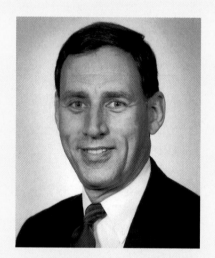

**Delos M. Cosgrove, M.D.**

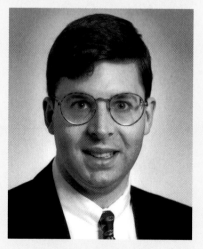

**A. Marc Gillinov, M.D.**

When a patient needs valvular heart surgery and does not require a coronary artery bypass graft, a variety of smaller incisions allow the mitral and aortic valves to be seen. These incisions generally fall into two categories: thoracotomy, or an incision in the side of the chest between the ribs, and partial sternotomy, or an incision in the middle of the chest that divides only a portion of the sternum. Using these smaller incisions to accomplish heart valve surgery is called minimally invasive heart valve surgery. At the Cleveland Clinic Foundation, heart valve surgery is performed through a 2.5-inch to 3.5-inch skin incision and a partial upper sternotomy. A large portion of the sternum is left intact, decreasing postoperative pain and hastening healing.

Since 1996, we have performed more than one thousand heart valve operations using this incision. The average patient age was fifty-six years, and the oldest patient was eighty-four years old. More than six hundred patients had mitral valve surgery, and nearly 90 percent of these patients had mitral valve repair. Three hundred patients had aortic valve procedures, including valve replacements with a variety of artificial valves and a considerable number of aortic valve repairs.

Overall, operative mortality was less than 1 percent, and wound infections occurred in only 0.3 percent of patients.

The average length of stay in intensive care was one day, and the average hospital stay was six days.

These results demonstrate that minimally invasive heart valve surgery can be performed very safely with a low risk of complications. There are many advantages to minimally invasive heart valve surgery. There is less blood loss, and patients generally report less postoperative discomfort.

Less time is spent in the intensive care unit and in the hospital, and recovery at home tends to be rapid.

The next decade is likely to bring even more ingenious approaches, including robotically assisted cardiac valve surgery. These advances promise refinements to minimally invasive heart valve surgery, further reducing hospital stays and increasing patient satisfaction.

# TISSUE ENGINEERING OF CARDIAC VALVES AND ARTERIES

By

John Mayer, M.D.

Professor of Surgery
Harvard Medical School

Senior Associate in Cardiac Surgery
Boston Children's Hospital
Boston, Massachusetts

TISSUE ENGINEERING unites engineering and biology in an attempt to develop replacement tissues. Normal tissues draw much of their strength and flexibility from specialized proteins and polysaccharide-protein complexes that are produced by their cells. Although it has been possible to grow specific types of cells in the lab for some time, it is difficult to cause these cells to organize into the complex structures that are found in normal tissues or to produce normal structural proteins in an organized fashion.

To overcome this challenge, we are attempting to "grow" heart valves and large arteries by using biodegradable polymers as temporary scaffolds. These polymer scaffolds provide the structure and stability necessary for tissues to develop. Ideally, these scaffolds would degrade as the cells produce normal structural proteins and begin to replicate normal, organized tissue structures.

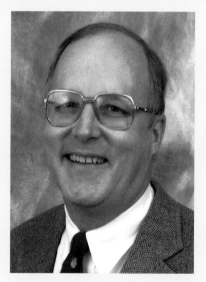

Diseases of the heart valves and large arteries account for about sixty thousand surgeries each year in the United States, including many replacement surgeries with synthetic substitutes. Ideally, any valve or artery substitute would function like the normal valve or artery, allowing blood to pass through it without narrowing or leakage, but it would also have the following characteristics: 1) durability, 2) growth potential, 3) compatibility with blood so that blood clots will not form on its surface, and 4) resistance to infection.

None of the currently available devices constructed from prosthetic or biological materials meets these criteria. Our concept, however, was to develop new valves or arteries from individual cells in the hope that these new tissues will have these desirable characteristics. The potential for growth is of particular importance to children with malformed or diseased valves or arteries.

Several projects have been undertaken in our laboratory to construct a heart valve leaflet and large arteries by using tissue engineering. We used cells from normal arteries that could be removed and separated into the various cell components. We found it was important to use the animal's own tissue as the source of the cells, thereby eliminating the possibility of immune rejection once the tissues were reimplanted. The cells were "expanded" in cultures by allowing them to divide, and then suspensions of the cells were mixed with the polymer scaffolds. The cell-polymer constructs were then incubated in culture for several more days before they were implanted as a valve replacement or an artery replacement. Valve leaflets and segments of large arteries functioned well for up to four months without structural failure or formation of blood clots on their surfaces. Importantly, when these structures were implanted into growing animals, they demonstrated growth. The tissues appeared to have relatively normal structure, and they produced the normal matrix proteins.

Despite these encouraging results, many questions remain to be resolved.

♥ First, all of these experiments have been carried out in animals, and it remains to be determined if human cells could be used to develop tissues in the same way.

♥ Second, the polymer used as the scaffold in these initial experiments is stiff, biodegradable polymer that may or may not have acceptable strength and flexibility ("handling") characteristics while still providing a hospitable environ-ment for the cells to develop into tissues.

♥ Third, the ideal source of the cells for the developing "tissues" has not been determined. In patients, it would be preferable to use veins rather than arteries as the initial source of the cells because veins are more plentiful and their removal does not compromise blood supply to normal tissues. We have some evidence that heart valves developed by using cells from the skin do not function as well as those developed with cells from the wall of the artery, but vein wall cells seem to work reasonably well.

♥ Fourth, because all of our experiments have been carried out in immature growing animals, it is not clear whether the cells that are used to form these "tissues" must be from immature animals. There is some reason to believe that fetal cells would be preferable. Because it is now possible to diagnose many forms of congenital heart disease while the embryo is still in utero, one might imagine using fetal cells to develop replacement valves or ar-teries while gestation is continuing. At birth, these replacement valves or arteries could be ready to be implanted.

♥ Fifth, it is not clear whether the "tissues" should be implanted while they are still dependent on the polymer scaffold for their physical integrity or if they should be allowed to develop further in culture before implantation into the body. One of our current ideas is that if the developing tissues are subjected to physical forces and/or chemical signals while in the laboratory, it may be possible to guide their development further before implantation into the body. Our understanding of how these developing tissues will respond to any number of physical and chemical signals remains very limited.

Tissue engineering is one new approach to solving the problem of creating replacement tissues for use as heart valves or arteries. Although initial animal studies have been encouraging, numerous questions must be resolved before we embark on clinical trials in humans.

# DIET PILLS AND HEART VALVE PROBLEMS

## By
## Larry Stephenson, M.D.

ON OCTOBER 8, 1999, AN article appeared on the front page of *The New York Times* with the headline, "Fen-Phen Maker to Pay Billions in Settlement of Diet-Injury Cases." This article is hopefully the final chapter in the story of the popular diet drugs, which were removed from the market after they were linked to heart valve problems. According to *The New York Times*, anybody with a pill-related heart valve injury could receive as much as $1.5 million.

"Some six million people took the diet drugs, Pondimin, American Home Products brand name for fenfluramine, the 'fen' in Fen-Phen, and Redux, a similar drug.

"The drugs were hailed earlier in the decade as miracle pills for obesity, as an alternative to pure diet and exercise. Diet centers actively promoted the pills to the obese and even to people who wanted to lose a few pounds. In 1996, doctors wrote

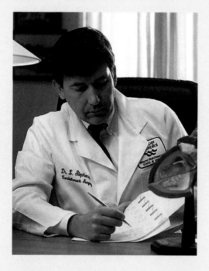

*eighteen million prescriptions for the two drugs.*

*"But in September 1997, the company removed the drugs from the market at the request of the Food and Drug Administration after studies linked them to heart valve damage."*

What is the specific problem caused by these drugs?

In the August 28, 1997, issue of *The New England Journal of Medicine*, a group of doctors from the Mayo Clinic reported on twenty-four women who had taken

Fen-Phen and had no previous history of heart disease. These women were evaluated at an average of one year after their initial treatment with Fen-Phen. All had leaky heart valves. Two required surgical repair of their mitral valves, two, replacement of their mitral valves, and one patient, replacement of her aortic valve and mitral valve and repair of her tricuspid valve.

In their report, the doctors from the Mayo Clinic concluded, "These cases arouse concern that therapy may be associated with valvular heart disease. Candidates for fenfluramine-phenteramine therapy should be informed about serious potential adverse effects, including pulmonary hypertension and valvular heart disease."

The following year, another article appeared in *The New England Journal of Medicine* by a group of doctors from Minneapolis who had studied more than two hundred patients who had received Fen-Phen therapy compared with a group who had not. They found that a greater percentage of the patients receiving Fen-Phen had cardiac valve abnormalities than those who had not taken the drug.

In the same issue of *The New England Journal of Medicine*, a group of doctors from Georgetown University in Washington, D.C., reported on a study of patients taking dexfenfluramine (a related drug) in which they found a small increase in the prevalence of aortic and mitral valve leakage.

Over the next year, twelve additional articles and letters to the editors appeared in *The New England Journal of Medicine* dealing with a possible link between appetite suppressants and valvular heart disease as well as a relation between high blood pressure in the pulmonary arteries and these drugs. There was considerable controversy among these doctors as to what the chances were of developing heart valve disease problems after Fen-Phen therapy.

Perhaps Dr. Richard B. Devereux from New York Hospital-Cornell Medical Center summed it up best by stating:

*"What advice should we offer patients based on these findings?*

*"First, all patients who receive fenfluramine or dexfenfluramine should be examined clinically. Echocardiography should be recommended for those who have a heart murmur or other evidence of valvular disease, as well as those who received one of the drugs for three or more months or at high doses....*

*"Second, standard prophylaxis against endocarditis (heart infections) should be recommended to patients with a heart murmur, those with 'silent' moderate or severe regurgitation ... and those with mild regurgitation....*

*"Third, in view of the delay in recognizing the association between the use of appetite suppressants and cardiac-valve abnormalities, caution should be urged in the long-term use of other agents that act on serotonergic mechanisms, albeit by different pathways [meaning drugs that have similarities in the way they work].*

*"Finally, it is important to remember that in patients who meet the FDA criteria for cardiac-valve abnormalities on echocardiography performed soon after the discontinuation of appetite suppressants, there is a possibility (ranging from as low as 5 percent to as high as 67 percent) that the abnormality is a naturally occurring phenomenon and not a consequence of drug use."*

The bottom line is, anyone who has taken these drugs should be checked by their doctor for symptoms of heart valve disease and/or pulmonary artery hypertension. If symptoms are present, a cardiologist will do a further evaluation.

The good news at this point is that the majority of patients who have taken these drugs seem to be doing quite well and have trivial, if any, heart problems.

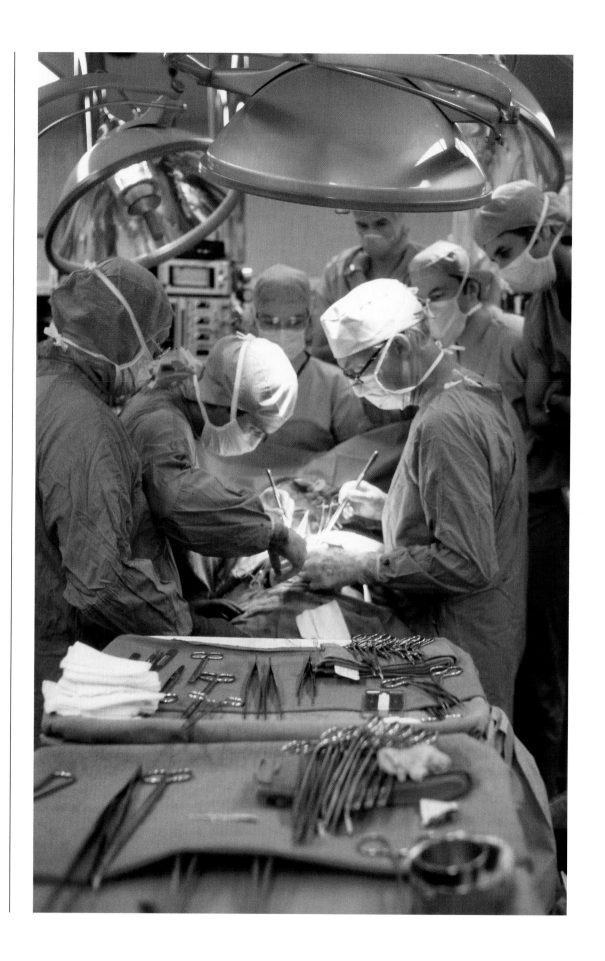

Transplantation techniques remain the gold standard for advanced heart failure treatment. Pictured is Dr. Bruce Reitz, right, performing a heart-lung transplant.

## CHAPTER ELEVEN

# ADVANCED HEART FAILURE: TRANSPLANTS, HEART ASSIST DEVICES, AND THE FUTURE

HEART TRANSPLANTATION IS THE gold standard surgical treatment for patients with advanced heart failure. Unfortunately, there is a worldwide scarcity of donors for heart transplants. Over the past ten years, the number of heart transplants performed in the United States has remained relatively stable at between twenty-five hundred and thirty-five hundred annually. If there were enough donor organs, it is estimated that more than fifteen thousand, and perhaps as many as thirty thousand, heart transplants would be done each year. Patients of any age could theoretically undergo a heart transplant, but because of the scarcity of donors and a somewhat higher rate of complications after surgery, patients more than sixty-five years of age are generally not eligible.

 ### The History of Heart Transplants

The technique for transplanting the heart and lungs did not rely exclusively on the heart-lung machine. The first transplantation was reported in 1905 by Drs. Alexis Carrel and Charles Guthrie. While at the University of Chicago, the pair implanted the heart of a small dog into the neck of a larger dog by joining the heart of the smaller dog to the jugular vein and carotid artery of the larger animal. The animal's blood was not anticoagulated, and the experiment ended about two hours after circulation was established because of a blood clot in the cavities of the transplanted heart.

In 1950, Dr. Vladimir Demikhov, the great Soviet surgical researcher, described more than twenty different techniques for heart transplantation and published various techniques for heart and lung transplantation. He was even able to remove an animal's own heart and replace it with the heart from another animal before the heart-lung machine was developed. This was accomplished by placing the donor heart above the dog's own heart, and then with a series of tubes and connectors, rerouting the blood until he had the donor heart functioning in the appropriate position and the other heart removed. One of his dogs climbed the steps of the Kremlin on the sixth postoperative day but died shortly afterwards of rejection.

By 1960, Drs. Richard Lauer and Norman Shumway in the United States had established the foundation for heart transplantation as it is performed today.

Their method had also been used by Sir Russell Brock in England and Demikhov in the Soviet Union but became popular only after Lauer and Shumway reported it publicly. Shortly thereafter, Dr. James Hardy at the University of Mississippi attempted the first human heart transplantation. Because no human donor organ was available at the time, a large chimpanzee's heart was used. It was unable to support the circulation.

The first human-to-human heart transplant occurred December 3, 1967, at Groote Schuur Hospital in Capetown, South Africa. A surgical team headed by Dr. Christiaan Barnard transplanted the heart of a donor, who had been certified dead after there was no heart activity for five minutes, into a fifty-four-year-old man named Louis Washkansky, whose heart had been irreparably dam-

aged by repeated heart attacks. This first transplant captivated the world's imagination, and Barnard's name quickly became one of the most recognizable names in medicine. Interestingly, Barnard himself did not think the operation was revolutionary. Not a single picture was taken during the entire procedure. In a recent interview, Barnard talked about the conditions that led to the first transplant:

*"Heart transplantation was successful because it was virtually just another heart operation. We had experience in major heart surgery. We knew how to prepare a patient for it. We know how to care for a patient during such an operation and how to care for the patient postoperatively. All we had to do was work out the surgical technique*

# ♥ THE FIRST HEART TRANSPLANT

DR. CHRISTIAAN BARNARD WILL always be remembered as the heart surgeon who performed the first successful heart transplant using a human donor heart. He attended medical school at the University of Cape Town, South Africa, where he received training in general surgery. Then, in 1956, he received a two-year scholarship to study surgery at the University of Minnesota in Minneapolis.

"I actually went to Minneapolis to study general surgery," Barnard recalled. "I was working in a laboratory one day in general surgery when I walked past one of the labs where Dr. Vince Gott was working with a heart-lung machine. [Gott later became professor and cardiac surgeon-in-charge at Johns Hopkins University.] He looked up and said, 'Listen, I'm working and I need a pair

of hands. Do you mind scrubbing and giving me some help?'

"It immediately fascinated me that we now had the ability to work inside the heart. I switched to cardiac surgery, and that's how I got involved in heart surgery. I trained under Dr. C. Walton Lillehei in Minneapolis, and I often went to Rochester, Minnesota, to watch Dr. John Kirklin work."

When his training was over, Barnard returned to South Africa, where he performed the world's first human-to-human heart transplant. In 1999, Barnard recalled that famous operation:

*"When I was ready to take the heart out of the donor, who was brain dead, I disconnected the respirator and waited until the heart went into ventricular fibrillation (a fatal rhythm)*

Dr. Christiaan Barnard earned worldwide fame when he performed the first human-to-human heart transplant in South Africa in 1967.

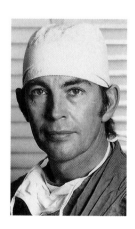

*and see how we were going to monitor and treat rejection."*

Indeed, cardiac surgeons were clearly successfully tackling the demands of heart transplantation. Only three days after Barnard's first transplant, the second human heart transplant using a human donor was performed on a child by Dr. Adrian Kantrowitz in Brooklyn, New York. Kantrowitz' patient died of a bleeding complication within the first twenty-four hours.

Washkansky, meanwhile, died on the eighteenth postoperative day. At autopsy, the heart appeared normal, but pneumonia was present, possibly because of the methods used to treat rejection.

Barnard performed his second heart transplant on Philip Blaiberg on January 2, 1968. Blaiberg was discharged from the hospital and became a celebrity for the several months he lived after the transplant. This highly visible success signaled that a heart transplantation was possible for humans suffering from end-stage heart disease.

In the first year after Barnard's first heart transplant, about one hundred heart transplants were performed by cardiac surgeons around the world. However, by the end of 1968, most groups abandoned heart transplantation because of the extremely high mortality related to rejection. Despite the lack of interest, Shumway, Lauer, Barnard, and a few others persevered both clinically and in the laboratory. Their eventual discovery of better drugs for suppression of the immune system response established heart transplantation as we know it today.

*before I opened the chest and took out the heart.*

*"The only moment that was an eerie moment was when I had taken the heart out of the recipient. That was the first time that I saw a human being without a heart but alive because he was kept alive by the heart-lung machine. That was the only moment of the operation I really, really remember.*

*"We did not consider the operation a big event. We realized we were doing a different operation, but we had done different operations before. We did not take a single photograph of the operation. In fact, I didn't even inform the hospital authorities that I was doing the operation that night. I only told them afterwards, and we didn't have press or anybody around. It was only the next day that the media found out that we'd done the operation."*

The celebrity surrounding that event changed his life and, in his own words, he found the publicity surrounding that event "disturbing for two reasons. It interfered quite significantly with my practice of surgery because there were always media around, and it also interfered with my family life."

After this famous transplant, however, Barnard was often on the leading edge of organ transplantation. Even before the heart transplant, he performed the first kidney transplantation in Africa and, later on, the third heart-lung transplantation in the world. He also performed the world's first **heterotopic transplant** (sometimes called the "piggy-back transplant"), an operation during which a donor heart is placed next to the patient's heart and the two work in parallel. This operation, which is still used today, was developed for circumstances when the donor heart was either questionable or too small.

**Heterotopic Transplant:**
A transplant of an organ or tissue, usually from one person to another, when the organ or tissue is not put in the location where it normally resides.

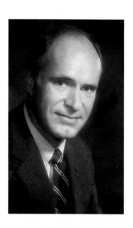

Dr. Bruce Reitz performed the world's first successful heart-lung transplant in 1981. His first patient, Mary Gohlke, was a long-term survivor.

# ♥ THE FIRST SUCCESSFUL HEART-LUNG TRANSPLANT

D R. BRUCE REITZ GRADUATED from medical school in 1970 in an environment that had been electrified by the first heart transplant.

"After Dr. Christiaan Barnard did that procedure, that's the kind of thing I was reading about every day as a medical student, and it really stimulated me," Reitz said. By the mid-1970s, working with Dr. Norman Shumway, Reitz was involved in a heart-lung transplantation program at Stanford University.

"Shumway suggested that I look at transplanting heart and lungs together," Reitz said. "He had done some work years ago, with a little bit of success. So we added a few things that got some successful results in the laboratory."

Building on this early work, Reitz performed the world's first successful heart-lung transplant. He recalled:

*"Well, it was really a unique high-point of my career. First of all, it is a project that we had started in the lab about five years before. We had gone through some development phases and then through a phase when things started to click, and cyclosporine was an extremely ex-*

*citing compound that was so promising. Then we had thought that it was ready for patients, and I had Shumway's complete support and encouragement. Then to actually do the operation — Shumway was assisting me — was a really terrific experience.*

*"When you take it all out like that (heart and lungs) and put it in, there are actually fewer connections. There's basically the blood coming into the heart and the blood going out that has to be hooked up, but the whole circulation to the lung and back to the heart remains attached, and you just connect the airway."*

His first patient, and the world's first patient to have a successful heart-lung transplantation, was a woman named Mary Gohlke, who suffered from a lung disease that had damaged her heart. "We were fortunate because we had a good patient who needed it, and she got better and was a terrific spokesperson for transplantation," Reitz remembered.

Reitz' team also discovered that the risk of rejection remains the same for a complete heart-lung transplant as for a heart transplant.

 **Heart and Lung Transplants**

Almost fifteen years after the first heart transplant, a team of doctors headed by Dr. Bruce Reitz began a clinical trial to transplant both the heart and the lungs. Operating at Stanford University in 1981, the team's first patient was dis-

charged from the hospital in good condition and was still healthy more than five years after the transplant.

This clinical success was partially due to the discovery of a potent antirejection drug. **Cyclosporine** was discovered by workers at the Sandoz Laboratory in Basel, Switzerland, in

**Cyclosporine**: A drug used to help prevent organ rejection in patients who have transplants.

1970. Ten years later, it was introduced at Stanford for cardiac transplantation. The incidence of rejection and infection was not reduced. However, these two major complications of heart and heart-lung transplantation were less severe with cyclosporine. The availability of cyclosporine stimulated the development of many transplant programs around the world in the mid-1980s.

Today, some patients who might have previously received a heart-lung transplant now undergo a single or double lung transplant, and the heart is repaired, if practical. Dr. Joel Cooper and his colleagues at the University of Toronto in the early 1980s led the way to human lung transplantation as we know it today.

### Heart Transplants

Heart transplants are recommended for patients with advanced heart fail-ure. Because donors are hard to locate, candidates for heart transplant have to meet certain standards. They should be psychologically stable. Their other organ systems, such as their kidneys, liver, and lungs, should be in good condition. It is possible, however, for some patients with severe lung disease and heart disease to undergo heart/lung transplantation. Candidates for heart transplantation cannot have long-standing insulin-dependent diabetes with organ damage. They are screened for most types of cancers because the drugs they will need to take after the transplant to help suppress rejection can actually cause certain cancers to grow rapidly. There are certain blood disorders that are also affected by these drugs. The drugs can suppress some blood elements and worsen these disorders. Patients generally are not considered qualified candidates if they have active infections because the immuno-

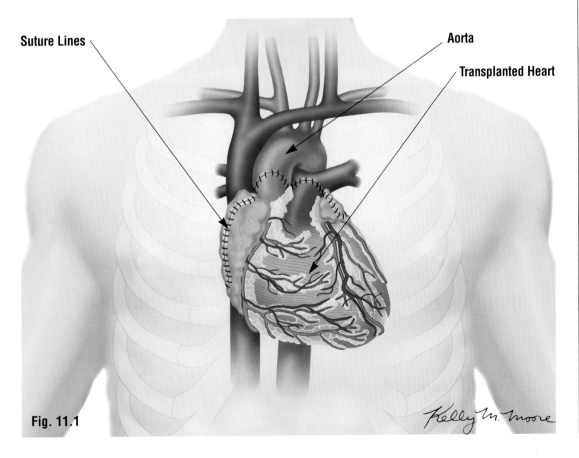

**Suture Lines**

**Aorta**

**Transplanted Heart**

**Fig. 11.1**

**Fig. 11.1:**
During heart transplantation, surgeons leave part of the native heart to sew onto the new, donor heart. The stitches show where the attachments are made during the operation.

suppression drugs make the body's immune system less effective in fighting infections and therefore can allow the infections to become worse.

Once it is determined that patients are candidates for a heart transplant, they are put on a waiting list for a donor heart that matches their blood and tissue type. When a match is found, the patient is admitted to the hospital.

The heart usually comes from a donor who has been in a traumatic accident and suffered fatal head injury and whose lung function was sustained by a ventilator. Frequently, the transplant team will have to go to another city or state, often traveling by private jet to retrieve the donor heart. The heart is removed from the donor. It is kept alive by using one of a number of techniques while it's brought back to the hospital where the transplant will take place. When the team bringing the donor heart is within a half hour of the hospital, the transplant patient is anesthetized and the chest is opened. When the team arrives with the heart, the patient is connected to the heart-lung machine. The diseased heart is then removed, and the new heart is sewn in (Fig. 11.1).

Portions of the transplant recipient's own left atrium with the four pulmonary veins and portions of the right atrium with the superior and inferior vena cava are not removed. The healthy donor heart is then sewn in. The left atrium and then the right atrium are connected to the remnants of the recipient's left and right atria. Next, the aorta and pulmonary arteries are connected. The clamp on the aorta is removed so the heart-lung machine, which had been supplying the body with oxygenated blood, can get blood to the recipient's new heart, and it will begin to beat.

After the chest is closed, the patient goes to the intensive care unit and usually spends at least a couple of days there followed by several more days in the hospital.

A number of powerful drugs are used to suppress organ rejection immediately after the surgery. When patients goes home, they will typically be taking cyclosporine, prednisone, and azathioprine or tacrolimus. These drugs have side effects that can be harmful, and they have to be monitored carefully. In a successful transplant, some of these can be eliminated after a few weeks.

In an attempt to diagnose rejection even before there is clinical evidence, the patient must undergo regular heart **biopsy**. This is done with a special catheter that is introduced through a vein in the neck to obtain a small biopsy specimen of the transplanted heart muscle.

Most rejection episodes can be treated successfully with medications, but sometimes when they are severe the patient's circulation needs to be supported with a mechanical heart assist pump or even a second heart transplant.

The chance of surviving heart transplant surgery and leaving the hospital is greater than 90 percent. The chance that the patient will be alive one year after the transplant is about 85 percent, and there is about a 4 percent mortality rate per year after that as the survival rates decrease owing to complications related to the rejection process. Nonetheless, some patients now are alive twenty years after a heart transplant. Some patients have had more than one heart transplant during that period. Many heart transplant patients return to work and live a relatively normal life after their surgery.

Research continues on using animals as donors for human hearts. At this point, the rejection process continues to be much more severe when an animal's tissues are transplanted into an animal of a different species, for example, a dog's organ transplanted into a cat. If the rejection problem can be solved through research, organ shortage would no longer be a problem because animals such as pigs could be bred for organ donation.

**Biopsy:**
The process of removing tissue from a patient for examination.

### Heart Assist and Artificial Hearts

Beyond heart transplantation, physicians have a number of mechanical options to assist failing hearts. One particularly useful device is called the **intra-aortic balloon pump**, which is used temporarily to treat patients with failing hearts and more commonly to help wean some patients from the heart-lung machine.

### Intra-Aortic Balloon Pump

The intra-aortic balloon pump consists of an external pump unit, a catheter slightly larger than a piece of spaghetti, and an inflatable balloon that's about the shape and size of a bratwurst (Fig. 11.2).

The catheter and the balloon pump are usually inserted into the femoral artery in the groin area and guided up into the aorta. The outside end of the catheter is attached to an external pump. The balloon is then synchronized to inflate and deflate with the cardiac cycle. This action pumps blood and helps the failing heart in a number of ways. For this machine to work appropriately, the heart has to do some of the work, but the device is capable of doing about 20 percent of the heart's work. In many cases, it can make the difference between life and death.

# ♥ ADRIAN KANTROWITZ: INTRA-AORTIC BALLON PUMP

DR. ADRIAN KANTROWITZ'S MANY contributions to heart surgery — early pacemakers and heart transplantation, for instance — include the most practical heart assist device in use today: the intra-aortic balloon pump. This novel device likely saves more than one hundred thousand lives every year worldwide.

Kantrowitz developed the device with his brother Arthur, a Ph.D. physicist and former rocket scientist. Shortly after returning from service in World War II, Kantrowitz worked in the laboratory at Case Western Reserve University in Cleveland. There, he coauthored a paper with his brother on arterial counterpulsation.

*"We showed you could increase coronary blood flow and unload the left ventricle. We published this as a theoretical thing because I couldn't figure out how to do it practically. Then Dr.* *Dwight Harken, professor of surgery at Harvard Medical School, did his work.... It was really Harken who put the word to it — counterpulsation.*

*"But the problem was you couldn't move enough blood. You had to move it through a small tube. My brother and I thought the way to do it was to put a balloon in — we literally thought of a balloon. We discussed this at our mother's house."*

They soon learned that Dr. Willem Kolff had published a paper in which he actually tried a balloon pump in human cadavers but never in living humans. The brothers then developed a device that, in 1967, Kantrowitz tested in living humans.

"These were patients who were in cardiogenic shock," Kantrowitz recalls. The results in their first three patients were published in the *Journal of the American Medical Association* in 1968.

Dr. Adrian Kantrowitz, working with his brother, developed the **intra-aortic balloon pump**, which is used to help support the circulation with weakened hearts.

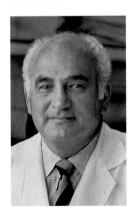

Fig. 11.2: **The Intra-Aortic Balloon Pump:** This device is placed into the aorta and inflates rhythmically to help maintain blood pressure in the heart and arterial system. It is a temporary, but very valuable, therapy for weakened hearts.

Fig. 11.2

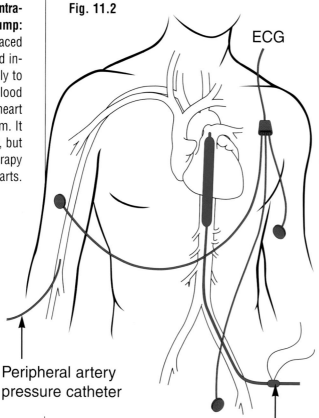

ECG

Peripheral artery pressure catheter

Attached to external pump and power source

The concept of aortic counterpulsation (as used with the intra-aortic balloon pump) was first described by Dr. Dwight Harken in 1958. In 1962, Dr. Willem Kolff's group introduced a balloon catheter into the aorta of an animal. One year later, Kantrowitz and associates reported the first use of the intra-aortic balloon pump in three patients. All were in shock but improved during balloon pumping. One survived to leave the hospital.

Nowadays, most hospitals in the United States and virtually all large hospitals around the world, particularly those that have a cardiac center, use the intra-aortic balloon pump. According to Kantrowitz, the intra-aortic balloon pump is used in the United States in about one hundred thousand patients every year.

Kantrowitz's team has also been approved by the FDA to surgically implant a permanent version of the intra-aortic balloon pump in a limited number of select patients.

 **Artificial Hearts**

Doctors also continue to work with the concept of implanting totally artificial hearts, which would alleviate the shortage of donor organs. Before this becomes a practical reality, however, there are several obstacles that need to be overcome.

The heart was first replaced with a mechanical device by Dr. Tetsuzo Akutsu and Kolff at the Cleveland Clinic in 1957. Working in animals, these two researchers implanted an artificial heart in a living dog. The animal survived for ninety minutes.

In 1966, a team of Houston doctors under the leadership of Dr. Michael DeBakey used a left ventricular assist device in a woman who could not be weaned from the heart-lung machine after having two heart valves replaced. After ten days of circulatory assistance with the pump, she was weaned successfully from the device and recovered. This woman was probably the first patient to be weaned from a heart assist device and leave the hospital alive.

The first artificial heart in a human was implanted in 1969 by Denton Cooley, who used it as a bridge to heart transplantation for a patient who would most likely have died if Cooley hadn't used it to support the patient's failing heart until a donor heart was found. Cooley's team performed the operation on a patient who could not be weaned from the heart-lung machine after heart surgery. After sixty-four hours of support with the artificial heart, heart transplantation was performed, but the patient died of an infection thirty-two hours after the heart transplant.

The first two patients successfully bridged (kept alive by a mechanical heart assist device) to heart transplantation were bridged at almost the same time and in the same metropolitan area but by different surgical teams. On September 5, 1984, in San Francisco, Dr. Don Hill implanted a Pierce-Donachy left ventricular assist device in a patient in cardiogenic shock. The patient's heart was replaced successfully two days afterward, and the patient was later discharged. Two days later, a team of surgeons at Stanford University successfully replaced the heart of a patient who had been maintained with an electrically driven Novacor assist device.

### Artificial Hearts Today

The first implantation of an artificial heart, called the Jarvik-7, that was meant to be permanent (as opposed to a bridge to heart transplantation) was performed

## ♥ DENTON COOLEY

DR. DENTON COOLEY, WHO WAS one of the physicians working toward successful heart transplantation in the late 1960s, vividly remembers the excitement at the dawn of heart transplantation:

*"Many of us in the United States, maybe four or five surgeons that I know of, were challenged by the idea of a heart transplant. I'm not sure what stopped the others. But what delayed me was trying to identify a donor. I could not quite understand how we were going to get a good donor heart."*

In 1968 and 1969, with those hurdles overcome, Cooley performed twenty-two heart transplants.

"Nothing for me could compare with the excitement of that first cardiac transplantation I did in 1968," he said in a recent interview. "It was very thrilling, but I felt a lot of pressure. I've never been more exhilarated than I was to see that heart begin to work and see the patient recover."

Although Cooley was at the very cutting edge of early transplantation, the first human-to-human heart transplantation was performed by another doctor, who shouldered the immense responsibility of showing that the concept was practical. "It is to Dr. Christiaan Barnard's enduring credit that he showed a beating human heart could be removed from one individual and implanted into another," Cooley said. "Prior to that, we weren't quite certain of the ethics of taking out a beating heart because in those days, we always thought that life continued until the heart stopped beating. We didn't quite understand the fact that sometimes with brain injuries, the heart would keep working long after the patient was clinically dead."

Since that first transplant, technology and medicine have made great leaps in the treatment of failing hearts, including ventricular assist devices, pacemakers, and defibrillators. Said Cooley:

*"If we had the donors, I think we would be able to forget about the mechanical replacement of the heart. But we're never going to have enough donors to meet the need. So we have to have some mechanical support devices, although many of these devices will be used as a bridge to transplantation."*

Dr. Denton Cooley performed twenty-two heart transplantations in 1968 and 1969, making him the most prolific transplantation surgeon in the world at that time.

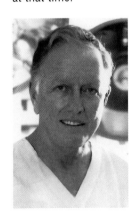

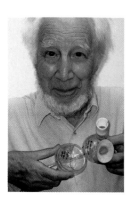

Dr. Willem Kolff was a true pioneer in artificial organ technology. His models for artificial hearts inspired the original Jarvik hearts that were implanted into human patients in the mid-1980s.

# ♠THE MECHANICAL HEART

AFTER THE HEART-LUNG MAchine had proved that people could live while being supported by a machine, it was a short and logical jump to a completely artificial heart. Working first at the Cleveland Clinic and later at the University of Utah, Dr. Willem Kolff became one of the leading doctors in the development of artificial hearts and other organs. Kolff, in fact, had invented the artificial kidney in the 1940s in Nazi-occupied Holland.

"I went to Berk EnamelWorks and spoke to Mr. Berk and explained the principal of the rotating drum artificial kidney to him," Kolff recently remembered about that first artificial kidney.

"Berk EnamelWorks began making artificial kidneys for me. When it came time to pay, it turned out they were only allowed to work for the German Wermacht, that is, the German army, so I never got a bill. We would, of course, have gone to concentration camps if we had."

Kolff used fifteen artificial kidneys during the war, and this invention went on to provide long-term benefits for thousands of patients. Like a real kidney, the artificial kidney is connected to the patient's circulation, except that it is done through small tubes. When blood flows through the machine, it cleanses the blood of the waste products that

by a group including Kolff, Dr. William DeVries, and Dr. Robert Jarvik at the University of Utah in 1982. By 1985, they had implanted the Jarvik heart in four patients, and one survived for 620 days after implantation. The Jarvik-7 heart was based on long-standing research by Kolff and his team at the University of Utah and earlier at the Cleveland Clinic.

All of these mechanical artificial heart devices required tubes running through the skin to an external power source and drive unit. Although the machines that powered the hearts were external and relatively large, they also had smaller portable drive units so patients could get up and walk around.

Over time, all of their patients suffered complications related to their artificial hearts, including blood clots and infections, which are particularly prone to occur with these types of devices. Any device that breaks the skin's natural barrier poses a danger of infection because the skin is such an effective barrier against bacteria. When tubes and wires go through the skin, bacteria can

eventually get into the body and infect these devices.

One of the patients who had such a device — Barney Clark — became somewhat of a celebrity. His device functioned for more than a year. One might consider these short-lived clinical research trials as failures. Nevertheless, much important information was learned and shared from having these devices in humans (as opposed to animals). At the University of Utah and other centers, laboratory research continues on various types of artificial hearts and ventricular assist devices.

Currently, however, there are no implantable artificial hearts being placed in humans worldwide.

**Ventricular Assist Devices**

Short of a totally artificial heart, the FDA has approved devices that are designed to help the heart's ventricles pump blood, called ventricular assist devices (Fig. 11.3). In most cases, these devices are used only as a bridge to heart the patient's own kidneys would normally remove. Renal dialysis, or mechanical blood cleansing, is now used all over the world to treat patients with kidney failure and is based on concepts initially developed by Kolff. In fact, Kolff estimates that approximately half a million people in the United States alone are treated each year with renal dialysis.

After the war was over, Kolff moved to the Cleveland Clinic, where he began researching the heart-lung machine and artificial hearts. In 1957, he and a colleague, Dr. Tetsuzo Akutsu, removed the heart from a dog and implanted the first artificial heart, which kept the dog alive for ninety minutes with its circulation totally supported by the device. Although the device was implanted,

tubes ran through the skin to the power source.

Soon after this, Kolff moved to the University of Utah, where he began to build an artificial organ program. It was in this program and under Kolff's leadership that Dr. Robert Jarvik began his research into the artificial heart that would later bear his name and be implanted into Barney Clark in 1982.

"Although it was not a clinical success, the procedure was an important milestone," remembered Kolff. "We knew from animals that we could sustain the circulation, but from Barney Clark, we learned that he still loved his family, that his mind was okay, that his sense of humor was okay, that he still wanted to serve his fellow man. All of the important things were retained."

**Fig. 11.3**:
The Jarvik 2000, a left ventricular assist device, is used to aid a failing left ventricle. It is thumb-sized. The controller and battery are the size of a portable telephone and worn externally.

transplantation and usually remain implanted for a few days up to several weeks. However, some patients have had these ventricular assist devices for more than a year.

When the devices are used as a bridge to heart transplantation, the results are good. The devices do not appear to affect long-term survival after heart transplantation, which is about the same in patients who needed the devices as in those who did not.

At some centers in Europe, ventricular assist devices are being implanted in patients who are not being considered for heart transplantation. Doctors are hoping that the sick heart will recover during several months, at which point the device can be removed. So far, however, it's been found that most of these patients do not recover enough to allow the devices to be removed.

One major drawback of the assist device is that it requires tubes that run through the skin to external power sources. Portable machines allow the

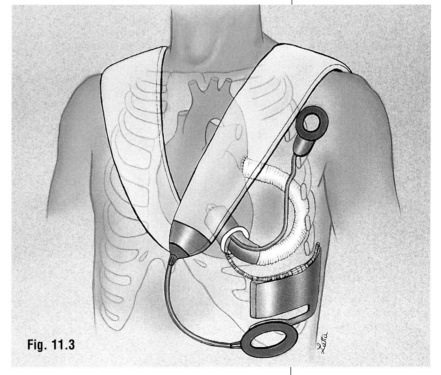

Fig. 11.3

patients to be fairly active or mobile so they can improve their physical condition over time. Unfortunately, infection often occurs over time with this type of device because of the tubes and wires that have to cross the skin barrier.

Patients who are having mechanical assist devices implanted on a permanent basis should consider this as clinical research. It's likely that with time and research, there will eventually be assist devices and artificial hearts commonly available at all hospitals where heart surgery is performed. Some will most likely be totally implantable so no tubes or wires will cross the skin. The surgery done to implant these devices will become routine.

### Batista Procedure

Dr. Randas Batista, a heart surgeon in Brazil, has recently developed a heart surgery procedure for certain patients with substantially enlarged, failing hearts. In the Batista procedure, the doctor removes a piece of the enlarged left ventricle and sews the remaining edges of the cavity back together (Fig. 11.4). After the size of the chamber is reduced, the left ventricle seems to function better and more efficiently. Batista has often found, however, that he has to either repair or replace the mitral valve because part of the muscle that controls it frequently has to be removed as part of the procedure.

The early mortality for this procedure, both in Brazil and in centers in this country, has been about 20 percent. By about

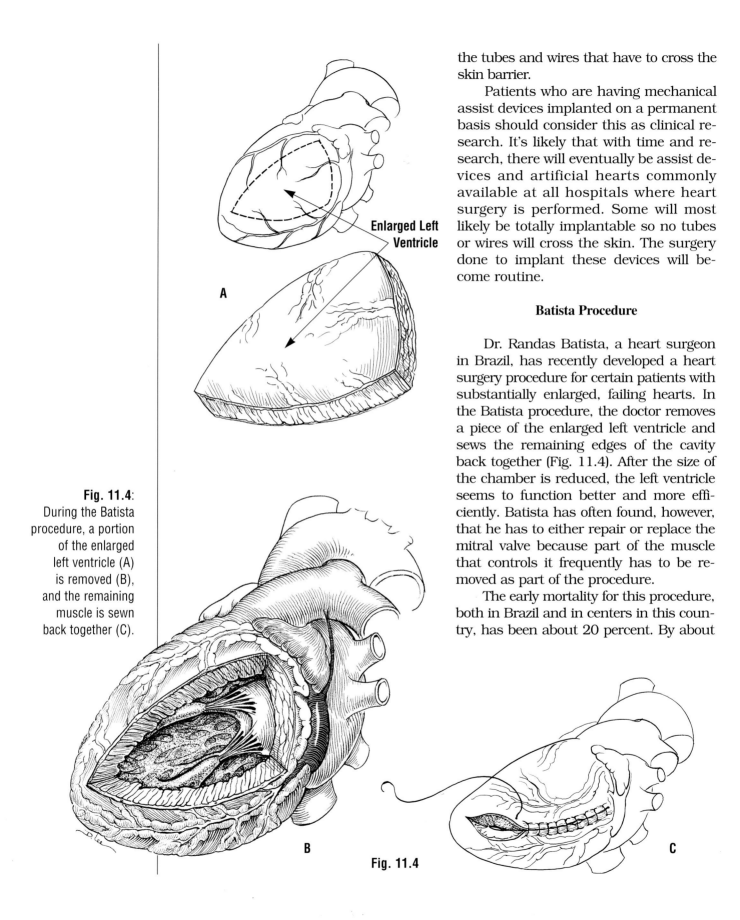

**Enlarged Left Ventricle**

A

**Fig. 11.4**:
During the Batista procedure, a portion of the enlarged left ventricle (A) is removed (B), and the remaining muscle is sewn back together (C).

B

**Fig. 11.4**

C

two years after the procedure, about 40 percent to 50 percent of the patients die; however, some of the patients who survive the procedure seem to do quite well and are relieved of their symptoms of heart failure for at least two years after the procedure. At this point, it is unclear how these patients will do long term or if the heart will expand again.

More information needs to be obtained, particularly from long-term follow-up, before this operation can be recommended as a routine form of surgery for treating patients with considerable heart failure.

### Skeletal Muscle Cardiac Assist

The final form of heart assist involves neither mechanical devices nor donated organs but uses part of the patient's own anatomy to bolster the heart's function. This approach was pioneered in animals by Kantrowitz in 1959 when he wrapped the diaphragm muscle around the heart and stimulated the muscle to contract in synchrony with the animal's heart. This worked, but only for several seconds until the muscle fatigued.

The problem of muscle fatigue was solved in 1969 when Drs. Stanley Salmons and Greta Vrbova from London, England, discovered that certain types of skeletal muscles, which are attached to the bones in our arms, legs, and elsewhere, could be electrically conditioned and made more fatigue resistant.

This observation led me and colleagues at the University of Pennsylvania to develop an electrical conditioning protocol for fiber transformation of animal muscles. Meanwhile, Dr. Ray Chiu and associates at McGill University developed the concept of burst stimulation to increase the force of muscle contraction.

These advances in muscle conditioning prompted several surgeons to wrap the back muscle, or latissimus dorsi, around the failing ventricles and stimulate the muscle to contract during contraction of the heart muscle. This procedure, which is known as **cardiomyoplasty**, was first performed in a human by Dr. Alain Carpentier in 1985.

**Cardiomyoplasty**: A surgical procedure using a muscle, usually the latissimus dorsi muscle in the back, to wrap around a failing heart. The muscle is then electrically stimulated so it will contract in synchrony with the failing heart and hopefully improve the signs and symptoms of heart failure.

# CARDIOMYOPLASTY AND AORTOMYOPLASTY

By
Michael A. Acker, M.D.

Cardiothoracic Surgeon
Associate Professor of Surgery, Division of Cardiothoracic Surgery
University of Pennsylvania
Philadelphia, Pennsylvania

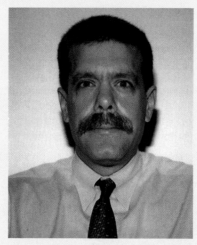

AN ALTERNATE FORM OF cardiac assistance is known as dynamic cardiomyoplasty (DCMP), a promising but unproven surgical treatment for patients with end-stage heart failure (Fig. 11.5). The procedure was first performed in a human by Drs. Alain Carpentier and Juan Carlos Chachques of Paris, France, in 1985.

It involves freeing up a back muscle called the latissimus dorsi. The main blood supply and nerve supply are left intact. The muscle is then placed inside the chest and wrapped around the heart, where it is stimulated with a pacemaker for several weeks to make it more fatigue resistant. After this period, the muscle is stimulated with a special type of pacemaker so it contracts in synchrony with the heart in hopes of helping the function of the patient's own failing heart muscle.

Over the last fourteen years, more than one thousand patients worldwide have had dynamic cardiomyoplasty performed. The vast majority have demonstrated substantial improvement in symptoms of heart failure.

Despite this dramatic improvement, however, consistent evidence of improvement in heart function has not been found. Also, there is no good evidence that patients undergoing this procedure live longer than similar patients who have not had dynamic cardiomyoplasty. Lack of clear survival advantage and ongoing misunderstanding of the procedure's mechanism of action has so far hindered dynamic cardiomyoplasty's acceptance as a treatment alternative for patients with end-stage heart failure.

In more than six hundred cardiomyoplasty patients implanted with Medtronic electrical stimulators, clinical improvement in signs and symptoms of heart failure has been noted in 80 percent to 85 percent of surgery survivors. Improvement in symptoms of heart failure usually begins within the first six months after the surgery. In addition, the number of hospitalizations for heart failure decrease. A similar clinical improvement was found in a Phase II trial of cardiomyoplasty in the United States conducted under the auspices of the FDA.

During the recently completed Phase III trial, patients undergoing cardiomyoplasty had an operative mortality of less than 3 percent.

Today, the sickest patients who have heart failure symptoms at rest or who are confined to bed or to sitting in a chair are considered at too high a risk for

192

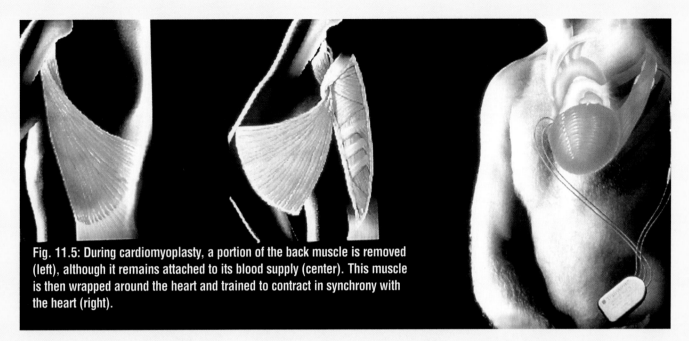

Fig. 11.5: During cardiomyoplasty, a portion of the back muscle is removed (left), although it remains attached to its blood supply (center). This muscle is then wrapped around the heart and trained to contract in synchrony with the heart (right).

cardiomyoplasty, so those patients are more likely to be referred for a heart transplant.

The Phase III randomized, clinical trial, again under the auspices of the FDA, commenced in June 1995 and was finished near the end of 1998. Slightly more than one hundred patients entered the study. It was a study designed to determine the safety of cardiomyoplasty as a treatment for heart failure due to dilated cardiomyopathy or ischemic cardiomyopathy (secondary to coronary artery blockages). In both dilated cardiomyopathy and ischemic cardiomyopathy, the main problem is that the heart muscle itself is failing. The study was designed to provide a clearer picture of the role of cardiomyoplasty as a treatment alternative for patients with end-stage heart failure.

Legitimate doubts about the efficacy of dynamic cardiomyoplasty remain. Although patients improve and have less severe symptoms of heart failure, no consistent improvement in heart function or survival benefit has been demonstrated.

Although many heart failure patients can be managed effectively with medicine alone, there are clearly many other patients receiving medical therapy whose quality of life and exercise capacity have worsened yet who are not sick enough to be considered for transplantation. It is clear that a more potent treatment alternative for these patients must be sought. Unfortunately, recruitment into this Phase III randomized trial, which perhaps would have been the definitive study, was too slow to allow definitive data to be collected.

With the trial's termination in the United States, cardiomyoplasty's potential clinical benefit may never be totally known. Its ultimate role in the treatment of heart failure depended on the outcome of a properly designed, controlled study with a minimum of four hundred patients. Clinical cardiomyoplasty has ceased being done in the United States, although in Europe, the procedure is still performed. The lessons learned from cardiomyoplasty, however, may still prove to be of greater significance.

## Aortomyoplasty

A similar surgical procedure, in which the skeletal muscle is wrapped directly around the aorta, is called aortomyoplasty (Fig. 11.6). This operation has been performed in more than twenty-eight humans worldwide and shows some promise.

The difference between aortomyoplasty and cardiomyoplasty is that the latissimus is wrapped around the aorta instead of the heart. In some of these procedures, it has been wrapped around the ascending aorta just as it comes out of the heart. In other procedures, it's wrapped around the descending aorta after the major blood vessels to the head and to the upper extremities branch off it.

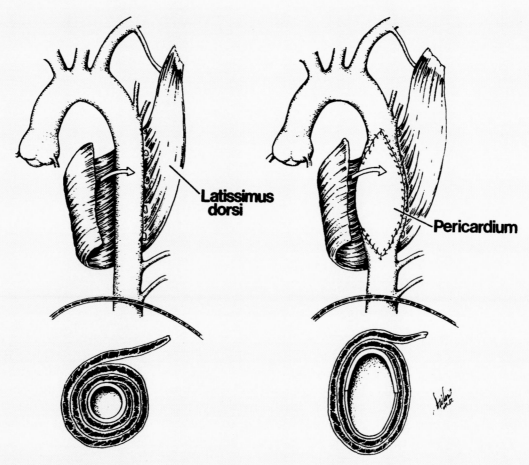

**Fig. 11.6:** During aortomyoplasty, a section of back muscle is wrapped around the aorta and trained to contract, easing the work load on the heart. In some cases, the aorta is also enlarged with pericardium.

Because the two procedures work on different parts of the anatomy, the muscle is trained to contract at different times. In cardiomyoplasty, the muscle is stimulated to contract at the same time as the heart ventricles. In aortomyoplasty, the latissimus muscle is stimulated to contract while the heart ventricles are relaxing. If the muscle was stimulated to contract to compress the aorta at the same time the heart ventricles were contracting, it would be working against the heart because they'd both be trying to pump blood in different directions at the same time.

One advantage this procedure has over cardiomyoplasty is that the sick heart itself does not need to be manipulated. In some cases, the heart is so large that the latissimus muscle cannot even be wrapped around it. In this case, cardiomyoplasty would not be performed, but an aortomyoplasty could be performed.

Although there are reports that patients with failing hearts have benefited from this procedure, it should be considered experimental, particularly until more long-term information is obtained.

# BUILDING A HEART PUMP FROM YOUR BACK MUSCLE

By
## Charles Bridges, M.D., D.Sc.
Cardiothoracic Surgeon

Assistant Professor of Surgery
Division of Cardiothoracic Surgery
University of Pennsylvania
Philadelphia, Pennsylvania

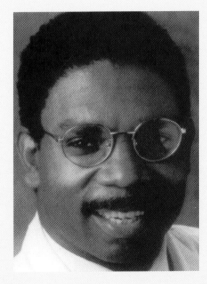

PHYSICIANS ARE CURRENTLy considering an alternative method of assist for congestive heart failure called the skeletal muscle ventricle procedure. In this novel approach, a pumping chamber is formed from the latissimus dorsi, which is a muscle located in the back that has been freed up and moved to the chest. The muscle is formed into a "pump" about the same size and shape as the left ventricle.

After the muscle pump is made, it is electrically stimulated for several weeks to make it fatigue resistant. During a second operation, the new pump is connected to the circulation and used as an assistive pump to help the heart.

These pumps have not been used in humans, although the results have been extremely encouraging in animals. In fact, one of these pumps has pumped blood effectively in the circulation of a laboratory animal for more than four years. In other cases, these pumps have been connected to the circulation with valves similar to those in the heart and have pumped blood for more than a year.

One of the advantages of a skeletal muscle ventricle compared with heart assist devices is that everything is implantable, including the special stimulators (which are identical to those used in cardiomyoplasty and aortomyoplasty). The procedure also has potential advantages over cardiomyoplasty and aortomyoplasty in that almost all of the latissimus muscle is used for the pumping action, and therefore, much more effective support of the circulation can be obtained. In addition, the potential advantage of the procedure over a heart transplant is the absence of rejection because the patient's own tissues are used.

Although the research is promising, the procedure is not yet ready for human trials.

# State of the Art in Mechanical Heart Assist Devices

O. Howard Frazier, M.D.

Professor of Surgery
University of Texas
and
Surgeon
The Texas Heart Institute
Houston, Texas

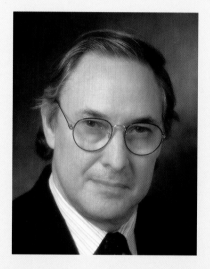

HEART TRANSPLANTATION has remained the best available option for some patients with terminal heart failure since its introduction in 1967. Despite this encouraging fact, however, the survival rate after transplantation is limited, and there is a wide gap between the number of available donor hearts and the number of patients who need them. Because of these limitations, researchers are always looking for better ways to help patients dying of heart failure. These efforts include the development of mechanical circulatory devices such as the total artificial heart and the left ventricular assist device (LVAD).

Patients usually die of heart failure because the left ventricle, the heart's primary pumping chamber, does not function properly. Researchers therefore have directed their efforts at developing the LVAD, which takes over the function of the left ventricle. In the early 1970s, research efforts, supported by the Device and Technology Division of the National Heart, Lung, and Blood Institute (NHLBI), were directed toward producing devices for long-term support (greater than two years).

The pumps were also used for short-term support in the hope that they would provide the necessary time for recovery of heart function. These pumps were pulsatile: The pump's action created a pulse similar to that of the natural heart and could draw blood from either the left ventricle or the left atrium and discharge it into the aorta.

In 1978, the Texas Heart Institute began using LVADs as bridges to transplantation. The devices were able to support patients during the time gap between imminent heart failure and heart transplantation. A similar device was implanted in 1984 at Stanford and again in 1986 at the Texas Heart Institute. Today, these large devices require an external connection to a battery pack. Despite this inconvenience, these devices have successfully supported many patients who otherwise would have died.

Over time, researchers observed that hearts that were supported by the LVAD and allowed to rest for longer time periods actually recovered some cardiac function; some patients have avoided transplant altogether. In turn, transplant surgeons have come to realize that long-term LVAD support improves the function of the body's other organs, leading to better outcomes when and if patients undergo transplantation. In the future, such devices may be

196

implanted permanently in some patients as an alternative to cardiac transplantation.

Alternative designs for mechanical circulatory devices are also being investigated. These include continuous flow pumps, which are considerably smaller than other assist devices currently in use. There is no need for valves because the blood flow is continuous.

The first temporary continuous flow pump, the Hemopump®, was successfully used in 1988 at the Texas Heart Institute. Continuous flow pumps offer great promise of widespread application, and the first clinical trials of the newest version were scheduled to begin in 1999.

In some cases, the heart is so damaged by disease that adequate support can only be obtained with a total artificial heart. Earlier versions of the total artificial heart included two single pumps, one to replace the right ventricle and one to replace the left ventricle, and the power source was outside the body. The first totally artificial heart was implanted at the Texas Heart Institute in 1969, followed by an-

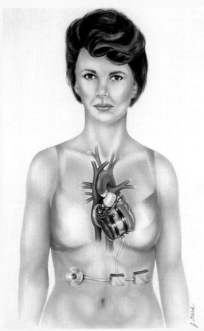

*The Abiomed total artificial heart.*

other implantation in 1982. Other implantations of permanent artificial hearts soon followed. These implantations were fraught with complications, and the devices and power consoles were large and cumbersome.

However, continued NHLBI funding from the mid-1980s enabled researchers to develop a smaller implantable device in which electrical power is transmitted across rather than

through the skin. These pumps are quieter and appear to be less likely to create the blood clots that plagued recipients of the earlier devices. Because this newly developed totally artificial heart can be nearly, if not completely, implanted under the skin, the risk of infection should be lower. These artificial hearts are currently being tested at the Texas Heart Institute and at Penn State, Hershey. They are almost ready for initial clinical trials and should be ready to implant in patients by the early part of the twenty-first century.

Many advances have been made in the field of mechanical circulatory support, and future generations of these devices hold great promise. Although heart transplantation remains an alternative for a select group of patients, it is currently not available to the vast majority of patients who are dying from heart failure. In the next millennium, a long-term device should be widely available for the treatment of heart disease and terminal heart failure, hopefully sparing many of these patients from an untimely death.

# CARDIAC RECONSTRUCTION FOR HEART FAILURE

By

## Patrick M. McCarthy, M.D.

Cardiothoracic Surgeon

The Cleveland Clinic Foundation
Department of Cardiothoracic Surgery
Cleveland, Ohio

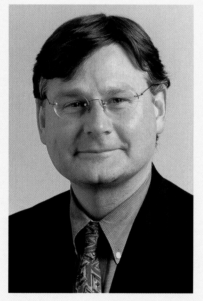

FOR DECADES HEART SURgeons have opened the left ventricle to "reconstruct" the damaged heart muscle. This has typically been used for cardiac aneurysms, or areas of scarred heart muscle that bulge out when the heart contracts and cause heart failure, blood clot formation, and heart rhythm problems. In recent years, this operation has been extended beyond classic aneurysms to include patients who have damaged hearts from heart attacks and in whom the weakened heart can be improved by reconstructing the heart muscle. In most instances, the scar is removed or reconstructed, blocked heart arteries are bypassed, and leaky valves are repaired.

A highly celebrated Brazilian surgeon, Dr. Randas Batista, extended this concept to hearts damaged not just from heart attacks but also from viral illnesses, valve problems, and a parasitic disease common in Brazil. The "Batista procedure" was popularized in the United States on many television network shows such as 20/20, NOVA, The Learning Channel, CNN, and all the network news stations. In this procedure, some of the heart muscle in these "flabby" hearts is removed, resulting in significant improvement in cardiac function in some patients. However, long-term follow-up is limited, and the results are unpredictable. Some patients had excellent results for years, whereas in others, treatment failed, and their weakened hearts required heart transplantation.

At the Cleveland Clinic, we have been working on reconstructing the heart with both the Batista procedure and also using methods for hearts scarred from heart attacks. These scarred hearts generally improve significantly after reconstruction often coupled with coronary bypass surgery and frequently with valve surgery.

Although the number of Batista procedures performed now is far less than two years ago, we think that it was a useful step along the way. We are currently developing a device that can recreate the improvements seen with the Batista procedure, but without having to use the heart-lung machine, open the heart, and cut out and remove a large portion of the heart muscle. This new device should pose a much lower risk than the Batista procedure and provide a more predictable success rate.

# GENE THERAPY

## By
## Todd K. Rosengart, M.D., F.A.C.S.

Cardiothoracic Surgeon

Associate Professor of Surgery
Cornell University
New York, New York

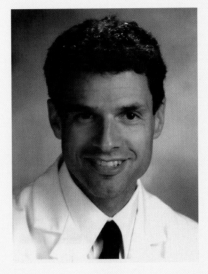

THERAPEUTIC ANGIOGEN-esis is a promising new treatment for artery blockages typically caused by atherosclerosis. Angiogenesis means the "formation of new blood vessels." In angiogenesis, a naturally occurring protein called a growth factor, or angiogen, is used to stimulate blood vessel growth. This enhances blood flow to tissues that are jeopardized by a blockage.

In the laboratory, therapeutic angiogenesis has been shown to help blood vessels develop. Among other actions, angiogenesis might reduce the effects of atherosclerosis, enhance wound healing, and promote tissue growth. It may be particularly useful for patients with such severe or widespread atherosclerotic disease that they cannot be fully helped by conventional therapies like angioplasty or bypass surgery.

Besides using growth protein, we are also considering gene therapy. To do this, we transfer genes directly into a targeted tissue, where the gene "turns on"

DNA that causes cells to produce the proteins that cause growth of new blood vessels. Genes can be transferred on genetically engineered viral particles. The adenovirus (Ad) is one such viral particle that efficiently transfers genes to tissues such as the myocardium, or heart muscle. Genes transferred by Ad remain in the tissue they are sent to and are active for only one or two weeks. This is important because it potentially prevents the overproduction of a protein that

might cause abnormal blood vessel growth.

We have so far tested the Ad protein transfer technique in twenty-one patients. These patients had not responded to coronary bypass surgery or coronary balloon dilatation because of the severity of their coronary artery disease. To date, the gene therapy appears to be well tolerated, and we plan to move into larger-scale human studies. Similar positive results have been reported by other investigators using a "naked" DNA segment that was not incorporated into a viral particle like Ad.

It is unknown which, if any, gene therapy strategy will work best, or whether they will be superior to the use of angiogenic proteins themselves instead of the genes for these proteins. Finally, it is unknown which, if any, of the many angiogenic proteins will work best, or which delivery method will be most beneficial. Preliminary studies and the promise of future advancements are, however, very encouraging.

# THE FUTURE IN ARTIFICIAL HEART TECHNOLOGY

By

Stephen Westaby, B.Sc., M.S., F.R.C.S.

Cardiothoracic Surgeon

Oxford Heart Centre
John Radcliffe Hospital
Oxford University
Oxford, England

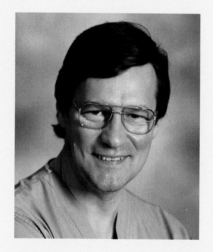

CURRENTLY, THERE ARE more than three million heart failure patients in the United States, with more than four-hundred thousand new cases every year. Treatment of heart attack has come a long way. Today, physicians are able to use clot-busting drugs and catheters to save thousands of lives. There is, however, an unfortunate consequence of this rapid advance. Some of these people who are saved, particularly patients with coronary artery disease, develop heart failure.

Because transplantation is limited, physicians have turned to mechanical hearts, a concept that has captured the imagination of cardiac surgeons, the public, and the media alike. Although there are no fully implantable mechanical hearts available, physicians do have mechanical treatment options for end-stage heart disease.

In fact, within the next ten years, a miniaturized blood pump is destined to become the treatment of choice to relieve symp-

toms and prolong life in older heart failure patients. Physicians have recently discovered that "resting" the heart with such a blood pump may promote recovery in some patients. This raises the possibility that circulatory support can be used as a therapy in conjunction with other treatments.

## Left Ventricular Assist Devices

The totally artificial heart, which received much publicity in the 1970s and 1980s, was conceptually flawed. These unwieldy devices were acceptable as a

bridge to transplantation (when meant to keep patients alive until they could receive a heart transplant) but were never a long-term solution. To be successful, an artificial heart must be more than a reliable blood pump; it must be forgettable. That was something the big artificial hearts could never be.

In recent years, however, physicians have realized that whole-heart replacement may not be necessary. After all, more than 90 percent of heart failure patients can be sustained with left ventricular support alone.

Currently, left ventricular assist devices are used mainly as a bridge to transplantation. The modern left ventricular assist device consists of a blood sac that is compressed by a pusherplate mechanism that is either electrically or air driven. Artificial heart valves direct the blood flow. This system mimics the human left ventricle by providing pulsatile blood flow while taking the burden of pumping off the patient's heart. This is a workable solution and saves many lives, but the serious problems of pump size, noise, driveline infection, and stroke remain. Nevertheless, some patients have had these devices in place for up to four years and enjoyed an acceptable quality of life. This has encouraged us to use the left ventricular assist device for long-term support in patients who are not eligible for transplantation.

## The Next Generation of Assist Devices

The ideal treatment for chronic severe heart failure must be reliable, cost effective, easy to manage at home, and capable of providing adequate circulation. Keeping these goals in sight, another generation of heart assist devices called axial flow impeller pumps is on the horizon. These are compact, silent, nonpulsing blood pumps that provide up to eight quarts of flow per minute.

Among these is the thumb-sized Jarvik-2000, which fits within the failing left ventricle and pumps blood to the aorta. The impeller revolves at up to eighteen thousand rpm, moving blood so rapidly that the red cells remain undamaged. The controller and batteries are the size of a portable telephone and fit easily onto a normal belt.

Other ingenious blood pumps are under development, including some with magnetically suspended rotors. These fully implantable, miniature artificial hearts will greatly increase our

ability to treat heart failure, although we do not know their reliability and complication rate.

A recent revelation has been the effect of chronic rest on the failing left ventricle. For years, we have known that prolonged bed-rest, which reduces heart function, results in improvement. However, the benefits are limited by the negative effects of inactivity on the limb muscles, blood vessel tone, and nervous system.

Ideally, patients would be able to exercise their bodies while their hearts rested. This is now possible with long-term implantable blood pumps. When we compare the heart muscle at the time of blood pump insertion to the muscle during transplantation, there is often a shift in heart muscle cells towards normal, both in shape and function. This discovery that recovering hearts were being removed at transplantation, coupled with the shortage in donors, led to the use of blood pumps to induce heart recovery.

Although the benefits of this therapy are obvious, there are certain requirements that must be met before this strategy has a chance for success. The first is a user-friendly blood pump for patients of all sizes. This must be simple to implant and remove, without the risk of infection, and easy to control. Second, it must be implanted before the heart degenerates to a point at which the heart failure cannot be reversed.

In our limited experience with this approach, certain factors

are apparent that separate those with sustainable heart recovery from others who will slip back into heart failure. Patients with long-lasting recovery tend to be younger, have a shorter history of heart failure, show a more rapid improvement in heart performance, and require a shorter period of blood pump support.

The type of heart disease is also important to recovery. Coronary artery disease patients with large areas of dead muscle will not recover. However, young patients with viral infections involving the heart can often be supported with a blood pump until the inflammatory process completely resolves. Even those who require external cardiac massage and a heart-lung machine during blood pump insertion can be restored to nearly normal cardiac function.

## A Look at the Future

The scope of mechanical heart failure therapy is developing rapidly as new blood pumps emerge from the bioengineering laboratories. These will eventually be used as often for heart failure as the pacemaker is for rhythm problems. The major issues are not ethical but economic. In the further future, new drugs, gene therapy, and tissue engineering with the patient's own heart muscle cells will be used to promote recovery of the patient's heart in conjunction with periods of mechanical circulatory support.

# Heart Cell Transplantation for the Failing Heart

By
Terrence M. Yau, M.D., M.Sc.,
Ren-Ke Li, M.D., Ph.D.,
Richard D. Weisel, M.D., and
Donald A.G. Mickle, M.D.
Department of Surgery and Laboratory Medicine and Pathology
University of Toronto
Toronto, Ontario, Canada

AN ESTIMATED 465,000 PAtients in the United States are diagnosed with congestive heart failure each year. For those patients with mild heart failure, medicine can often relieve their symptoms and improve their quality of life. However, for patients with severe heart failure, medicine may be insufficient, and heart transplantation may offer the potential for a better, longer life. Unfortunately, there is a limited supply of donor hearts, and less than 10 percent of patients needing a heart transplant will actually receive one.

This dilemma — what to do for patients with severe heart failure who are unable to receive heart transplants — stimulated our interest in heart cell transplantation, an exciting new field with the potential to improve the quality of life and lengthen the lives of patients who suffer from heart failure. We hope we can begin the first trials of heart cell transplantation in human patients within the next two years.

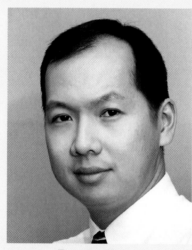

**Terrence M. Yau**

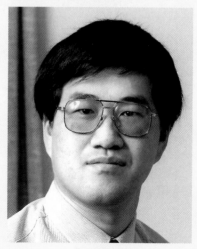

**Ren-Ke Li**

So far, our research group has succeeded in growing animal and human heart cells in cell culture, outside the body. It is a very painstaking and exacting process that was previously thought to be impossible. However, over the course of ten years, we have developed techniques that permit these cells to grow and reproduce in a culture dish while retaining most of the characteristics of heart muscle cells.

When transplanted into rat hearts that have been scarred by injury to the heart's main pumping chamber, the transplanted cells formed a block of muscle tissue within the scar tissue that can be easily identified under a microscope. Consequently, hearts that had been injected with the cultured muscle cells had better pumping function than those injected with only the solution the cells were grown in but not the cells themselves.

On the basis of this finding, we realized that injecting cultured heart muscle cells into an injured heart had the potential to restore function. However, we also found that the rats developed an immune response to the transplanted cells, which were taken from a different rat, and the cells were gradually destroyed over about six months.

To avoid this immune response, we have taken heart muscle cells from one animal, grown them in the laboratory, and transplanted them back into the same animal. These cells, because they are recognized by the animal as its own cells, do not cause an immune response and are not destroyed. Again, these transplanted heart muscle cells improved heart function and blood flow to that area of the heart.

Within the next one to two years, we hope we will be able to use a similar approach in human patients undergoing heart surgery. At the time of their heart catheterization, patients with poor heart function would have a very small amount of heart muscle tissue removed. This tissue would be grown in the laboratory over several weeks to obtain a much greater number of cells. Then, during heart surgery, the cultured heart cells would be transplanted back into the patient's

heart. The resulting improved heart function will hopefully result in a greater exercise capacity, better quality of life, and longer life expectancy.

This form of therapy does not apply only to heart muscle cells. We have also examined the role of muscle cells from other parts of the body, the cells responsible for making fibrous tissue, and the cells that form blood vessels. When blood vessel cells were transplanted into the scar tissue, we found that the number of blood vessels in the area tripled.

Our research suggested that a combination of heart muscle cells, to improve heart function, and blood vessel cells, to improve blood flow to the heart, might be the best solution for failing hearts with inadequate blood flow. This is exactly the situation seen in many patients with advanced atherosclerosis.

We are also using our experience in culturing heart muscle cells to build a graft material that could be used to repair heart defects in children with congenital heart disease. The graft materials currently available for repair of these defects have no living cells and therefore do not grow after implantation. Inevitably, the

child outgrows the graft and usually requires a second or third operation to replace it. Each successive operation carries a greater risk.

A graft that grows with the child and does not require additional operations would be a significant advance. We have been able to grow heart muscle cells in a three-dimensional mesh, which is gradually dissolved by the body, leaving only the cells. When this mesh is seeded with heart muscle cells and implanted into the legs of rats, the graft can be seen to beat rhythmically just like normal heart muscle.

We hope to someday build a graft that can be used to repair heart defects and that will grow with the child. Although much more work is necessary to develop this kind of graft, our initial results have been very encouraging.

Heart cell transplantation is an exciting new technology with the potential to improve heart function and blood flow in patients with advanced heart failure and extensive atherosclerosis. It may also lead to the development of living graft materials that can be used to repair heart defects in children, avoiding the need for second or third operations.

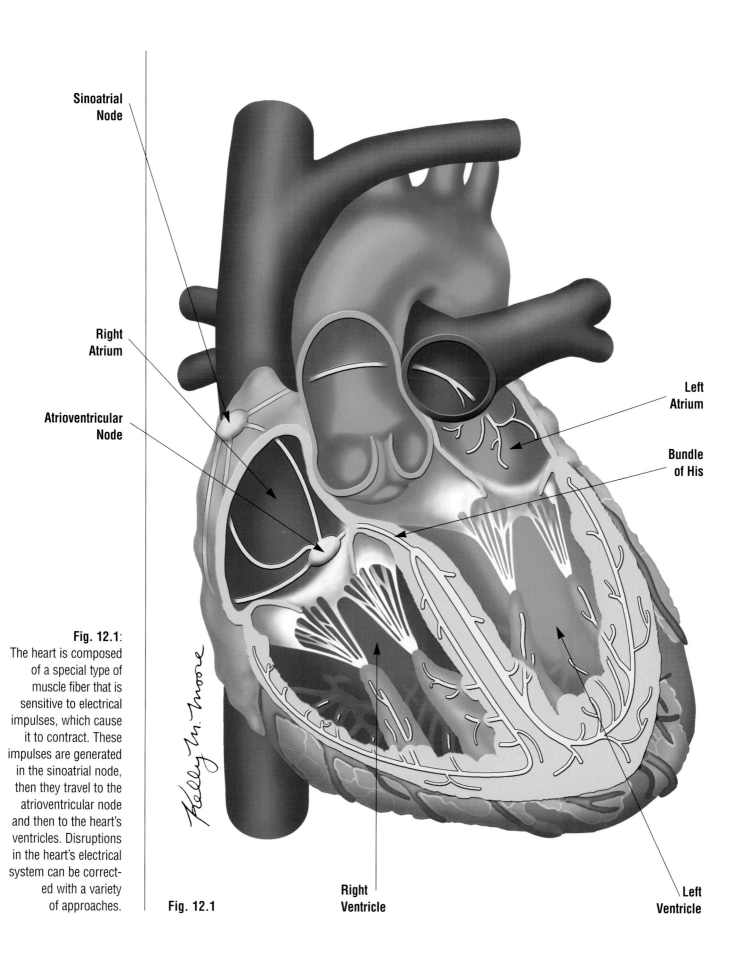

**Sinoatrial Node**

**Right Atrium**

**Atrioventricular Node**

**Left Atrium**

**Bundle of His**

**Fig. 12.1:**
The heart is composed of a special type of muscle fiber that is sensitive to electrical impulses, which cause it to contract. These impulses are generated in the sinoatrial node, then they travel to the atrioventricular node and then to the heart's ventricles. Disruptions in the heart's electrical system can be corrected with a variety of approaches.

**Fig. 12.1**

**Right Ventricle**

**Left Ventricle**

204

# ARRHYTHMIAS, PACEMAKERS, AND DEFIBRILLATORS

EVERYBODY HAS AN IRREGULAR heartbeat now and then, and not all types of irregular heartbeats, or **arrhythmias,** are necessarily bad. They can range in severity from simply a nuisance to life threatening, especially those that originate from the heart ventricles.

In most cases, an arrhythmia is caused by a faulty electrical conduction system, or pacemaker cells, in the heart muscle. Abnormal heart rhythms may interfere with the heart's pumping function and therefore may cause fatigue, lightheadedness, a sensation of uneasiness, or sometimes even passing out, particularly if the heart rate is very slow or very fast. Some patients can develop angina-type chest pain from a decreased flow of oxygenated blood to the coronary arteries or from very rapid heart rates.

The normal heart rhythm is called **sinus rhythm**. If there is a problem with the heart rhythm, patients may be referred to a cardiologist who specializes in heart rhythms called a cardiac electrophysiologist. Patients may undergo studies of their heart rhythm called EPS (electrophysiology studies). In this case, wires are guided into the heart through blood vessels in the groin or arm to study its electrical system.

If someone suffers from an arrhythmia, they may need treatment with medication or even an implantable electrical device such as a **pacemaker** or **defibrillator**. These devices monitor the heart's rhythm and intervene in case of certain types of irregularity. There are many companies worldwide that produce heart pacemakers, and each company makes several different types that approach different heart rhythm problems with various design strategies.

###  Pacemakers

The first successful electrical pacing probably took place in Australia in the 1920s when two doctors supposedly revived a stillborn baby. By the 1950s, doctors were able to control the heart rate in dogs by using external pacemakers.

The real advent in pacing as we know it today, however, is credited to Dr. Paul Zoll from Harvard Medical School. In 1952, he used an external pacemaker on two patients suffering from recurring, prolonged episodes of ventricular standstill (heart ventricles not contracting, therefore not pumping blood). The first patient was a seventy-year-old man with complete

**Arrhythmia:**
Any abnormal heart rhythm. Also called dysrhythmia.

**Sinus Rhythm:**
The normal rhythm of the heart that is stimulated by the sinoatrial node.

**Pacemaker:**
A small, battery-powered device implanted in the chest wall to send electrical impulses to the heart, causing it to contract in a rhythmic fashion. Mechanical pacemakers are used when the body's natural pacemaker is not functioning properly.

**Defibrillator:**
A device used to electrically shock the heart into a more normal rhythm.

**Sinoatrial Node:**
Also referred to as the sinus node and S-A node. This is the true pacemaker of the heart, located at the junction of the right atrium and superior vena cava. These cells rhythmically discharge electrical impulses that cause the heart to contract. This impulse also travels to the A-V node, and then to the ventricles, causing them to contract.

**Atrioventricular Node:**
Also called the A-V node. A specialized nerve-type tissue located in the wall of the right ventricle. It receives electrical impulses from the sinoatrial node, then relays the impulse to the ventricles, which causes them to contract.

heart block, meaning the atrial heartbeats could not get through to pace the ventricles. The patient had been revived with thirty-four separate intracardiac injections (sticking a needle connected to a syringe through the chest straight into the heart!) of adrenalin given during four hours. Zoll applied electric shocks, two milliseconds long, through the chest wall at frequencies of twenty-five to sixty shocks per minute and increased the intensity of the shocks until ventricular responses were observed. After twenty-five minutes, however, the response became weaker, and the patient died. Many subsequent patients, however, survived.

Shortly afterward, Dr. C. Walton Lillehei and associates reported on a series of patients whose hearts needed pacing after open heart operations at the University of Minnesota. The major difference between Zoll's pacing and Lillehei's was that Zoll used large external electrodes placed on the patient's chest wall, whereas Lillehei attached electrodes directly to the heart during the operation and connected these electrodes to an external power source. In this way, he could pace the heart with much less current, and it was not painful to the patient, in contrast with Zoll's shocks permeating the skin and chest wall. It was also a more efficient way to stimulate the heart. The survival rate of Lillehei's patients with surgically induced heart block, a complication of heart surgery, was substantially improved with the pacemaker.

Only a few years later, Rune Elmquist and Dr. Ake Senning in Sweden developed a prototype of the first totally implantable pacemaker. It had a battery that was small enough for a pocket under the skin and electrodes that were connected directly to the heart. The first unit was implanted in a patient in 1958.

Drs. William Chardack, Andrew Cage, and Wilson Greatbatch from the University of Buffalo School of Medicine in Buffalo, New York, are perhaps better known for their development of a totally implantable pacemaker. In 1961, they reported on a series of fifteen patients in whom they placed the totally implantable pacemakers they had developed.

In these early days, implantable pacemakers were not synchronized with the heart rhythm. They delivered an electrical impulse independent of the underlying cardiac rhythm. During the past forty years, however, enormous progress has been made in cardiac pacing. The number of individuals with artificial pacemakers is unknown. However, estimates indicate that about five hundred thousand Americans are living with a pacemaker, and that each year another one hundred thousand or more patients require permanent pacemakers in the United States alone.

### Heart Pacemakers

The most common need for heart pacemakers today occurs when there is an inappropriate slowing of the **sinoatrial node**, or S-A node, which is located in the right atrium and is responsible for generating a normal heart rhythm. Electrical impulses travel from the S-A node through the atrium and arrive at the **atrioventricular node**, or A-V node, which is located at about the junction of the right atrium and right ventricle. From there, the impulse travels through another electrical system that activates the right and left ventricles and stimulates them to contract (Fig. 12.1).

If the A-V node is diseased, the electrical impulse cannot get through to the ventricles. In this case, the A-V node is often able to generate its own electrical impulse, but this impulse tends to occur at a slower rate than that of the S-A node, and the rhythm is not in synchrony with the atrial rhythm. Thus, the atria may contract at one rate, and the ventricles may contract at a slower rate. In fact, the ventricles may not contract at all.

# THE FIRST PRACTICAL PACEMAKER

C. WALTON LILLEHEI'S FIRST battery-powered pacemakers were built by Earl Bakken, an engineer and medical equipment repairman at the University of Minnesota.

Bakken gained interest in electricity and medicine from the Mary Shelley novel *Frankenstein; or, The Modern Prometheus.* In the book, Dr. Frankenstein rejuvenates an inert body with electricity. As a boy, Bakken imagined using the same treatment on sick people.

*"Later, while in graduate school at the University of Minnesota, I started wandering over to the hospital. I got acquainted with people in the labs and the EKG department, and was asked to help repair some equipment. That's when the idea came to set up Medtronic in 1949 as an electronic repair service in the field of medicine."*

Shortly afterward, he met Lillehei, who was working on cross circulation for cardiopulmonary bypass, and sold the surgical team some equipment.

"They wanted lots of monitoring for both the parent and the child, which I was glad to sell them," Bakken said. "Then they wanted to be sure it was running right, so they wanted me in surgery with them. Lillehei used to say I was the only engineer whom he could get to come into surgery; the other engineers wouldn't do it. So I got to know all the residents and interns who later went on to become the heads of surgery all across the country, all around the world."

During the operations, Lillehei was using big, externally powered pacemakers. Although these helped some children who developed heart block, they had the major drawback of needing to be plugged into a wall socket. When the patient needed to be moved, Lillehei's team ran extension cords down the hospital corridors to keep the pacemakers working — even going so far as dropping cords down elevator shafts.

During a 1957 blackout, the pacemakers stopped working in several patients and, according to Bakken's recollection, one child died. Lillehei turned to Bakken and asked him to develop a back-up system. Bakken recently told how this request sparked development of the modern pacemaker:

*"I envisioned that because the pacemaker was a large AC unit sitting on a cart, we could put an automobile battery on the lower shelf.... If the power failed, the battery would keep it going for several hours. Automobile batteries were six-volt back then. An invertor could change that to a fifteen-volt pulse.*

*"I went back to my garage to think about building that. Then it dawned on me. Why go through all that big cart full of apparatus and end up with a little fifteen-volt pulse? In fact, further work showed we didn't need more than five volts. So that's when I built the first battery-operated, wearable, transistorized pacemaker."*

The pacemaker electrodes were attached to the heart, and the wires ran through the skin to the relatively small battery-powered unit. Bakken's pacemaker provided the foundation for modern pacemakers and also spurred the development of Medtronic into a one of the world's largest medical device companies.

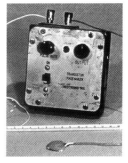

The first wearable, transistorized, battery-powered pacemaker, above, was developed in 1957 by Earl Bakken, middle. The Chardack-Greatbatch pacemaker, below, is a later-generation implantable device.

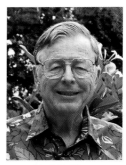

**Earl Bakken**

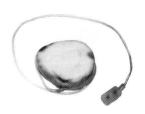

Obviously, if this happens, it is a very serious situation.

### The Single-Chamber Pacemaker

The simplest type of pacemaker is called a VVI and is designed to pace the ventricle (Fig. 12.2). It senses the ventricle's electrical activity and is inhibited from pacing if the heart rate is faster than a preset rate. The first "V" in VVI means the heart's ventricle is paced, the second "V" means the heart's electrical activity in the ventricle is sensed by the pacemaker, and the "I" refers to the mechanism by which the pacemaker is turned on and off.

The most common way we connect pacemaker leads is to thread them through a vein in the shoulder area to the right atrium and into the right ventricle, then connect them to what's called a pulse generator (the brains and battery of the system) located in a pocket under the skin.

These pacemakers' electrical impulses can be set so that if the ventricle is naturally contracting at an acceptable rate (usually around sixty or seventy beats per minute, or bpm), the pacemaker will simply monitor the heart rhythm. However, if the patient's heart rate drops below a preset number of beats per minute, the pacemaker takes over. For example, the pacemaker could be programmed so that if the ventricular rate is seventy bpm or faster, the pacemaker remains in "standby" mode. If the rate drops below seventy bpm, the pacemaker kicks in and delivers electrical impulses at the preset rate. This rate is whatever the physician decides to set and varies from patient to patient. The pacemaker does

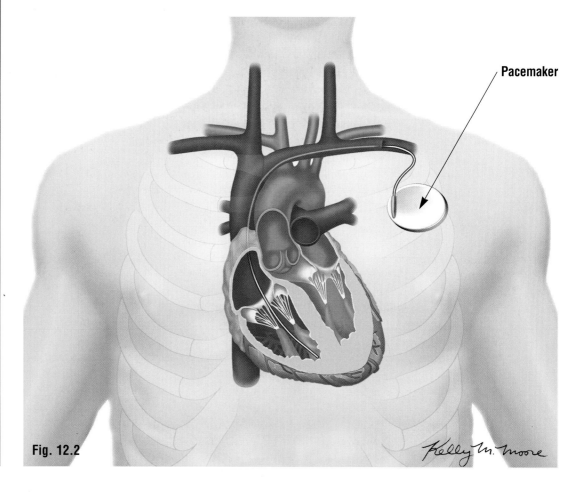

**Pacemaker**

**Fig. 12.2**:
A VVI pacemaker, or single-chamber pacemaker, is designed to pace the ventricle. It is set to send an electrical impulse only when the ventricular contractions slow to an unacceptable rate.

**Fig. 12.2**

*Kelly M. Moore*

# DENTON COOLEY: BUILDING HIS OWN DEFIBRILLATOR

WHEN DENTON COOLEY WAS A surgical resident at Johns Hopkins Hospital in the 1940s, it was not uncommon for seriously ill infants and children with congenital heart defects to develop ventricular fibrillation, a fatal rhythm of the heart's ventricles, during surgery. The usual treatment was to give various medications in hope that the heart rhythm would change back to normal. Sometimes it did not work, and the patient died.

Cooley recently remembered that during the surgery to close a patent ductus arteriosus, or abnormal communication between the aorta and pulmonary artery, the child's heart went into ventricular fibrillation and could not be returned to normal rhythm. Cooley was extremely discouraged by this. He went to see Dr. William Kouwenhouven, who was chairman of the department of electri-

cal engineering and who had been working with cardiac resuscitation for electrocution victims. They spoke about building a defibrillator for the operating room.

Subsequently, based on an article by Dr. Donald Hooker and Kouwenhouven and another by Dr. Claude Beck, Cooley built his own defibrillator with the help of the hospital's machine shop. Unlike most other defibrillators that were used by placing the electrodes on the patient's chest, Cooley's defibrillator allowed the electrodes to be placed directly on the patient's heart in the operating room. It cost about $90 of Cooley's own money to build.

"The defibrillator was used at Johns Hopkins in the operating room for about ten years until commercial devices were available," Cooley said. "My salary then, as a fourth-year surgical resident, was $25 a month."

not actually wait a full minute and count seventy beats before activation. Rather, it measures the time interval between heart electrical impulses so if the next heart impulse is slow to arrive, the pacemaker has already taken over.

Usually patients do not know when their heart is being paced and when it is not. They can sometimes tell when the pacemaker switches on or off, however, just like some people can feel when their heart skips a beat or the heart rhythm changes.

Sometimes the leads or wires can also be attached directly to the surface of the heart, as opposed to threaded inside

the ventricles. This requires a surgical incision, usually in the chest or upper abdomen, so the leads can be fastened to the surface of the heart. This might be done in a patient needing a pacemaker whose chest is already open during a heart operation. Leads might be connected directly to the surface of the heart if the patient has an infection in the bloodstream or an artificial heart valve replacing the tricuspid valve.

More sophisticated ventricular pacemakers have a feature that can sense your physical activity level and actually increase the heart rate so more oxygenated blood is pumped to the body tissues. This is helpful in active patients. These devices usually sense changes in body heat or increases in skeletal muscle activity.

### Dual-Chamber Pacemakers

The next most common type of pacemaker stimulates and monitors both the ventricles and the atria (Fig. 12.3). This more sophisticated pacemaker is called a DDD pacemaker (each D stands for dual: it can pace both the atria and the ventricles; it can sense the electrical activity in both the atria and the ventricles; and there are dual methods to make sure it turns on or off at the correct time). In addition to the lead connected to the ventricle, it also requires an electrode connected to the atrium. This additional electrode is also introduced through a vein and threaded into the right atrium. The other end of the lead is connected to the pacemaker.

A DDD pacemaker has certain advantages. It will be able to sense your S-A node rhythm and pace the ventricles in harmony with the atria. If you're resting, the S-A node rate may only be sixty bpm, but, if you're active, it may be one hundred. The pacemaker will sense the appropriate S-A node rate and deliver a corresponding impulse to the ventricle. If the S-A node is pacing the atria at an undesirably slow rate, it can also take over and pace the atria. This type of pacemaker allows the ventricles and atria to coordinate their activity.

The DDD pacemakers can be equipped with an additional feature that senses

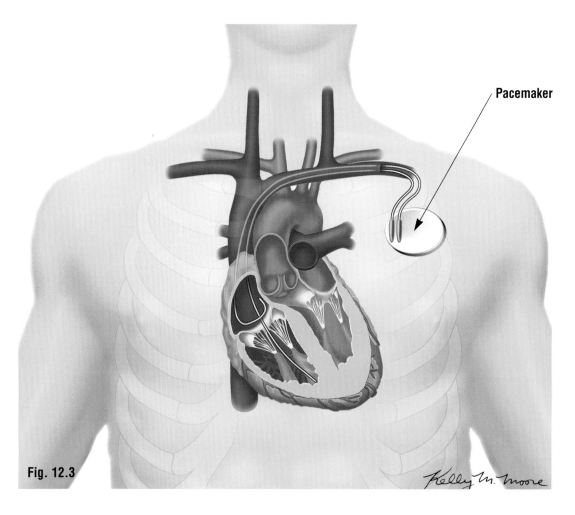

**Pacemaker**

**Fig. 12.3**:
Dual-chamber pacemakers can monitor and pace both the ventricles and the atria.

**Fig. 12.3**

*Kelly M. Moore*

# ♥AKE SENNING AND THE FIRST IMPLANTABLE PACEMAKER

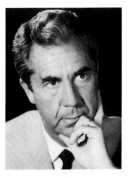

Dr. Ake Senning placed the first totally implantable pacemaker, which he developed with a Swedish engineer.

SWEDISH DOCTOR AKE SENNING became a doctor by default. Although he had wanted to be an engineer, his mother urged him towards medicine. That summer in the 1930s when he was signing up for school, he went on a motorcycle holiday and missed the deadline to apply for technical school. With that option closed, Senning pursued medicine. In 1949, he was invited to join the thoracic clinic of the renowned surgeon Dr. Clarence Crafoord, where he was assigned to develop a heart-lung machine.

There, another young surgeon, who also would distinguish himself in cardiac surgery, Dr. Viking Bjork, was also working on a heart-lung machine of his own design. At one point, Senning remembered in a recent interview, he even visited Dr. John Kirklin's lab at the Mayo Clinic to see the first-generation heart-lung machine and, through an accident, had blood sprayed all over a new suit (the suit was saved).

Senning gained experience with external pacemakers during his heart-lung machine experiments when, in some cases, he had to stimulate the heart with electricity to regain a beat.

"In 1955, a friend of mine came from the United States," Senning said. "He had a small pacemaker. When I saw this, I thought, 'We can make it smaller.'" But Senning was concerned about infection because the wires had to run through the skin to the external pacemaker. Senning started with external pacemakers, but many became infected. The next step was to work towards an implantable pacemaker.

By 1957, Senning and his colleagues had developed what they hoped would become a workable internal pacemaker. But there was skepticism: "The cardiologist said there was no indication; a patient with A-V block can live at least two years. And then you had the priest, who said if you have a heart that God stopped, you shouldn't try to start it!"

Then an agitated woman came to him and pleaded with him to implant a pacemaker in her husband. He had been hospitalized for months and was having twenty to thirty cardiac arrests every day. Senning told her their pacemaker was not ready for human implantation. She replied, "So make one!"

Senning referred her to the engineer Rune Elmquist, who was working on the experimental pacemaker. That day, the woman drove back and forth several times between Elmquist's office and Senning's.

Shortly thereafter, on October 8, 1958, Senning received his pacemaker and placed it in his patient. It functioned for eight hours, then stopped. Senning replaced it with another, which failed several days later. Eventually, the patient survived more than twenty-five years and during that period had several more pacemaker implants.

One of Senning's other major contributions to cardiac surgery was the Senning operation, which he reported on in 1959. This was the first corrective operation for a congenital heart defect called transposition of the great arteries, which until then was usually fatal within the first year of life.

an increase in physical activity. If the S-A node does not increase its rate with increased physical activity like walking or running, the pacemaker can be programmed to increase the heart rate so more blood is pumped.

There are numerous variations on the VVI and DDD types of pacemakers, but these are the basic principles on which these pacemakers work.

### Pacemakers for Atrial Tachyarrhythmias

Some pacemakers are designed for patients who have episodes of abnormally fast heartbeats that are generated in the atria. If these fast beats in the S-A node or other areas in the atria reach the range of one-hundred sixty to more than two hundred beats per minute and are transmitted to the ventricles, causing them to contract at an abnormally fast rate, the heart

becomes inefficient, and you may become lightheaded or even pass out from less oxygenated blood getting to the brain.

A kind of pacemaker called an anti-tachyarrhythmia pacemaker can sense these rhythms, take them over, and pace the atria into a more normal rhythm. Tachy means fast; arrhythmia means abnormal heart rhythm.

### Surgery for Pacemakers

Pacemakers are usually implanted by either heart surgeons or cardiologists. The surgery is done in the operating room, cardiac catheterization laboratory, or electrophysiology laboratory. The pacemakers are usually implanted after local anesthesia is induced with the patient awake. The skin is washed and painted with soap; then sterile drapes are placed over the patient and around the area where the inci-

**Tachycardia:**
An abnormally fast heart rate, usually more than one-hundred beats per minute.

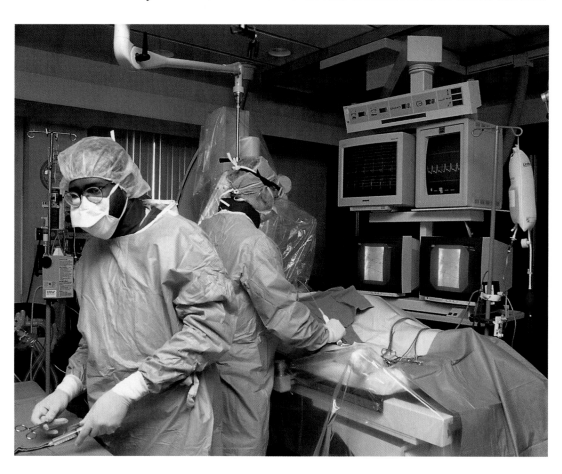

During an electrophysiology study, physicians are able to locate the exact source of abnormal heart rhythms. This procedure is performed with catheters that are guided into the heart through the groin or arm.

sion will be made. A local anesthetic, usually lidocaine or xylocaine, is injected under the skin in the shoulder area just below the collar bone. Next, an incision is made through the skin about two to two-and-a-half inches long and down to the muscle layer. The tissue is freed up just above the muscle layer to make a pocket for the pulse generator. The size of pacemakers is variable, but they can be as small as a quarter or a silver dollar and a bit thicker. Next, using one of several techniques, a vein in that area is located, and one or two leads are threaded through it into the heart.

The surgery to install pacemakers can take anywhere from a half hour up to more than two hours depending on how difficult it is to get the leads into the best spot in the ventricle and atrium (for the DDD type) for the best pacing and sensing thresholds. Every patient's anatomy is a little different, and the exact best spot to place the lead in the atrium or ventricle can vary from patient to patient, which can account in part for the relative difficulty of insertion in some patients.

Once the wire leads are connected to the pulse generator, the pulse generator is placed under the skin and a fat layer in the shoulder area, and the wound is closed. The pulse generator has a battery and a small, sophisticated computer. Most pacemakers (computer plus battery) are small enough so they are not noticeable under the skin.

The settings of the pacemaker are adjusted through the skin so that no needles or objects need to break the skin barrier. The device used to program your pacemaker is somewhat like your remote control television programmer. The batteries in the pulse generator usually need to be changed about every seven to ten years. When the pulse generators are changed, generally the leads are left in place, but tests are done to check them.

My patients usually go home later that day or the next morning with a prescription for some minor pain medicine, which is usually needed for only a few days. Pacemakers require routine follow-up to ensure proper function and to assess battery longevity.

# MANAGING ARRHYTHMIAS

By

## Marc D. Meissner, M.D., C.M., F.A.C.C, F.A.C.P.

Associate Professor of Internal Medicine
Cardiac Electrophysiologist and Cardiologist
Detroit Medical Center
Wayne State University

and

## Randy A. Lieberman, M.D.

Assistant Professor of Internal Medicine
Cardiac Electrophysiologist and Cardiologist
Detroit Medical Center
Wayne State University
Director, Detroit Medical Center Electrophysiology

THE HEART'S PUMPING action, which creates the pulse, is generated by a burst of electrical energy that activates specialized cells in the heart muscle. Normally, this electrical activity originates in a structure called the sinus node (or sinoatrial or S-A node), which is located in the right atrium. From there, it spreads across the atria, causing them to contract, or beat.

After stimulating the atria, the impulse travels along a bridge of special conducting tissue called the A-V node to the ventricles. Similarly to the atria, ventricles pump in response to the electricity, thus sending blood out to the organs.

Any abnormalities in this electrical circuit affect the heartbeat. These may give rise to abnormal heart rhythms, called arrhythmias. The heart may beat too slowly (bradycardia), or it may beat to quickly (tachycardia). In some instances, slow heartbeats are normal, such as during sleep or in well-trained athletes. Likewise, fast

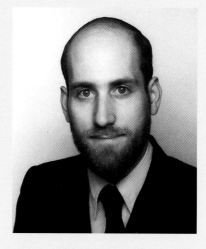

**Marc D. Meissner**

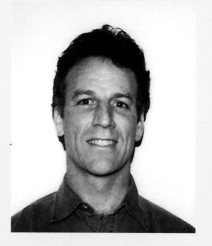

**Randy A. Lieberman**

heartbeats can be normal in some circumstances, such as with exercise, excitement, or high fevers.

In other cases, however, the electrical impulse itself is slowed or blocked and leads to an abnormally slow heartbeat, which may result in heart block. These slow heartbeats may require a pacemaker to correct them. The A-V node is the most common place for the electrical impulse to be blocked.

Tachycardias, or rapid heartbeats, may originate from either the atria or the ventricles and can be treated with various techniques.

Finally, arrhythmias can occur both in people whose hearts are otherwise normal and in those whose hearts have structural abnormalities.

### Treatment Approaches: Medication and Electrophysiology

Antiarrhythmic medications are designed to suppress or prevent irregular heartbeats. They can be used to slow a fast heart-beat but do not necessarily eliminate it. Although medications can be very effective, they may have side effects as well as a problem known as proarrhythmia. This means that antiarrhythmic medications may actually worsen heart rhythms. Patients with the sickest and weakest hearts are most prone to this complication, and a cardiac electrophysiologist (a cardiologist who specializes in heart rhythms) should decide whether the potential benefits of drug treatment outweigh the risks.

Many tachycardias, or fast heartbeats, can be cured by electrophysiology procedures. These are performed by cardiac electrophysiologists, generally in an outpatient setting. A very small area inside the heart, about the size of a pen tip, is cauterized, or burned. This is done to eliminate the focus that may be triggering the abnormal rhythm, or to break a circuit that allows a tachyarrhythmia to start or to maintain itself.

This procedure is done with catheters that are threaded through a blood vessel in the groin or arm, and patients are generally able to go home the same day or early the next day. Increasingly sophisticated computers, catheters, and methods of viewing the heart are already beginning to improve an already impressive cure rate and are increasing efficiency and safety.

## Implantable Defibrillators

Implantable cardioverter defibrillators (ICDs) are another tool that focuses on electricity in the heart. These are implanted into a patient's body and automatically detect life-threatening arrhythmias (Fig. 12.4). When one occurs, the device shocks the patient back to a more normal heart rhythm, much like a built-in EMS squad!

These novel implantable devices were invented by Dr. Michel Mirowski in 1969 and first used in patients at Johns Hopkins Hospital in 1980. Cardiac patients owe much to his vision, ingenuity, dogged perseverance, brilliance, and caring. Deeply saddened by the sudden death of his friend and mentor, Mirowski felt there had to be a better and faster way to resuscitate patients who suffered a sudden cardiac death, as can occur, for example, during a heart attack.

---

**Fig. 12.4**: The implantable defibrillator device acts like an EMS squad. It senses the heart rhythm, and if the heart develops a harmful rhythm, it delivers a mild shock to the ventricles and returns the heartrate to a normal level.

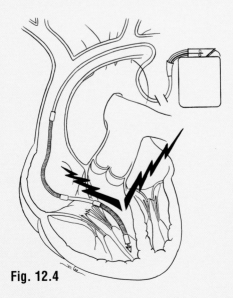

Fig. 12.4

Since the early prototypes, amazing technological advances have been made. Today, ICDs are only slightly larger than pacemakers and can be implanted exactly like them. Programming is performed with a wand that "talks" via telemetric transmission to the pulse generator (computer and battery). The implantation can be completed in about an hour or less, and patients can often go home soon after surgery.

### Tachyarrhythmias

*Atrial Fibrillation*

There are several types of atrial arrhythmias. The most common is called atrial fibrillation, in which the atria beat extremely rapidly (at more than six hundred beats per minute) and somewhat chaotically. This may cause a fast and irregular overall heart beat. Atrial fibrillation occurs more often in the elderly and in patients with hypertension, diabetes, or enlarged atria. It may also be caused by special situations such as an overactive thyroid, serious infection, or open heart surgery.

This condition is not always accompanied by visible symptoms. Only some may feel irregularity in their pulse. Whether there are symptoms or not, the biggest concern is the risk of stroke. For this reason, such patients generally receive anticoagulants, such as coumadin, to minimize stroke risk. Aspirin is the second-best treatment.

At the very least, it is important to control the heart rate in atrial fibrillation. Physicians may opt to try to restore a normal rhythm. As with other forms of abnormal heartbeat, this can often be done with antiarrhythmic medications.

The physician may try to restore the normal heart rhythm with electricity in a process called electrical cardioversion. Patients are sedated, and a shock is delivered through special pads placed on the patient's chest and/or back. This does not damage the heart and is not painful; it is often very helpful in treating atrial fibrillation.

Much progress has been made in understanding atrial fibrillation. It appears that a certain group of patients may have a trigger spot that sets off their atrial fibrillation. These may be cured with a catheter-based technique that inactivates the abnormal area.

Implantable defibrillators are also used to shock patients out of atrial fibrillation. Patients with such devices may choose when they want the device to terminate their arrhythmias (when they have bothersome symptoms), or they may elect to have the device automatically terminate the arrhyth-

mias. Finally, permanent pacing from two different sites in the atrium at the same time may help prevent or decrease the number of atrial fibrillation recurrences.

Atrial flutter is a different kind of atrial arrhythmia. It consists of a rapid and regular beating of the atria. Although electrical cardioversion can be very effective, atrial flutter can also be terminated by rapid pacing inside the heart. An exciting advance has been ablation, or the destruction of the electrical pathway with a catheter, which provides a cure in more than 90 percent of patients. Even when a total cure is not achieved, the patients may have far fewer recurrences of the flutter, particularly if they are also using anti-arrhythmic medication

### Atrial Tachycardia

Atrial tachycardia is a condition in which a rapid rhythm originates in one or both of the atria. Wolff-Parkinson-White (WPW) syndrome, named after the men who first described it, is a pattern

of this condition that can be seen on the ECG. Not every person born with WPW has an arrhythmia problem. However, the potential exists for an abnormal rhythm to occur. Ablation has an extremely high chance of curing the condition and is the treatment of choice in most of these patients.

Finally, patients may have isolated "skipped" heartbeats (one or two at a time) relating to electrical impulses coming from different areas of the heart without a sustained arrhythmia. Frequently, no therapy is required. On other occasions, the patient may wish to discuss with his or her physician what the approach should be. These are rarely, if ever, life threatening or problematic.

### Ventricular Arrhythmias

Ventricular arrhythmias, which involve the main pumping chambers of the heart, tend to be more serious than atrial arrhythmias. The three main ventricular arrhythmias include premature ventricular complexes (PVCs),

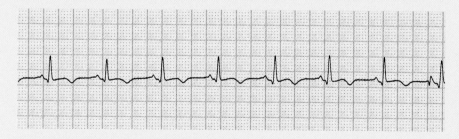

These recordings of the heart's rhythm were recorded on an ECG machine. A normal cardiac cycle, left, includes the spike typical of ventricular contraction. The heart strip below depicts atrial fibrillation. The ventricular rhythm is also irregular.

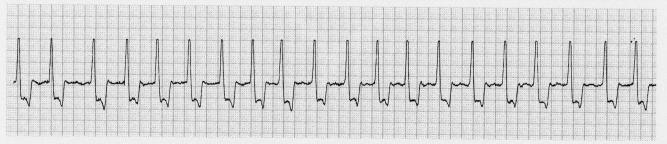

ventricular tachycardia, and ventricular fibrillation.

Premature ventricular complexes refer to beats originating from the ventricles. They may or may not indicate a serious cardiac problem, and each patient should have his or her situation individually assessed. Some people are completely unaware of their PVCs; others are very symptomatic. The approach may vary from no treatment to anti-arrhythmia drugs to ablation when appropriate.

Ventricular tachycardia is an abnormal rhythm originating in the ventricles, which often beat faster than one hundred beats per minute. It can occur in structurally normal or abnormal hearts. The rate, duration (number of beats in a row), ECG appearance, and symptoms can also vary, both within a given person and among people. As with atrial arrhythmia, some people appear to be born with the predisposition for ventricular tachyarrhythmias. Others develop this predisposition.

Management of ventricular tachyarrhythmia can be very complex, and many clinical factors need to be considered. In some cases, anti-arrhythmia medication provides good control. In other cases, ablation is the best approach. Currently, implantable cardioverter defibrillators can provide life-saving treatment for patients with potentially or actually life-threatening ventricular tachyarrhythmia.

Ventricular fibrillation is an extremely rapid, often chaotic rhythm of the ventricles. It is a very serious and often fatal condition because the heart cannot effectively pump blood to the body. Unless rapidly corrected by an electrical shock (such as from an EMS team or an external or internal defibrillator), death will follow. For most patients who have been successfully resuscitated from ventricular fibrillation, the treatment of choice is implantation of an ICD.

## General Observations

When dealing with the vast and complicated field of arrhythmia, each person's situation should be evaluated on a case by case basis. However, some general observations do apply.

Symptoms: Some people with arrhythmias do not feel them; others do. The same person may notice some arrhythmias and not others; symptoms may vary and can include palpitations (feeling certain heart beats), skipped beats or fluttering sensations, fatigue, dizziness, lightheadedness, or even loss of consciousness. The factors accounting for this variability are complex and not always understood. The presence or absence of other cardiac medical problems may play a role in some cases. An abnormal ECG or irregular or unusually fast pulse may be the first clue of an arrhythmia. Some people have symptoms but when monitored have no arrhythmias.

Triggers: Many people do not notice a pattern or trigger to their arrhythmias. For some people, drinking excess caffeine or alcohol may be a trigger, in addition to eating certain foods.

Cause: Some people are born with very subtle electrical abnormalities in their hearts, which may not be noticed by using methods such as the ECG, echocardiography, or other tests. Many such people go through life without ever having an arrhythmia. Still others develop a problem later in life. It is not well understood why this occurs.

An electrical problem can develop as a result of an abnormality or damage (such as after a heart attack, after heart valves are damaged from rheumatic fever, or after heart muscle is damaged from another cause — high blood pressure, a viral infection, etc.).

Natural history: In some people, the frequency of an arrhythmia may change spontaneously with age; more often than not, there is no clear pattern or trend in the frequency of arrhythmia recurrences. In some cases, an arrhythmia such as atrial fibrillation will recur and persist. Many factors, including certain medications, may affect what would have been the natural history of the arrhythmia.

## The Future

Advances in understanding of arrhythmias make this an exciting time in arrhythmia management. Many lives have already been saved and improved. For example, studies are presently evaluating the use of specialized pacing techniques (e.g., pacing of both ventricles at the same time) to help patients with congestive heart failure. Heading into the next millennium, we anticipate even more exciting developments.

# SURGERY FOR THE IRREGULAR HEARTBEAT

By

James L. Cox, M.D.
Professor and Chairman
Cardiovascular and Thoracic Surgery

Surgical Director
Georgetown University Cardiovascular Institute
Georgetown University Medical Center
Washington, D.C.

IRREGULARITIES OF THE heartbeat (cardiac arrhythmias) are the most common maladies affecting the heart. Because the heart does not pump blood as efficiently when it has an irregular heartbeat, patients with cardiac arrhythmias usually complain of tiredness and shortness of breath, especially with physical exertion. More serious cardiac arrhythmias may result in heart failure, strokes, and death. Fortunately, many cardiac arrhythmias can be successfully treated with medicines or catheters. However, when arrhythmias are not responsive to drug therapy and cannot be treated with catheters, heart surgery may be required if the symptoms are particularly severe or life threatening.

One of the unique problems facing surgeons who operate on the heart for cardiac arrhythmias is that the arrhythmia cannot be seen. In the past, it was necessary to place tiny electrodes on the heart to record abnormalities in the heart's electrical

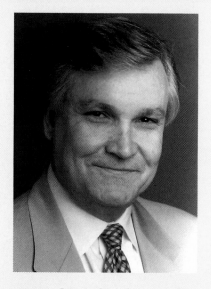

activity. Once the abnormalities were identified and located, the physician could apply the specific surgical procedure required to cure them.

The first such operation was performed for a simple arrhythmia in 1968. Although the surgical treatment of cardiac arrhythmias flourished in the 1970s and 1980s, catheter techniques were developed in 1990 that could cure virtually all arrhythmias that were not responsive to drug therapy. The one exception, unfortunately,

is the most common of all cardiac arrhythmias, atrial fibrillation.

Atrial fibrillation is a type of cardiac arrhythmia in which the electrical activity in both atria becomes chaotic, causing them to quiver (or fibrillate) rather than beat in a regular fashion. More importantly, it also results in severely irregular beating in the lower two pumping chambers, the left ventricle and the right ventricle. Because the left ventricle is the main pumping chamber of the heart, symptoms invariably develop when it pumps less efficiently than normal.

Many times, atrial fibrillation can be successfully treated with drugs and/or an electrical shock to the heart called cardioversion. Unfortunately, the drugs and cardioversion don't always work. This is particularly unfortunate because blood clots can form inside the left atrium as a result of atrial fibrillation and subsequently break off and pass through the bloodstream to the brain, where they cause a stroke. Recent studies have shown that about 2.2 million people in the United States suffer from atrial fibrillation and that seventy-five thousand strokes occur each year from this common cardiac arrhythmia.

After years of laboratory research, my research team, first working at Duke University, then at Washington University in St. Louis, developed a heart operation to cure atrial fibrillation. The procedure is referred to as the "maze procedure" and involves making several incisions in the right and left atria. The heart-lung machine is used during the surgery.

In 1987, we first used the maze procedure to treat a patient. During the past eleven years, this technique has proven to be essentially 100 percent successful. In addition, the maze procedure has been shown to eliminate the risk of stroke from atrial fibrillation, primarily because patients no longer have atrial fibrillation after the surgery.

Over the last two years, we have also developed a new minimally invasive surgical approach for the maze procedure that has resulted in much less pain and debilitation for patients. The recuperation time has been markedly reduced as well.

The maze procedure has now been applied in virtually all of the major national and international medical centers. Its use is particularly common in Japan, where several thousand patients have undergone the maze procedure for treatment of atrial fibrillation. When performed as originally described, the excellent results are reproducible by most cardiac surgeons. In our own institution, we are now performing nearly one hundred maze procedures per year. The average length of the operation is three hours, and the usual hospital stay is about one week. Most patients return to full-time activity, short of heavy physical exertion, about one month after surgery.

Although there is no catheter-based approach available that uses the maze procedure, numerous cardiologists around the world are working daily on this challenge. They are developing a technique for performing the maze procedure or some related procedure without surgery, even minimally invasive surgery. Thus far, these approaches have been highly experimental and largely unsuccessful or dangerous. Nevertheless, it is almost certain that in the near future some type of nonsurgical approach will be perfected that will be capable of curing this last, most common, and potentially dangerous cardiac arrhythmia.

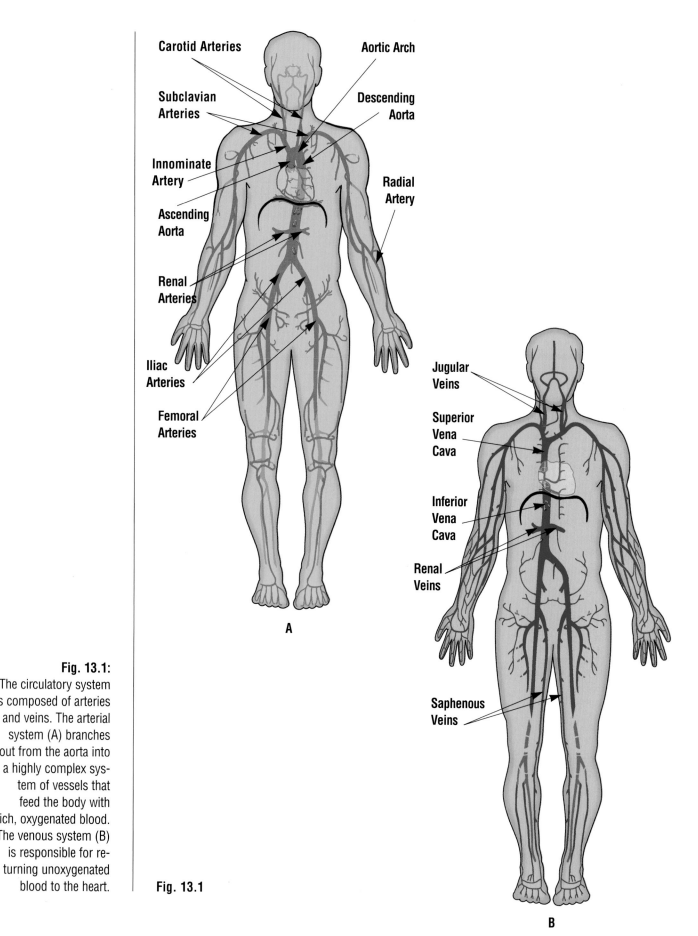

**Carotid Arteries**

**Aortic Arch**

**Subclavian Arteries**

**Descending Aorta**

**Innominate Artery**

**Radial Artery**

**Ascending Aorta**

**Renal Arteries**

**Iliac Arteries**

**Femoral Arteries**

A

**Jugular Veins**

**Superior Vena Cava**

**Inferior Vena Cava**

**Renal Veins**

**Saphenous Veins**

B

**Fig. 13.1:**
The circulatory system is composed of arteries and veins. The arterial system (A) branches out from the aorta into a highly complex system of vessels that feed the body with rich, oxygenated blood. The venous system (B) is responsible for returning unoxygenated blood to the heart.

**Fig. 13.1**

220

## CHAPTER THIRTEEN

# ANEURYSMS AND OTHER BLOOD VESSEL PROBLEMS

THE ARTERIAL SYSTEM CARRIES blood away from the heart to supply the rest of the body with nutrients and freshly oxygenated blood. The wide-ranging arterial delivery system looks much like the branches of a tree, with the main trunk, the aorta, branching directly off the heart (Fig. 13.1). The aorta is one of the body's most important blood vessels, and it is the largest. The aorta is twice the width of an average thumb and strong enough to absorb the entire blood pressure generated by the heart for the duration of life. Imagine a single pipe slightly more than one inch in diameter that carries more than fifteen hundred gallons of blood per day and remains in good repair after decades of continuous use. That is the aorta.

This main blood "highway" originates at the left ventricle, where the aortic valve regulates blood flow into the vessel. From there, the aorta first heads up toward the neck, then makes a U-turn, heading downward through the chest, usually just to the left of the body's midline, and into the abdomen. The region where the aorta makes the U-turn is called the aortic arch.

Immediately after it leaves the heart, the first branches arise from the aorta. These are the coronary arteries, and they supply the heart muscle itself with blood. The next arterial branch is the innominate artery, which originates in the aortic arch and divides into the right subclavian artery, going into the right arm, and the right carotid artery, which heads to the brain. The subclavian artery also gives off the right vertebral artery that goes to the brain.

The third arterial branch is the left carotid artery, which also goes to the brain. Next comes the left subclavian artery, which travels to the left arm and gives off the fourth artery that goes to the brain, the left vertebral artery.

As the aorta courses through the chest, numerous small branches split off to feed the chest muscles, the spinal cord, and other tissues. Just below the heart, a large breathing muscle called the diaphragm separates the contents of the chest from those of the abdomen. The aorta pierces this muscle to enter the abdomen, where the celiac artery branches off to supply the liver, spleen, and part of the stomach. Two mesenteric arteries also branch off in the abdomen and supply blood to the small and large intestines, and the renal arteries branch off and supply the kidneys.

# DACRON: MICHAEL DEBAKEY'S SURPRISE SUCCESS

DACRON GRAFTS HAPPENED TO be the best option for repairing the damaged aorta — but no one would have known that in the beginning, least of all the doctor who introduced them. Dr. Michael DeBakey recently told the story of how Dacron came to be the fabric of choice for arterial grafts:

*"It's an interesting story because another doctor had done studies with a material called Vinyon N, in which he showed that tissue would attach to it. That was what stimulated my thinking of using some kind of a plastic cloth material, and the most common material at that time was nylon.*

*"So I went to the department store to buy a yard of nylon, and it happened that they had just run out, but they said they had a new material*

*called Dacron. That was the first I heard of it, but I looked at it and felt it.*

*"I purchased several yards and cut them in different sizes to make tubes on my wife's sewing machine. I had been taught by my mother as a boy to sew, and I became an expert. These tubes proved highly successful in animals, and although we later obtained sheets of Orlon, Teflon, nylon, and Ivalon, none of these was as good as the original Dacron."*

In 1954, DeBakey was called on to treat a patient with an aneurysm of the abdominal aorta. He implanted the first Dacron graft and remembered that it "worked beautifully."

Thirty years after his early cases, DeBakey still had patients with the original Dacron grafts, although more modern versions of the grafts are used today.

---

In the lower abdomen, the aorta itself divides into the two large iliac arteries, which supply blood to the pelvis and genitalia. As they enter the legs, these become the femoral arteries, which give off various branches.

 ### The Development of Vascular Surgery

Blood vessel, or vascular, surgery followed a somewhat different pattern of development from heart surgery. In fact, doctors could suture and transplant vessels more than fifty years before the development of open heart surgery because the technique is not necessarily tied to the use of the heart-lung machine, al-

though today some of the major vascular surgical procedures use it.

Many early surgical techniques were pioneered by Dr. Alexis Carrel of Lyon, France. He later traveled to Chicago in 1905, where he and Dr. Charles Guthrie developed a way to join the ends of blood vessels (called **anastomosis**) and a technique to transplant arteries and veins and even organs. Although Carrel's work did not receive immediate attention from more mainstream doctors, he received the 1912 Nobel Prize in Physiology or Medicine for his work with blood vessel surgical techniques and organ transplantation.

World War II set the stage for the next leap forward in blood vessel surgery.

**Anastomosis:** When two blood vessels are connected. Usually done with stitching but can be done with stapling or other methods.

Blood vessels had of course been injured in previous wars, but World War II saw antibiotics, blood transfusions, and a much higher percentage of formally trained surgeons, factors necessary for vascular surgery to advance. Doctors began to use improved surgical techniques to repair injured blood vessels, and surgeons also successfully treated coarctation of the aorta, a congenital condition in which a portion of the aorta in a newborn child is abnormally narrow.

The 1950s, when the heart-lung machine was in development, were exciting years for blood vessel surgery. Early in the decade, surgeons began to report success in removing aortic aneurysms (Fig. 13.2) and replacing them with segments of aortas from human cadavers. An aneurysm is the abnormal "ballooning" of an artery or other blood vessel. During the Korean War, advancing vascular surgical techniques helped lower the amputation rate from 49.6 percent in World War II to 11.1 percent.

Many of these 1950s techniques in vessel grafting are still in use today for smaller arterial injuries. However, synthetic grafts have mostly replaced biological grafts for replacing larger-diameter arteries. These synthetic grafts were pioneered in 1952 by Dr. Arthur Voorhees at Columbia University, where a team of doctors developed cloth tubes to replace diseased arteries. Over the next ten years, the devices were improved by the introduction of the crimped graft and by Michael DeBakey's introduction of Dacron arterial grafts.

During the 1950s, DeBakey, Drs. Denton Cooley and E. Stanley Crawford, and other members of their team led the way in graft replacements of various segments of the thoracic aorta for aneurysm. Other operations had to wait for the development of the heart-lung machine. The replacement of the aortic arch was one of those and remained beyond the surgeon's knife until 1957, when the same Houston group removed an aortic arch aneurysm and replaced the diseased segment with a reconstituted aortic arch from a human cadaver.

### Aortic Aneurysms

About two-thirds of the time, aortic aneurysms are discovered accidentally on a routine chest x-ray. About 25 percent to 33 percent of patients with aortic aneurysms have some degree of pain or discomfort in the chest or neck related to the aneurysm expanding and pushing on adjacent structures, including nerves. Sometimes there are other symptoms related to the aneurysm pushing or stretching nearby organs or

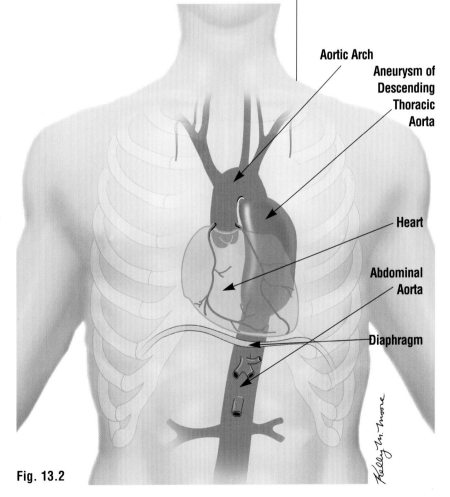

**Fig. 13.2:**
An aortic aneurysm occurs when a section of the major artery balloons out and weakens. It is a very dangerous condition that can be treated in a variety of ways.

Aortic Arch

Aneurysm of Descending Thoracic Aorta

Heart

Abdominal Aorta

Diaphragm

**Fig. 13.2**

tissue. If an aneurysm is suspected, doctors will obtain a CT of the chest and/or an MRI scan and/or an angiogram of the aorta. Any one of these tests usually confirms the diagnosis.

Aortic aneurysm is a dangerous condition that often requires surgery. It can occur anywhere in the aorta, including the ascending aorta, the aortic arch, the descending aorta, the abdominal aorta, or where the aorta divides and becomes the iliac arteries. Aneurysms tend to enlarge over time, and they are more likely to rupture as they get larger. If they rupture, death is likely to occur fairly quickly. Surgery is recommended if the aneurysm is moderate to large in size, or even if it is relatively small but enlarging quickly.

Surgery to repair an aortic aneurysm tends to become more challenging as the vessel nears the heart. If an aneurysm occurs in the ascending aorta, the heart-lung machine has to be used during graft replacement. If the aortic heart valve is also leaking, a heart surgeon may need to repair or replace it. During replacement of the ascending aorta, the coronary arteries may need to be detached. In that case, they can either be reimplanted directly into the synthetic graft, or they can be bypassed and the bypass graft sewn to the synthetic vascular graft (Fig. 13.3 and Fig. 13.4).

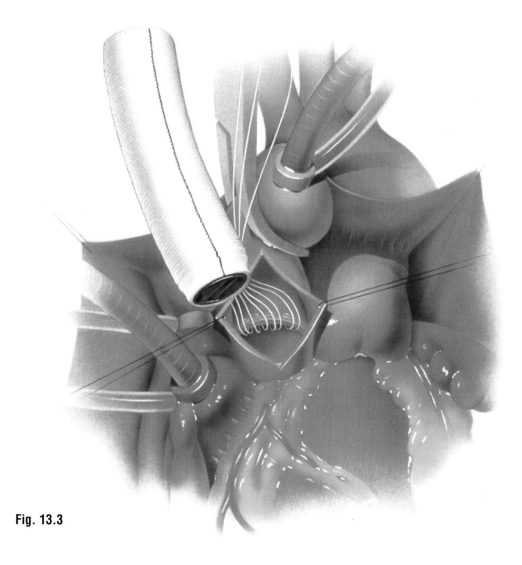

**Fig. 13.3:**
During placement of an arterial graft in the aorta, the diseased section of the ascending aorta and aortic valve is removed, then replaced with a synthetic tube and artificial valve.

**Fig. 13.3**

Patients who undergo elective surgery for aneurysms of the thoracic aorta have about a 90 percent chance of surviving the procedure, but the risk can be somewhat lower or higher depending on the exact circumstances, such as age, other medical conditions, and so forth. Most patients do well after the surgery and have about a 70 percent to 80 percent chance ten years later of being free of additional problems related to that aneurysm surgery.

If there is an aneurysm in the aortic arch, aortic aneurysm surgery is more serious and risky because of the vessels that arise to feed the brain. There are two common approaches to this kind of surgery. In the first, the heart-lung machine is used to cool the patient's body temperature to 20°C or even colder. The patient's head may be packed in ice, and while the aneurysm is replaced and the vessels going to the brain are reimplanted, the heart-lung machine is turned off. Keeping the patient cold slows the metabolism and thereby protects the brain. The patient is in a state of hypothermia during which there may be no circulation to the brain, the heart, or the rest of the body for several minutes and sometimes as long as an hour. There are other techniques with which the brain can be supplied with blood during these procedures.

For aneurysms of the descending aorta, various bypass techniques are usually used, and these depend on the surgeon's preference. If an aneurysm is in the abdomen, no special circulatory support is usually needed. The surgeon clamps each side of the aneurysm, opens it, and replaces that segment of the aorta with a synthetic graft, usually of Dacron. If the iliac arteries are involved, a graft divided into two limbs at one end like a pair of pants is used.

Sometimes more than one portion of the aorta is affected by the aneurysm. Some aortic aneurysms involve portions of the aorta in both the chest and the abdomen. These are called thoracoab-

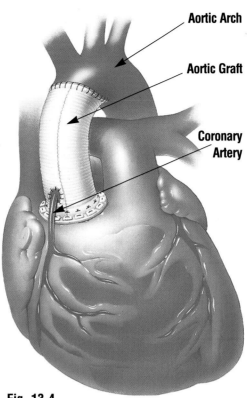

**Fig. 13.4**

**Aortic Arch**

**Aortic Graft**

**Coronary Artery**

**Fig. 13.4:**
The graft, which replaces a section of the aorta, resembles the aorta in both size and function. The coronary arteries are implanted onto the graft.

dominal aortic aneurysms. When these aneurysms are replaced with synthetic grafts, the many arteries that branch off the aorta in that area will usually be sewn back onto the synthetic graft.

### Catheter or Stent Treatment of Aortic Aneurysms

During the last several years, stents have been developed to treat aortic aneurysms. These are somewhat similar to the stents used to open a blockage in a coronary artery but much longer. These devices have been used to treat aortic aneurysms in both the abdominal aorta and the thoracic aorta.

The stents are coiled and attached to a catheter that is inserted into an artery in the leg. When the stent reaches the aortic aneurysm, a balloon on the catheter is inflated, which causes the stent to uncoil and form a new channel for the blood, and theoretically cures the aneurysm.

These procedures are being done at relatively few centers. They are still considered experimental and are done with the approval and supervision of the Food and Drug Administration (FDA). The results are encouraging, but these procedures are not yet widely available at most centers performing vascular surgery. Hopefully, as research with these techniques advances, stent procedures for the treatment of aortic aneurysms will become routine and may spare patients major surgery.

### Aortic Dissection

**Aortic dissection** is a condition in which the layers of the aorta separate and begin to come apart, or unravel (Fig. 13.5). There are three layers to the aorta and other arteries. The innermost layer is called the intima. There is a middle layer called the media, and the outer layer is the adventitia. When a dissection occurs, these layers separate. The dissections can start in almost any portion of the aorta and can progress either upstream or downstream. As the tear progresses, it can shear off the aorta's arterial branches, and in some cases the various branches of the aorta are no longer able to supply blood to the organs and tissue beyond that point. This is a serious situation.

Severe chest pain is a cardinal symptom of aortic dissection and occurs in about 90 percent of patients. This pain can initially be confused with that of a heart attack. The location of the pain in the chest can vary depending on where in the aorta the dissection is located and can be in the breast, in the neck, or in the back. It is often described as a "ripping" or "tearing" type of pain. Other signs and symptoms can also be present depending on which organs are no longer getting enough blood. If the outer wall of the aorta ruptures, the patient will go into shock from blood loss, and death usually follows rapidly.

Sometimes the entire aorta, from the aortic valve to the iliac arteries, is involved. Usually, when treating an aortic dissection surgically, the area upstream is repaired. If the ascending aorta is involved, the portion up to and sometimes including the aortic arch is replaced with a synthetic graft.

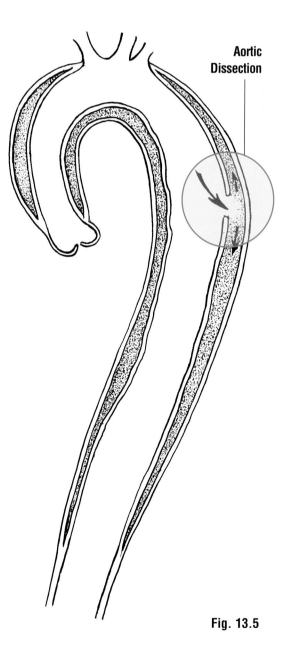

Aortic Dissection

**Fig. 13.5**

**Fig. 13.5:
Aortic Dissection:**
This condition occurs when the interior wall of the aorta begins to weaken and rupture. If caught early enough, it is a treatable condition.

226

Sometimes the aortic valve also needs to be repaired or replaced.

If the dissection is acute (the aorta has just dissected), the risk of death or severe complications during surgical repair can be quite high. There is also the risk of paraplegia (being paralyzed from the waist down). Without surgery, however, the risk of death and complications is generally higher.

If the dissection starts in the descending aorta and does not involve the ascending aorta, this condition can frequently be treated with medicine to lower blood pressure. Surgery can often be avoided for aortic dissections of the descending aorta only.

### Traumatic Aortic Rupture

The aorta can also rupture as a result of trauma, particularly as a result of a car accident in which a person is not wearing a seat belt and hits the chest on the steering wheel. In this case, urgent or emergency surgery is required to repair the tear.

Patients who make it to the hospital alive are those in whom the tear is contained by the adventitia, or outer aortic wall. However, these tears usually need to be repaired relatively soon because there is a high likelihood of the tear rupturing through the adventitia within the first few days after it occurs. In some cases, the tear can be repaired with simple stitches. In many cases, however, the injured portion of the aorta has to be replaced with a Dacron graft. Any time surgery is performed on the aorta, particularly the descending aorta in the chest, there's a chance that a patient may become paraplegic, or paralyzed from the waist down, as a result of the surgery because this is where the blood vessels going to the spinal cord branch off. There are certain techniques that lower the chances of becoming paralyzed, but even in the best hands, this complication occurs.

### Atherosclerotic Disease of the Aorta and its Branches

As with the coronary arteries, which can become blocked from atherosclerotic material, the aorta itself can become extensively atherosclerosed (Fig. 13.6). Although, because it is a large vessel, it will not usually become totally blocked, its various branches can become blocked and may need to be bypassed.

In some cases, the atherosclerotic material can be cleaned out of the branches of the aorta (but usually not out of the aorta itself). This procedure is called an endarterectomy. It is performed by opening the artery and using special instru-

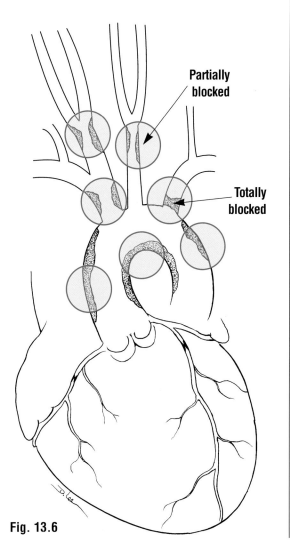

**Partially blocked**

**Totally blocked**

Fig. 13.6

**Fig. 13.6:** Atherosclerotic material can build up in the aorta's major branches. This can be treated with surgery.

ments to "peel out" the atherosclerotic plaque. Often, the intima, or inner lining of the arterial wall, is removed with this clump of material. The artery wall is then stitched back together. Where the blockage is, how extensive it is, and a number of other factors affect whether the surgeon will choose to bypass the blockage, replace a segment of artery, or perform an endarterectomy. The carotid arteries are particularly suitable for endarterectomy.

When arteries in the leg become clogged, this may cause pain when walking. This is analogous to the angina or chest pain that occurs when there's not enough blood getting to the heart muscle. In this case, the muscles in the leg ache and throb. Patients may have to stop walking and rest until the pain subsides. This condition is called **claudication**, and the pain can come on with minimal exercise or only after prolonged periods of walking or running.

If the arteries to the legs are blocked, a doctor may be able to dilate these arteries with a balloon catheter. If not, an endarterectomy may need to be performed, or segments may need to be replaced or bypassed. This depends on the location of the blockage and other factors.

If the arteries in the leg are severely blocked in all of their subbranches, the area of the leg downstream could actually die and develop gangrene. In certain cases, toes or a portion of the foot or leg may even have to be amputated. Fortunately, in most cases, this is not necessary because of the surgical arterial revascularization techniques that are currently available. In general, if an artery is injured or damaged, it's best to try to fix it or replace it.

### Venous Disease

Veins are blood vessels that return blood to the heart, and the atherosclerotic process tends to spare them. Veins also have better collateral channels (accessory blood vessels or routes), so if a vein does become blocked, the blood can usually flow in another direction around the blockage and still get back to the heart.

### Blood Clots in Veins

Blood clots can form in the veins just under the skin in the leg or arm (Fig. 13.7). When this occurs, the skin over the vein is often tender and inflamed. The clotted vein under the skin usually feels like a cord. This condition is called superficial thrombophlebitis (superficial, for just under the surface; thrombo for blood clot; phleb for vein; itis for inflammation). This is not generally a serious condition but more of a nuisance. If it occurs in an arm vein while in the hospital, it can be related to an intravenous catheter that had been in the vein for several days. Most of the time, this problem is self-limiting and is treated with aspirin or other drugs that block the activity of the platelets in the blood. If there is considerable inflammation involving skin around the vein, antibiotics may also be prescribed.

Deep vein thrombosis, or DVT, occurs when veins deep in the tissue of the leg or pelvis become blocked with blood clots. It may be caused by lying in bed, crossing your legs for prolonged periods, or other factors. It can result in painful inflammation around the vein. Depending on where the blockage is, patients may need anticoagulant drugs to prevent the clot from getting larger or possibly even drugs that can dissolve the clot. If the clot breaks loose and travels through the heart to the lungs, patients will likely be treated with anticoagulant medicine such as coumadin for many weeks or longer.

Occasionally, veins that have blockages are bypassed, or the clot is removed. With the larger veins, particularly when the vein is injured, a surgeon may repair

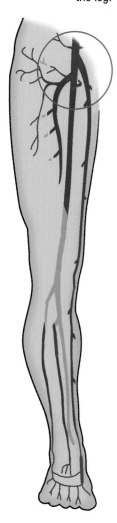

**Claudication:**
Pain, numbness or tiredness in the leg caused when the muscles are not getting enough oxygenated blood.

**Fig. 13.7:**
Clots can also occur in the veins of the leg.

the vein or bypass the injured area, but under most circumstances, bypasses of veins are not performed, and reconstruction of veins is not commonly done because veins have numerous backup, or collateral, channels. If one portion becomes blocked, the other portions can take over. In addition, atherosclerosis generally does not affect the veins.

If clots continue to develop or if patients cannot take an anticoagulant because they have a bleeding disorder or bleeding ulcers, they may need a filter inserted in the inferior vena cava. Blood clot filters come in different shapes, and all are inserted through a catheter. They prevent larger clots from getting through the vena cava and traveling to the lungs, where they can cause shortness of breath. If the clot is big enough, it may actually block the blood flow to the lungs and could be fatal. When a blood clot goes to the lungs, this is called a **pulmonary embolus**. Most blood clots that travel to the lungs can be dissolved with drugs, but sometimes they need to be removed surgically.

### Varicose Veins

A varicose vein is one that has become enlarged and somewhat twisted. Typically, this condition involves the veins in the legs, particularly those just beneath the skin. The valves in the veins become incompetent. These veins become engorged and can look very unsightly. They can also clot off and can be very painful. This can occur during pregnancy. Exercising will ease the burden on the veins. Patients can wear elastic stockings, especially if their occupation requires long periods of standing. They should lose excess weight as well.

There are a number of techniques that can be used to treat varicose veins. The veins can be injected with a chemical agent which causes them to collapse permanently. This is called sclerotherapy, which is a relatively simple and effective way to treat varicose veins. Some of the risks of sclerotherapy include brown spots at the injection sites, clot development in the superficial veins, and a reaction to the injected chemicals. Sometimes, new bursts of small red or purple veins called spider veins occur as a result of the chemical injections. Spider veins can often be removed with laser therapy. In some cases, varicose veins may have to be removed through a surgical procedure, which is referred to as vein stripping. Fortunately, the procedure is straightforward and low in risk.

### Venous Insufficiency

Venous insufficiency is a condition in which the valves in the veins in the legs become damaged and incompetent. As a result of this, the legs may swell, particularly in the ankle areas. This is a relatively common condition. It cannot be cured, but there are things that can be done to lessen the problem. Patients need to wear support stockings. Certain exercises help. Long periods of standing should be avoided; when sitting in a chair, patients should elevate their legs. Sometimes other types of treatments are necessary.

In more advanced cases, the skin in the calf and ankle area may break down, and sores called venous stasis ulcers form. There are various treatments available for this condition. In some cases, surgery can be done to repair or replace the damaged valves in the vein.

**Pulmonary Embolism:** This happens when an abnormal piece of material (embolus), such as a blood clot, lodges in one of the blood vessels in the lungs, usually causing damage and possible shortness of breath.

# STENT-GRAFTS:
# AVOIDING MAJOR AORTIC SURGERY

By
## D. Craig Miller, M.D.
Thelma and Henry Doelger Professor of Cardiovascular Surgery
Stanford University
Stanford, California

THE CONVENTIONAL SURgery to repair an aneurysm of the descending portion of the thoracic aorta is a major operation. It requires a large incision between the ribs on the left side of the chest and has a substantial risk of death or serious complications, including stroke and lower body paralysis. After surgery, the hospital stay can range from one to two weeks followed by months of convalescence and rehabilitation. It is much more complex and risky surgery than coronary artery bypass graft or heart valve surgery.

Our surgically treated aneurysm patients are very grateful to be alive and free of the risk of aneurysm rupture but usually don't get back to feeling normal until three or more months after the operation. Despite this difficulty, surgical treatment of thoracic aorta aneurysms has saved innumerable lives since the late 1950s — and otherwise these aneurysms are almost universally fatal. Similar to a "blister" on a

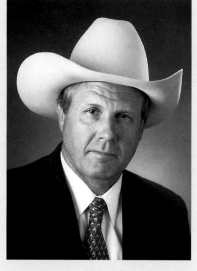

worn-out car tire, the aneurysm may blow out unpredictably.

Unfortunately, most of the aneurysms do not cause symptoms, such as back or chest pain, until they are very large. They are commonly discovered only serendipitously, for instance when a chest x-ray is ordered to evaluate other symptoms. Patients with thoracic aortic aneurysms often do not have any warning that they have a life-threatening aortic problem until something catastrophic occurs.

Thanks to better diagnostic tests (mostly imaging techniques such as CT, MRI scans, and echocardiography) and longer life spans, the number of patients diagnosed with an aneurysm of the thoracic aorta has grown rapidly over the last decade. Patients at the highest risk of having an aneurysm are middle-aged to elderly people who have a history of high blood pressure; younger individuals born with "weak" aortas that they inherited; and those with a family history of aortic aneurysm or aortic dissection.

In the last two decades, minimally invasive techniques, often using catheters and smaller incisions, have been developed to treat more heart and cardiovascular problems. This treatment results in less pain and trauma to the patient and shorter hospital stays. Indeed, many heart and peripheral arterial problems that ten years ago required a week in the hospital can now be treated on an outpatient basis.

Because the surgery done to repair thoracic aortic aneurysms is so traumatic and the recovery process so long compared with that for many other cardiovascular problems, there is good reason to use minimally invasive techniques. Conventional surgical treatment of aneurysms requires replacing the weakened segment of the aorta with a Dacron tube graft.

To accomplish this using minimally invasive techniques and without opening the chest, the aneurysm must be covered with a tube placed inside the aorta. This blocks the high-pressure blood flow from entering the thin, weakened aneurysmal segment and eliminates the chance of aortic rupture. This inner graft, or "sleeve," must be anchored firmly on either end so it cannot migrate over time.

This device is called a "stent-graft," or covered stent. In a stent graft, an expanding metal stent is used to anchor the synthetic tube graft to the normal aortic wall. This stent is unlike the more commonly used uncovered stents, which are open metal frameworks that crush plaque against the arterial wall and open a bigger channel for more blood flow.

At Stanford University Medical School, we have been exploring the use of endovascular, or in-vessel, stent-grafts to treat various types of aneurysms of the descending thoracic aorta (Fig. 13.8) since 1992. To the surprise of some and the utter amazement of others, these pioneering efforts have been fairly successful. The clinical feasibility of using stent-grafts for descending thoracic aortic aneurysms has

been firmly established, even though the learning curve was fairly steep. We learned which specific types of aneurysms are best suited to stent-grafting, which patients could be treated successfully, and many essential technical points about gaining access to the aorta, device design, and stent-graft deployment.

We conducted the first large-scale clinical trial of descending thoracic aortic endovascular stent-graft repair in 103 patients between 1992 and 1997 at Stanford University. The average age of the patients was sixty-nine years. Importantly, 60 percent of cases were judged by a cardiovascular surgeon to be otherwise inoperable.

In this preliminary first-generation study, a primitive self-expanding stent-graft device was used. This "home brew" stent-graft used self-expanding stainless steel covered with woven Dacron. The device was semirigid and quite large in diameter (10mm–15 mm, or more than one-half inch). Various types of aneurysms were treated, including atherosclerotic/degenerative aneurysms, a few aortic dissections, and others. Although the stent-graft was intended to be inserted in the groin by using a small incision and general anesthesia, the large size of this early device and/or arterial blockages in the pelvis and abdomen made this possible in only 58 percent of cases. A larger incision in the left flank was therefore necessary in 30 percent.

Immediate serious complications included fatal aortic perforation in one patient, obstruction of the aortic arch due to buckling of the stent graft in another, stent-

graft misdeployment outside the target zone in 3 percent, and a major peripheral arterial injury in 4 percent. The early mortality was 9 percent, which was quite good considering how old and sick many of these patients were.

Early neurological complications, which are the most dreaded complications of this type of major surgery, included paraplegia (paralysis of the legs and lower body) in 3 percent and stroke in 7 percent. The incidence of paralysis was similar to that for open surgical repair. The only risk factor associated with a higher probability of paraplegia was "more difficult surgical access," i.e., the need to insert the stent-graft via the abdominal aorta. We believe the stroke was caused by debris coming loose from the aorta and traveling to the brain in five of the seven cases, but two strokes were due to cerebral hemorrhage. No risk factors for stroke were identified.

The link between the design of our primitive device and stroke is indirectly substantiated by our more recent (1998) experience in an FDA Phase I trial in twenty-three carefully selected patients. We used a new commercial stent-graft called the Thoracic Excluder, built by W.L. Gore and Associates, Inc. In the entire FDA Phase I trial, which included twenty-eight patients, there were no strokes and no cases of paraplegia. We attribute this primarily to advanced design features, but more careful selection of patients could have also played a role. Nonetheless, the ability to avoid using large, stiff catheters and hardware inside the atherosclerotic ascending aorta and arch

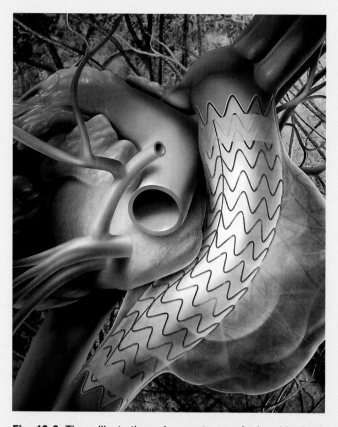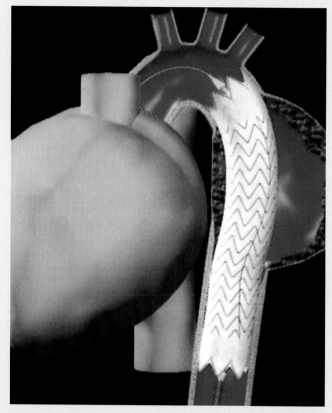

**Fig. 13.8:** These illustrations show a stent-graft placed in the descending thoracic aorta. After the stent-graft has been placed inside the aneurysm, which can be seen bulging out to the right, blood flow can no longer enter the aneurysm sac. The aneurysm, which becomes a "blind pouch," then clots, and over time, it is hoped this blood clot will turn into scar tissue and the aneurysm sac will shrink. *(Illustration courtesy of W.L. Gore and Associates, Inc.)*

is a key advance. Additionally, this new stent-graft conforms more easily to the curved aortic arch, is more flexible, and is considerably smaller. This gives us reason to expect that the incidence of stroke in the future will be much lower than before.

Given that 60 percent of the initial 103 cases treated with stent-grafts at Stanford University were deemed inoperable, our five-year clinical experience with the first-generation device indicates that endovascular stent-grafting of descending thoracic aortic aneurysms is feasible and relatively safe. The more refined devices available today cause

much less trauma and enable more precise stent-graft deployment, which should further reduce the risks and make this procedure more reliable. These major design and technical advances, coupled with the lessons we have learned and more refined patient selection, should mean the results will be even better in the future.

Nonetheless, caution is necessary because very long-term follow-up is required before we can be completely confident this approach is a permanent solution. Only ten years or more of observation of greater numbers of patients will determine if

stent-grafting is a durable and effective alternative approach to preventing aneurysm rupture. Until these long-term results are available, our Stanford multidisciplinary group believes younger, low-surgical-risk patients should opt for conventional open surgical graft replacement, which has a forty-year proven track record and is the gold standard. Conversely, stent-grafts are a reasonable option for patients who are not surgical candidates owing to advanced age or other coexisting medical problems and who otherwise cannot be offered any form of treatment.

# SURGERY OF THE THORACIC AORTA

By

## Nicholas T. Kouchoukos, M.D.

Cardiothoracic Surgeon
Missouri Baptist Hospital
St. Louis, Missouri

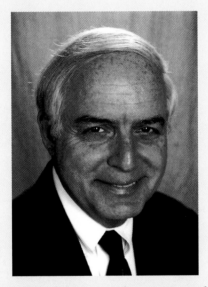

DURING THE LAST DECADE, extraordinary progress has been made in the treatment of aneurysms of the thoracic and thoracoabdominal aorta. We have better diagnostic techniques as well as improved substitutions for the aortic wall and safer systems to protect patients during surgery.

Currently, it is possible to safely cool the brain to low temperatures (12° to 15°C, or 54° to 59°F) by using the heart-lung machine. At these temperatures, the circulation can be totally stopped for up to forty-five minutes (and sometimes even longer) without producing detectable injury to the brain. This allows surgeons to remove diseased segments of the ascending aorta and aortic arch with a mortality in most instances of 10 percent or less and a correspondingly low incidence of brain damage.

Until recently, operations to replace long segments of the descending thoracic or thoracoabdominal aorta were associated with a high risk of death, a high risk of paralysis (up to 40 percent) of the legs (paraplegia), and a risk of kidney failure. Fortunately, however, this risk for this kind of aortic surgery has been lowered. Doctors support the circulation with a pump or a heart-lung machine, and in some instances cool the spinal cord and kidneys during operations. Surgery on these segments of the aorta can now be performed with a mortality of 10 percent or less and a risk of paralysis or kidney failure that does not exceed 5 percent.

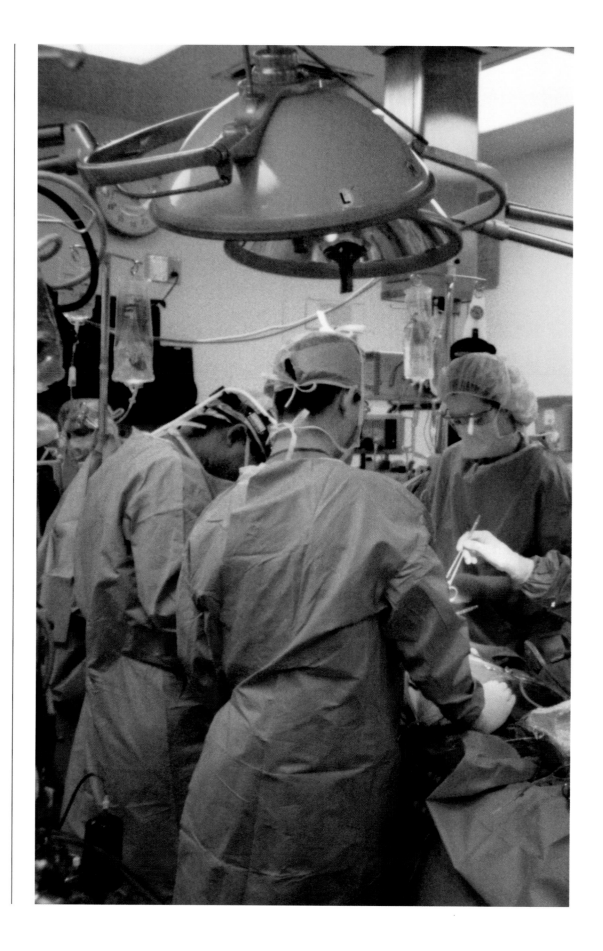

As techniques in heart surgery improve, it is possible to operate on older victims of heart disease. This raises new questions for both the patient and the family.

## CHAPTER FOURTEEN

# HEART SURGERY IN THE ELDERLY

AMERICA IS GROWING OLDER. According to data compiled in the 1980 census, 43 percent of all Americans alive then were expected to live to be eighty-eighty years old. In 1990, 7.4 million Americans — 3 percent of the population — were eighty years of age or older. In 2010, the corresponding estimate is that 4.3 percent, or 12 million, Americans will be octogenarians.

Heart disease is relatively more common among the elderly. By the age of seventy years, clinically diagnosed coronary artery disease is present in approximately 15 percent of men and 9 percent of women. Likewise, hypertension affects as much as 50 percent of the population by age seventy. Among octogenarians, approximately 40 percent of the population has cardiovascular disease; 18 percent to 20 percent of those people have coronary artery disease.

Reports in the medical literature vary as to the cut-off age for being classified as elderly. One report from Israel titled "Heart Valve Replacement in Elderly Patients" published in the medical journal *Geriatrics* as recently as 1970 included all patients more than forty-five years of age! As heart surgery has advanced,

however, age limits for performing heart surgery have been rolled back. In 1978, I coauthored a medical article published in the heart journal *Circulation* titled "Surgery Using Cardiopulmonary Bypass in the Elderly." At that time, our experience was with eighty-nine patients seventy years of age or older. To my knowledge, this was the first article to specifically deal with heart surgery in patients who were seventy years of age or older. Now it is likely that at least a third of the patients who undergo coronary artery bypass graft surgery are age sixty-five to seventy years or older.

As the age limit continued to advance, I coauthored an article published in *The New England Journal of Medicine* in 1988 entitled "Open Heart Surgery in the Octogenarian." In that article we again reviewed our results at the Hospital of the University of Pennsylvania, but this time examining one hundred consecutive patients who were eighty years of age or older. I believe this was one of the first two or three medical articles to specifically address heart surgery in those older patients. At that time the oldest patient operated on in our group was ninety-seven years old. When I did the follow-up evaluation, our ninety-seven-year-old lady was age 102. She was in good spirits and doing well.

I subsequently operated on another ninety-seven-year-old woman who had already had her heart valve dilated with a balloon catheter and had been on a mechanical ventilator two or three times because of episodes of severe shortness of breath. I replaced one heart valve, performed a coronary bypass, and installed a pacemaker. She became somewhat of a celebrity in the local news at hospital discharge.

Common sense dictates discretion when recommending major surgery in octogenarians. The aging process reduces the reserves of all organs. For example, these patients are more prone to develop strokes, kidney failure, and pneumonia after major operations. Some vital organs might lack sufficient reserve to absorb the stresses of major surgery. Moreover, these persons, having most of their lives behind them, may lack both the will and the incentive to endure the physical and mental exhaustion associated with major surgery. Generally, octogenarians do not seek open heart surgery; it is forced upon them by the onset or progression of cardiac disease. Operations become the best of the unattractive options.

The chances of complications after major surgery increase with age, particularly beyond age seventy-five years. There are, however, a considerable number of elderly patients with good minds who are limited only by their heart disease. I personally have observed a number of these elderly patients who were almost bedridden and after a relatively simple, straightforward heart operation were able to return to an active and fulfilling life, including in some cases mowing their own lawns, shopping, and so forth.

It is my opinion, however, that elderly patients should not be pushed into heart surgery, by either their family or their physician. As already pointed out, some patients age eighty years or more feel they have lived their life and will not choose to undergo a major heart operation under any circumstances. I believe their wishes should be respected. When some elderly patients are pushed into these operations by family or physicians, they sometimes lack the will to fight and to help the physicians and nurses get them through the surgery and postoperative recovery. Lacking the will and not doing what is necessary to recover make it more difficult and frustrating for the patient, the physicians, the nurses, and especially the family.

So what is the age limit at which one would not recommend performing a heart operation? The answer to that question varies. I believe most surgeons feel that patients should have a good mind and not be bedridden or incapacitated from diseases other than their heart problem. The likelihood that heart surgery can be performed to get the patients back on their feet is worth considering, regardless of age. The other factor that needs to be considered is that even though two patients may have been born on January 1, 1915, one person, in health and general attitude, could seem more like sixty-five years of age whereas the other may be more like one hundred years of age. The chronological and physiological ages of elderly patients can vary greatly. This, too, has to be considered by physicians when they consider whether to recommend heart surgery.

In some countries where the government controls health care, there have been official or unofficial age limits mandating who can and who cannot have heart surgery. This of course involves sensitive ethical and economic issues. Some countries can afford to offer expensive operations to elderly patients at high risk. Is there a level of risk that precludes operation? And if so, who will decide what it is? Is it ethical to refuse to perform high-risk operations when the alternatives have higher risks? Are surgeons justified in exercising preoperative selection criteria without including the patient in the decision-making process? Can patients demand operations? These and other questions deserve open discussion both within and outside the medical community.

On the basis of the heart surgery results published in the medical literature, surgical intervention can be a reasonable therapeutic option in elderly patients with advanced cardiac disease in whom alternative approaches have failed or are not feasible. Nonetheless, the risk of death and other complications is somewhat higher in these patients.

Although there is no particular medical reason to set an age limit for patients undergoing heart transplantation, there is in fact an age limit set by most heart transplant centers of about age sixty-five years or less. This age limit is arbitrary and not related to patient characteristics but rather to the scarcity of heart donors. The feeling is that younger patients who have more of their life ahead of them should receive the heart transplant.

### Coronary Artery Disease and Viagra

As male patients get older, the chance of developing coronary disease increases. The incidence of **erectile dysfunction** or impotence also increases with aging. Recently, a new medication called Viagra has become available to treat erectile dysfunction. Although effective, it should not be used with certain heart medications. Those of us who specialize in heart disease receive many questions regarding Viagra and sometimes questions on other treatment options for impotence from patients who shouldn't take Viagra. I have therefore asked my colleague, Dr. Chipriya B. Dhabuwala, who specializes in impotence and is a professor of urology at Wayne State University, to discuss Viagra as it relates to heart medication and to also discuss other treatment options available for erectile dysfunction.

### Erectile Dysfunction, Viagra, and Heart Disease

by C.B. Dhabuwala, MD
Professor of Urology
Wayne State University, Detroit, Michigan

Impotence, or erectile dysfunction, is the inability to achieve or maintain an erection for sexual intercourse. The incidence of erectile dysfunction increases with age. It is estimated that 20 to 30 million men suffer from erectile dysfunction in the United States.

### Mechanism of Erection

Erection is a complex process that begins with impulses of sexual arousal at the brain centers of sexual excitement. The impulses travel along nerves from the brain to the penis, where they cause secretion of a substance called nitric oxide. Nitric oxide sends signals that cause dilatation of blood vessels and increase blood flow to the penis. It is estimated that during the early stages of erection, the blood flow in the penis increases 2,000 percent to 4,000 percent. This increase in blood flow, along with the relaxation of the smooth muscles of the penis, causes the penis to increase in length and diameter (engorgement). The veins that normally drain the blood away from the penis are closed during erection. Any disturbance in the whole chain of events can contribute to erectile dysfunction.

### Causes of Erectile Dysfunction

The incidence of erectile dysfunction increases with age. Hardening of the arteries and blockage within the arteries is the most common cause of erection problems. Very often, blockage of the arteries of the penis occurs with blockage of the coro-

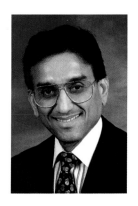

C.B. Dhabuwala, M.D.

**Erectile Dysfunction:** Also referred to as impotence. The inability to achieve or maintain an erection for sexual intercourse.

**Leriche's Syndrome:**
Involves blockages of the lower aorta as well as the arteries in the pelvis coming off the aorta, including the iliac arteries. It is characterized by claudication, which is pain, aching, and tiredness of the legs and buttocks. It is associated with erectile dysfunction.

**Guanosine Monophosphate (Cyclic GMP):**
A chemical neuromediator that helps to transmit messages through the nervous system.

nary arteries of the heart. In many individuals, the erection problem is followed a few years later by coronary artery disease and even heart attack. Blockage of the terminal aorta (**Leriche's syndrome**), internal iliac arteries, or internal pudendal arteries by the atherosclerotic process can also lead to erectile dysfunction.

There are many other reasons for erectile dysfunction. People with diabetes are at increased risk of developing erection problems. Several studies suggest that almost half the people suffering from diabetes develop erectile dysfunction. High blood pressure can lead to progressive thickening of the arteries of the penis and is associated with erection problems. Smoking cigarettes, excessive use of alcohol, and abuse of substances such as marijuana and cocaine are also associated with erection problems. Automobile and motorcycle accidents causing fracture of the pelvis can very often interrupt the blood supply or the nerve supply of the penis, leading to erection problems.

Other causes of erectile dysfunction include surgeries for cancer of the rectum or prostate cancer, which can damage the nerves that register sexual excitement. Certain medications used for treating high blood pressure, diseases of the nervous system such as multiple sclerosis and spinal cord injury, and even radiation therapy for prostate cancer can also lead to erectile dysfunction.

In younger individuals without any risk factors such as diabetes, high blood pressure, and cigarette smoking, the cause of erectile dysfunction is often psychological.

About 5 percent to 10 percent of men with erection problems have low levels of male hormones. Many men can be effectively treated with male hormones.

**Medical Treatment of Erectile Dysfunction**

Treatment of erectile dysfunction very often depends upon the cause of erectile

dysfunction. A person with hormone deficiency will respond best to hormone replacement. Erectile dysfunction due to the use of medications may respond to a change in the medications. Very often, replacing one medication with another may resolve erectile problems.

*Viagra, a Pill that Helps Men with Erectile Dysfunction*

Viagra, which is also called sildenafil, has provided a breakthrough in the oral treatment of erectile dysfunction. An erection normally occurs with the relaxation of the smooth muscles of the cavernous sinuses and an increase in blood flow to the penis. Nitric oxide produced in response to erotic stimuli acts through a secondary system involving cyclic GMP. This cyclic **guanosine monophosphate**, or GMP, relaxes the smooth muscles, which increases blood flow and penile erection. The human body naturally inactivates cyclic GMP. Viagra prevents this local inactivation of cyclic GMP, thereby enhancing the erection.

In clinical trials, Viagra-related improvement in erections occurred in 70 percent to 90 percent of patients. The pill is taken one hour before sexual activity. It is effective in enhancing penile erection in a wide variety of patients with erectile dysfunction.

*Viagra and Heart Patients*

The side effects reported with Viagra are usually mild to moderate in nature. These include a flushing sensation, indigestion, nasal congestion, some alteration in vision, diarrhea, and headache. Viagra should not be used by men with coronary artery disease who are taking medicine containing nitrates. Nitrates are found in many prescription medicines used to treat chest pain, or angina, due to coronary artery disease. These medicines include nitroglycerin sprays, ointments, pastes, or tablets that are swallowed, chewed, or dissolved in the mouth. Nitrodur, Imdur, and

Ismo are a few popular ones. If you are not sure whether any of your medications contain nitrates, or if you do not understand what nitrates are, consult your doctor or pharmacist.

Taking Viagra and nitrates can be dangerous. It can lead to a sudden decrease in blood pressure, dizziness, or even death.

Similarly, patients taking medicines to treat high blood pressure and patients who have had heart attacks should check with their doctors before using Viagra.

Some medicines like erythromycin and cimetidine can affect the metabolism of Viagra. Liver problems, kidney problems, or even old age can also affect the way Viagra is handled by the human body. One should never experiment with Viagra by borrowing a pill from a friend. It must always be used under medical supervision after an adequate history assessment and physical examination.

### Penile Injection Therapy

Besides Viagra, there are numerous other options for treating erectile dysfunction that are proven and have been used for some time. Medications such as papaverine and prostaglandin, for example, dilate blood vessels, increasing the blood flow and dilating the smooth muscles of the penis. These medications are best administered by a direct injection into the side of the penis using a very fine needle. After the injection, patients experience increase in the blood flow and an erection within fifteen to thirty minutes.

### Vacuum Devices

Vacuum devices are another treatment option. They consist of three common components: a plastic cylinder, a vacuum pump, and a constriction ring. The quality of erection produced by the vacuum device, however, is inferior to that of a normal erection. Numbness or a cold sensation of the penis occurs in nearly 75 percent of patients. This can be quite un-

comfortable. The tight rubber band used to maintain erection also leads to altered feelings of orgasm and may cause a blood clot to form under the skin. Similarly, tiny purplish spots may appear under the skin from microscopic hemorrhages.

### Surgical Treatment

There are three different types of surgical treatments available:

1. implantation of a penile prosthesis,
2. vein ligation for venous incompetence, and
3. vascular surgery for arterial blood flow abnormality.

#### Penile Prosthetic Implants

##### Semirigid Prosthesis

The surgical implantation of this semirigid device is simple. With this type of device, the penis is rigid all the time. However, during sexual activity it is possible to adjust the angle so the penis is at a right angle to the body. After sexual activity, the penis can be bent downwards.

##### Inflatable Penile Prosthesis

Unlike the semirigid prosthesis, with which the penis is rigid all the time, the inflatable penile prosthesis induces an erection at will. The three-piece inflatable penile prosthesis is one type of these devices. It produces an excellent and cosmetically attractive penile erection.

The inflatable cylinders are placed into the corpora cavernosa, and the pump is placed in the scrotum. The reservoir of fluid is implanted inside the pelvis. Very often, the entire operation can be performed through a one-inch incision on the scrotum. The hospital stay is usually less than twenty-four hours.

##### Postoperative Complications

The incidence of mechanical malfunction of the prosthesis has decreased greatly during the last several years because of better manufacturing methods and better materials. The vast majority of patients can expect trouble-free functioning of the implant for eight to ten years. If the implant develops any malfunction, such as fluid leakage, the whole implant or the leaking part can be replaced.

Another possible complication of penile implant surgery is infection. This occurs in 3 percent to 5 percent of patients. The prosthesis is usually removed to allow the infection to be controlled and is replaced at some other time. Other complications such as erosion and persistent pain are rare. Some patients complain of reduced penile length.

*Patient and Partner Satisfaction*

There is very high patient and partner satisfaction with the quality of erection and sex life after penile prosthesis placement. Penile prosthesis placement, when performed correctly, does not alter sensation during sexual intercourse, nor does it interfere with ejaculation or fertility.

*Surgery for Venous Incompetence*

Venous ligation surgery, or tying off veins that drain blood from the penis so the blood drains more slowly, was designed to improve penile erection. The outcome of this surgical intervention has been very poor.

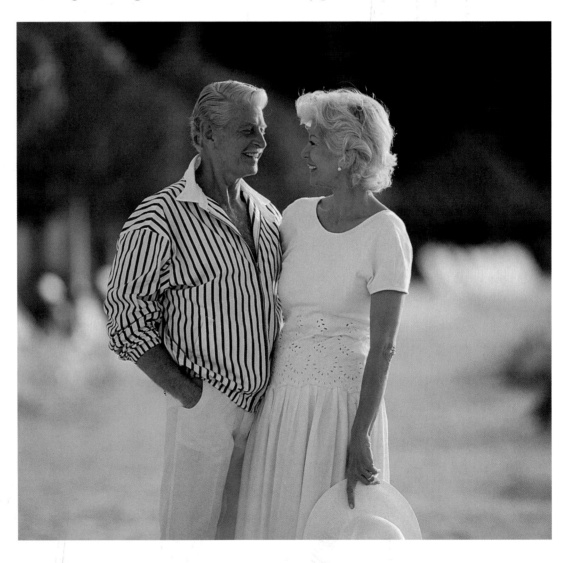

In many cases, erectile dysfunction, whether caused by heart disease or not, can be treated successfully and allow patients and their partners to return to a normal sex life.

*Surgical Arterial Revascularization*

Obstruction of penile blood flow can occur as a result of atherosclerosis in the terminal aorta, such as in Leriche's syndrome, which can produce erectile dysfunction. Similarly, obstruction of the internal iliac or internal pudendal arteries in the pelvis also leads to erectile dysfunction. Vascular disease occurring in the arteries of the penis as a result of diabetes or high blood pressure can also lead to erectile dysfunction. Arterial revascularization surgery in the aorta and iliac arteries may eliminate the original obstruction and lead to improved erectile function.

An alternative form of revascularization such as bypass surgery in the penis has been tried. Unfortunately, the long-term results of this type of bypass surgery are disappointing. Very careful patient selection combined with good surgical technique can sometimes lead to successful results.

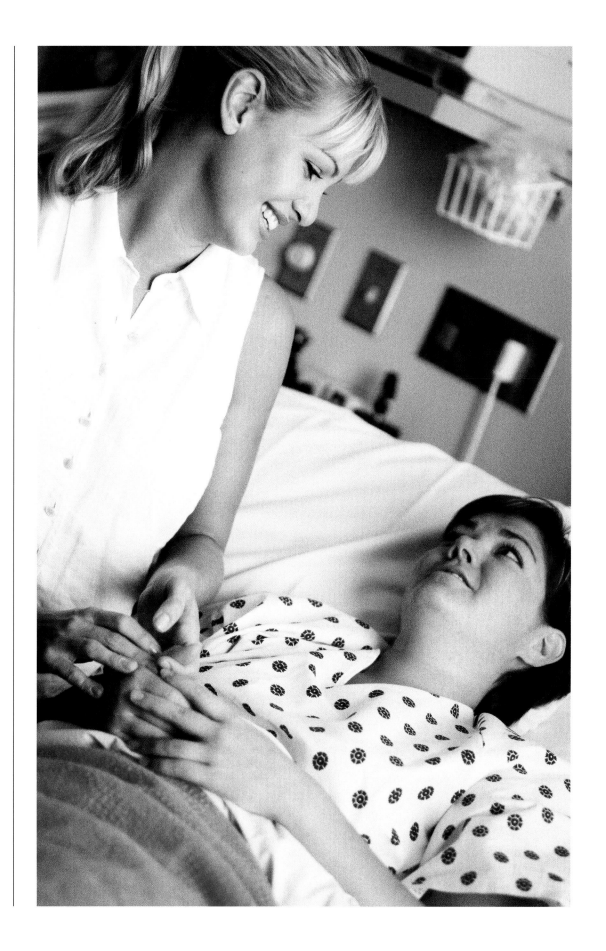

Most patients are discharged from the hospital between the fourth and the eighth day after their operation.

242

# RECOVERY AFTER HEART SURGERY AND A SECOND BYPASS OPERATION... WILL YOU NEED IT? WHEN?

RECOVERY AFTER HEART SURGERY begins when the patient leaves the operating room and arrives in the intensive care unit. By that time, the anesthesia is wearing off, and the patient begins to awaken. Patients are still connected to drainage bottles and monitoring devices, and a temporary pacemaker may also be used.

People usually start to wake up within an hour after their heart surgery and are soon able to follow simple commands such as "Move your foot, move your arm." When patients are alert and breathing on their own, and if the blood oxygenation level is appropriate, the endotracheal tube in the patient's throat and windpipe (trachea) is removed. This usually occurs anywhere from a few hours after heart surgery to the next morning. In some cases, with some cigarette smokers for example, the endotracheal tube may need to stay in longer.

Chest drainage tubes can usually be removed by the next day. Sometimes they're left in until the second morning after heart surgery.

Eating is also introduced gradually. If the patient is awake and alert, and his or her intestines are functioning, the standard fare is ice chips and water. From this point, progress toward a liquid diet is usually rapid.

By the morning after surgery, most patients are able to sit in a chair next to their bed. Depending on the progress and also, to some extent, the preferences of the heart surgery team, most patients are transferred from the intensive care unit, or ICU, late on the morning after the heart surgery.

### Transfer from the ICU

After transfer from the ICU to the hospital ward, also known as the "stepdown unit," the heart rhythm is still monitored at the nursing station. By the second postoperative day, most people are able to walk to the bathroom and down the hospital corridors with some assistance. By the third day after heart surgery, some people are ready for discharge. Others may have to stay for a few more days, and some will have to stay longer even, depending on the circumstances.

### Discharge Home

Today, most heart surgery patients are discharged between the fourth and the eighth postoperative day. Before discharge, they are given instructions regarding the various medications that are usually prescribed after heart surgery. For example, patients with considerable heart pumping dysfunction will fare better with ACE-inhibitor drugs. Patients with bypass grafts will likely need aspirin. Patients with abnormal heart rhythms may require medication to regulate their heartbeat. A dietician also instructs patients on appropriate diets. Many of the instructions the patients get before discharge deal with various activities they can and cannot do at home, and in a way this is more or less an informal cardiac rehabilitation program.

The most common form of incision during heart surgery is an incision down the middle of the breastbone, which is closed after the surgery with stainless steel wires. Although the wires stay in indefinitely, there is a period of healing after heart surgery that demands special attention. Recent heart surgery patients are instructed not to lift anything heavier than twenty pounds for four to six weeks. In some ways, this healing process is similar to that for a broken arm or leg bone, which takes about three months to heal.

There is usually little pain associated with this incision, called a midline sternotomy incision. Nerves come from the spinal cord out of the back bone and run around the ribs to the front, so there is not a concentration of nerves in the area. However, it is worth noting that everybody's pain threshold is different. On some days, the incision pain can be more noticeable than on others. In most cases, it is gone after three to four weeks, although in some patients, it may be present for two months or longer.

Typically, we recommend that patients avoid using excessive salt in the first few weeks after the surgery. Don't eat potato chips, pickles, and other salty foods, and don't add salt to food. After major operations, and particularly heart operations, the body has a tendency to retain salt and water. Because salt causes people to drink more liquids, the result can be edema, or swelling of the legs. It can also lead to fluid overload, a condition in which veins become engorged and the extra fluid backs up into the lungs. The patient then becomes short of breath.

Salt restriction is usually no longer necessary after about a month. It is, however, still necessary in some patients who are on certain medications and those who have high blood pressure or some degree of chronic heart failure.

### Surgical Wounds

When the patient leaves the hospital, the wound's skin edges are joined together, and the wound is in the process of healing. Wounds should not be scrubbed with a washcloth but gently cleaned with soap and water. In many cases, stainless steel staples are used to close the skin. If a patient goes home between the third and even the fifth postoperative day, the staples are usually left in, and arrangements are made for them to be removed later.

### Recovery at Home

After finally arriving home, most patients discover they are weaker than they thought they would be. This is typical. Hospitals are very sheltered environments, and, although confidence is gained walking up and down the hospital hallways, there are obstacles at home that weren't considered, like stairs and everyday movements.

Confidence usually returns fairly quickly as energy levels rise, but patients should strive to strike a balance between exercise and rest. Exercise itself is very good for a recovering heart patient if done very carefully at first and in moderation. It will help control blood pressure and blood sugar, burn excess calories, and lower body fat. Before any heavy exercise is possible, light stretching is a good idea. There are several effective stretches that will help the incision heal properly.

♥ Arm raises — forward: In a sitting position, straighten your arms, and raise them over your head.

♥ Pectoral stretches: In a sitting position, begin with your hands on top of your head, and push your elbows back until they are in line with your hands. Relax, bringing elbows slightly forward.

♥ Arm raises — side: In a sitting position with your arms at your sides, straighten your arms and raise them over your head. Keep your palms up.

♥ Sideways body bends: Place your feet about 1½ feet apart for balance while sitting in a chair. Bending slowly sideways at your waist, reach your right hand upward towards the ceiling and lower your left hand towards the floor on the left side of your chair. Hold for three seconds. Return slowly to sitting position.

After these light exercises have been performed, check your pulse.

Within a week or so, many patients have progressed to taking walks outside. Within a month, they can often walk a mile or two without difficulty. Driving, however, is not recommended for the first several weeks after heart surgery. I must admit, however, that one of my patients owned his own eighteen-wheeler tractor-trailer rig, and I found out when he came in for his routine postoperative visit five weeks after the heart surgery that he had gone back to driving his rig across the country a week after he returned home from his heart surgery. Clearly, we don't recommend this.

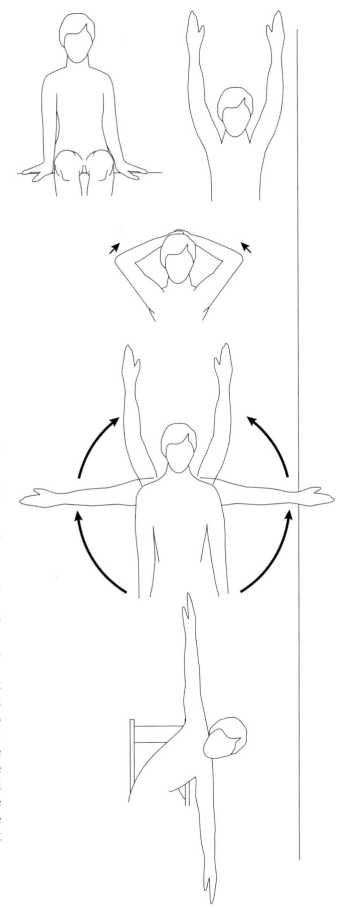

# LEARN HOW TO TAKE YOUR PULSE

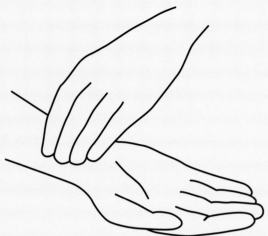

AFTER HEART SURGERY, FATIGUE and stress during exercise should always signal that a rest is needed. Before that, however, patients should check their pulse during exercise to make sure the heartbeat is staying within a reasonable limit.

It is important to remember that pulse rates vary from individual to individual. There is no "magic number" but rather a range of about sixty to one hundred beats per minute when the heart is at rest. The pulse rate is increased by exercise as well as emotional states like anger, fear, excitement, and anxiety.

Your pulse can be taken anywhere on the body where an artery near the surface can be compressed against a firm surface. Most commonly, doctors use the inner forearm (wrist), where the radial artery can be compressed against a bone in the forearm. There are some practical approaches to taking a pulse.

♥ Sit in a comfortable position.

♥ Place the index, second, and third fingers of one hand on the wrist of the other hand.

♥ Exert firm pressure.

♥ If you cannot feel a pulse, lighten the pressure. If that doesn't work, move up along the wrist until a pulse is located.

♥ Count the beats for ten seconds, then multiply by six. This is the "resting pulse" per minute.

♥ To determine a good "speed limit" for exercise, add three to the resting pulse. For example, if the resting pulse is fifteen (or 90 beats a minute), a reasonable exercise target would be 18 beats in a ten-second period (or 108 beats per minute).

The pulse should be checked in the middle and at the end of exercise. If it rises above a reasonable limit, take a break or slow down. This can be done with abdominal breathing exercises. During an abdominal breathing exercise, the hands are placed over the abdomen and a deep breath is drawn in through the nose, allowing the abdomen to rise under the fingers. Breathe out through the mouth while pushing in on the abdomen. Repeat this eight to ten times. This will lower your respiratory rate.

Usually, after five or six weeks, patients can begin driving again, but even this should be avoided if the patient is suffering from dizzy spells, blackouts, or light-headedness. When driving, it is a good idea to put a pillow between the seat belt and the incision to protect it.

Sexual activity can usually be resumed three or four weeks after heart surgery, depending on how the patient feels and how recovery is progressing.

Decreased appetite is common for the first several weeks after heart surgery, but appetite will gradually improve. Insomnia is experienced by some patients at times. Moodiness, irritability, and mild depression are not uncommon on some days of the recovery phase. Usually, over several weeks, these symptoms disappear, and patients will have the type of personality they had before heart surgery. A strong emotional support system is very helpful in getting through this period.

Even after several weeks of healing, excess stress should not be put on the breastbone. The arms are connected to the collarbones, which are anchored on the sternum. Any exercise that requires arm strength, including push-ups and lifting objects weighing more than twenty pounds, puts pressure on the breastbone and could cause it to become loose. For this reason, it is recommended that patients push with their body weight instead of pulling whenever possible.

Similarly, sports such as bowling, tennis, and golf should be avoided for the first three months. After that time, any of these activities can usually be resumed, although you should always check with your cardiologist before resuming these activities.

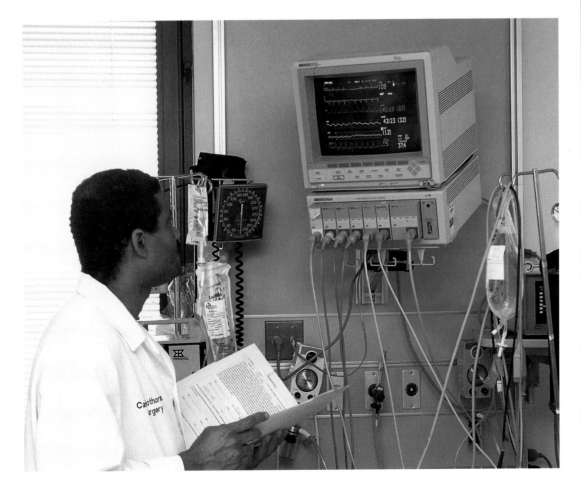

After their surgeries, patients are transferred to the intensive care unit, where they are constantly monitored.

### Recovery from Coronary Bypass Surgery

About three to eight weeks after heart surgery, some cardiologists recommend an **exercise stress test** for all of their patients. The stress test is performed as a baseline evaluation. The test may also be done to assess the patient's status in case of recurrent angina. This is not true for all doctors, however. Others perform the test only for those patients who may be doing activities that require more blood going to the heart. A good example is the patient who plans to run in a marathon or plans on playing tennis or perhaps patients who have the lives of many people in their hands, such as commercial pilots.

Repeated tests are also performed in patients with recurring or ongoing angina. If the exercise stress test result is normal, one can usually resume virtually any activity provided it is approved by a cardiologist. If it's abnormal, the cardiologist may recommend some limitation of activity or change in medication.

### Recovery from Heart Valve Surgery

Recovery from heart valve surgery is similar in many ways to recovery from coronary artery bypass surgery. The incision is similar, and the breastbone needs time to completely heal. Again, excess salt should also be avoided.

Some patients will be taking coumadin (warfarin), an **anticoagulant** or blood thinner. As long as coumadin is being taken, patients should avoid all vigorous contact sports such as rugby, soccer, and football. Dangerous sports like skydiving, in which one might receive blows to the head or begin bleeding, should also be avoided.

If the blood is not anticoagulated enough, blood clots can form on the heart valve or break off the valve and go to the brain, causing a stroke, or the valve itself could even clot off. If the anticoagulation level is too great, bleeding from the intestines or kidneys or even a stroke caused by bleeding into the brain could develop.

With heart valve surgery, the ventricle itself may be very thickened or enlarged as a result of the long-standing heart valve disease that was present before the valve surgery. In this case, the muscle tends to outgrow its blood supply, and although the valve has been fixed or replaced, the heart itself will likely take several months to recover. Patients should therefore avoid vigorous exercise such as running and playing tennis until these activities are approved by a cardiologist.

Stress tests are sometimes used after valve replacement that did not include coronary artery bypass grafting to assess postoperative exercise ability and heart rhythm during exercise. An echocardiogram is often recommended to see how the ventricles are recovering after the valve has been repaired or replaced.

Patients who have had heart valve surgery will need to undertake a regimen of antibiotics before and after dental surgery or additional surgical procedures.

### Cardiac Rehabilitation

Cardiac rehabilitation actually begins when one leaves the operating room. By the time patients arrive home, they are starting the second or third stage of cardiac rehabilitation, depending on whose definition of cardiac rehabilitation is used.

It is important to only gradually increase physical activities like walking. This promotes recovery. People who live in cold areas often do their walking in large shopping malls because extreme temperatures (less than 30°F and more than 90°F) should be avoided for the first month or so. During that period, patients

**Exercise Stress Test:**
A test during which a patient is connected to an electrocardiogram, or possibly other types of monitoring machines, and asked to walk on a treadmill or possibly pedal a stationary bicycle while being monitored.

**Anticoagulant:**
A drug that prevents or slows the blood clotting process. Also referred to as a blood thinner.

should avoid contact with people with colds and other types of illnesses that, if contracted, will cause coughing.

### Formal Cardiac Rehabilitation Programs after Heart Surgery or Heart Attacks

Some cardiologists feel strongly that all patients should be enrolled in a formal rehabilitation program. These programs typically last six to twelve weeks after heart surgery or heart attacks. Other cardiologists feel that the need to enter a formal cardiac rehabilitation program should be more individualized, and not all patients, particularly those that are already quite active, need to be enrolled.

These programs are typically located at a hospital, community center, or rehabilitation facility. They are designed to help build the patients' confidence. Patients are closely monitored for abnormal blood pressure and irregularities of the heartbeat by trained personnel in a group or class setting. They are taught to monitor their pulse rate and to look for signs of chest pain (angina type), particularly if they are coronary patients. Their activity level is slowly increased. During rehabilitation, they are educated about diet and other types of behavior modification that lead to a healthier lifestyle and a healthier heart.

### The Second Coronary Bypass Operation: Will I Need It? When?

I frequently hear comments from patients or their family members such as, "My neighbor told me these bypass opera-

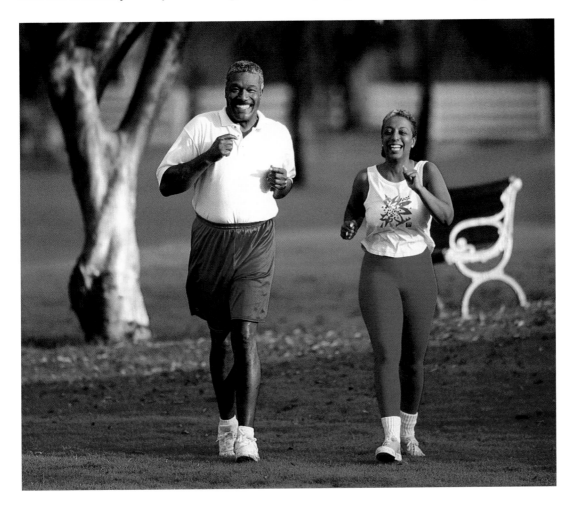

Moderate exercise after heart surgery is a very valuable tool in rehabilitation. The level of exercise, however, should be determined at first by a cardiologist.

tions have to be redone every three to four years. Is that true?" Patients are naturally very apprehensive about surgery to begin with, and when it comes to the possibility of having to repeat a procedure, they want to know the bottom line. Will they need a second bypass operation? If so, how long before it is needed?

The answer that heart surgeons and cardiologists would always like to give is, "Never!" The realistic answer, however, is more complicated. One can say, "Hopefully never," but the fact is that every patient is unique, and every situation depends upon a number of variables.

When arteries are used as the bypass grafts, they tend to stay open longer than veins. Sometimes, however, the patient's vessels considered for use as bypass grafts may not be in the best shape. This can influence how long the bypass stays open.

The arteries normally considered as candidates for grafts may be too small or diseased, or the amount of blood flow through them may make them unacceptable. Likewise, the diameter of the veins may be too big or too small, or the vein itself may have other abnormalities. The surgeon will not use arteries unless he or she feels they are acceptable, and he will try to use the best quality segments of vein available.

How long bypass grafts stay open also depends on the condition of the coronary arteries themselves. Ideally, the coronary artery that was originally bypassed was a relatively large artery, appearing to be normal except for one localized area of blockage. Unfortunately, sometimes we find coronary arteries that have multiple blockages, or the entire artery has significant atherosclerosis build-up. In addition, some arteries are only a millimeter or less in diameter (there are twenty-five millimeters in an inch). Sometimes the arteries are so brittle with calcium that it is difficult to find a spot to place a bypass graft, and some-

times the needle used to stitch the bypass to the coronary won't go through the coronary's calcified wall. Also, bypass grafts tend not to stay open as long in insulin-dependent diabetic patients and those with cholesterol disorders.

### Bypass Grafts Closing

If you have three, four, or more bypasses and one or two of them close, that does not necessarily mean you need a second bypass operation. In fact, if they all close, you still may not need a second operation. You might need a balloon angioplasty (PTCA) and maybe a stent. After bypass surgery, your cardiologist may have more treatment options. For example, if you need a balloon angioplasty, your doctor may be able to dilate either the coronary artery or the bypass graft. It may turn out that if the bypass fails, translaser myocardial revascularization (TMLR) may be a better option than a second bypass operation. This procedure can be done either with an operation or with catheters passed from an artery in the groin or arm into the heart.

### The Second Operation

In addition to all of these factors, doctors' criteria for recommending a second bypass operation can be somewhat different than they were for the first operation because the risk of a second bypass operation is usually higher than that of the first. The patient is older. The atherosclerotic coronary disease is usually more advanced. Some of the arteries and veins used to do the first bypass are no longer available for the second operation.

Adhesions will be present that formed after the first operation. This means that the surfaces of all the tissues will be stuck to each other so that it is more difficult and time consuming for the surgeon to expose the heart and coronaries or sometimes just to find the coronaries. Also, because of the adhesions, bypass grafts that are still functioning may be damaged while exposing the heart, which also adds to the complexity of the operation. The recovery after the second bypass operation, however, tends to be similar to the first.

So how risky is a second coronary bypass operation, and what are the chances of needing a second operation? The risk of not surviving a second operation varies depending on various factors, but in most cases is less than 10 percent.

What are the chances you will need a second coronary artery bypass operation? The field of cardiology, particularly interventional cardiology in which balloons and stents are used to treat coronary blockages, is advancing rapidly, as well as the specialty of cardiac surgery. My guess is that a person currently undergoing coronary bypass surgery has about a 10 percent chance of having a second coronary bypass operation. (A third bypass operation is uncommon, and having more than that is rare.)

Although unlikely, some patients need a second bypass operation within a year of the first. But for the majority of patients who will need a second bypass operation, it will most likely occur more than five years after their first and sometimes more than twenty years after it.

### You Can Help

Lifestyle after coronary surgery plays an important role in keeping bypass grafts open longer. Keeping your cholesterol in a safe range is important. If you are a smoker, quit. Watch your weight and exercise. Also, taking an aspirin a day makes platelets in your blood less sticky and probably helps to keep bypass grafts open longer.

# References for Selected Chapters

## Chapter One
## Dawn of Open Heart Surgery

Digliotti AM: Clinical use of artificial circulation with a note on intra-arterial transfusion. Bull Johns Hopkins Hosp 1951; 90:131.

Dodrill FD, Hill E, Gerisch RA: Some physiologic aspects of the artificial heart problem. J Thorac Surg 1952; 24:134.

Hill LL: A report of a case of successful suturing of the heart, and table of thirty-seven other cases of suturing by different operators with various terminations, and the conclusions drawn. Med Rec 1902; 2:846.

Kirklin JW: The middle 1950s and C Walton Lillehei. J Thorac Cardiovasc Surg 1989; 98:822.

Lillehei CW, Cohen M, Warden HE, et al: The direct vision intracardiac correction of congenital anomalies by controlled cross circulation. Surgery 1955; 38:11.

Lillehei CW, Cohen M, Warden HE, et al: The results of direct vision closure of ventricular septal defects in eight patients by means of controlled cross circulation. Surg Gynecol Obstet 1955; 101:446.

Rehn L: On penetrating cardiac injuries and cardiac suturing. Arc Klin Chir 1897; 55:315.

Ramaine-Davis, Ada: *John Gibbon and His Heart-Lung Machine*, University of Pennsylvania Press, Philadelphia, PA, 1991.

Shumacker, Harris B, Jr: *A Dream of the Heart: The Life of John H. Gibbon, Jr., Father of the Heart-lung Machine*, Pithian Press, Santa Barbara, CA 1999.

Shumacker, Harris B, Jr: *The Evolution of Cardiac Surgery*, Indiana University Press, Bloomington, IN, 1992, p. 13.

Spencer FC: Intellectual creativity in thoracic surgeons. J Thorac Cardiovasc Surg 1983; 86:167.

Stallworth, Clarke: "First heart operation performed…" The Birmingham News, Birmingham, Alabama, Sun., Nov. 9, 1975.

Stephenson, Larry W and Ruggiero, Renato: IN: *Heart Surgery Classics*, Adams Publishing Group, Ltd., Boston, MA, 1994, pp 121-141.

Williams DH: Stab wound of the heart and pericardium – recovery – patient alive three years afterwards. Med Rec 51: 1897; 437-39.

## Chapter Two
## The Normal Heart

### What You Should Know About Your Heart During Pregnancy
### *by Dr. Pam Gordon*

*Cardiac Problems in Pregnancy: Diagnosis and Management of Maternal and Fetal Disease*, eds Uri Elkayam and M. Gleicher. 2nd edition. New York: Dean R. Liss, Inc. 1990

Metcalfe, James, McAnulty, John H., and Ueland, Kurt: *Heart Disease and Pregnancy: Physiology and Management*. Little, Brown and Co., New York, NY, 1986.

*Pregnancy and Cardiovascular Disease*. Uri Elkayam, In *Heart Disease: A Textbook of Cardiovascular Medicine*, Eugene Braunwald, ed. Philadelphia: W.B. Saunders. 1997.

## Chapter Three
## Staying Healthy

### Nutrition for a Healthy Heart
### *by Dr. Morrison C. Bethea, M.C., F.A.C.S.*

Bao W., Srinivasan S.R., Berenson G.S.: Persistent elevation of plasma insulin levels is associated with increased cardiovascular risk in children and young adults: The Bogalusa heart study. Circulation 1996; 93:54-59

Despres J-P, Lamarche B, Muariege P, Cantin B, Dagenais GR, Moorjani S, Lupien P-J: Hyperinsulinemia as an independent risk factor for ischemic heart disease. N Engl J Med, 1996; 334;952-957

Frost G, Leeds AA, Dore CJ, Madeiros S, Brading S, Dornhost A: Glycaemic index as a determinant of serum HDL-cholesterol concentration. The Lancet, 1999;343:1045-48.

Ludwig D, Majzoub JA, Al-Zahrani A, Dallai GE, Blanco I, Roberts SB: High glycemic index foods, overeating, and obesity. (Abstract) Pediatrics, 1999;103(3);e26, p. 656.

### Wine, Alcohol, and Your Heart
### by Dr. R. Curtis Ellison

*Breast Cancer*

Fuchs CS, Stampfer MJ, Colditz GA, et al: Alcohol consumption and mortality among women. N Engl J Med 1995; 332:1245-1250.

Longnecker MP: Alcoholic beverage consumption in relation to risk of breast cancer: metaanalysis and review. Cancer Causes and Control 1994;5:73-82.

Longnecker MP: Invited commentary: The Framingham results on alcohol and breast cancer. Am J Epidemiol 1999;149:102-104.

Zhang Y. Kreger BE, Dorgan JF, et al: Alcohol consumption and risk of breast cancer: The Framingham Study revisited. Am J Epidemiol 1999;149:93-101.

*Coronary Heart Disease*

Pearson, TA: Alcohol and Heart Disease: Circulation 1996; 94:3023-3025.

Rimm, EB, Willen EC, Hu FB, et al: Folate and vitamin B6 from diet and supplements in relation to risk of coronary heart disease among women. JAMA 1996; 279:3598-364.

*Guidelines*

Cole P: The moral bases for public health interventions. Epidemiology 1995;6:78-83.

Sensible Drinking. The Report of an Inter-Departmental Working Group. Department of Health, United Kingdom. December, 1995.

*Total Mortality*

Coate D: Moderate drinking and coronary heart disease mortality: Evidence from NHANES I and the NHANES I follow-up. Am J Public Health 1993;83:888-890.

Gronbaek M, Deis A, Sorensen TIA, et al:. Influence of sex, age, body mass index, and smoking on alcohol intake and mortality. BMJ 1994;308:302-306.

Thun MJ, Peto R., Lopez AD, et al: Alcohol consumption and mortality among middle-aged and elderly U.S. adults. N Engl J Med 1997;337:1705-1714.

### Chapter Six
### What is Cardiac Catheterization?

Forssmann W: Catheterization of the right heart. Klin Wochenshr 1929; 8:2085.

Forssmann W: 21 Jahre Herzkatheterung, Rueckblick und Ausschau. Verh Dtsch Ges Kreislaufforschung 1951; 17:1.

Sones FM, Shirey EK: Cine coronary arteriography. Mod Concepts Cardiovasc Dis 1962; 31:735.

### Chapter Seven
### Heart Problems of
### Infants and Children

Anderson RC, Lillehei CW, Jester RG: Corrected transposition of the great vessels of the heart. Pediatrics 1957; 20:626.

Bailey LL, Gundry SR, Razzouk AJ, et al: Bless the babies: One hundred fifteen late survivors of heart transplantation during the first year of life. J Thorac Surg 1993; 105:805.

Blalock A, Taussig HB: The surgical treatment of malformations of the heart in which there is pulmonary stenosis or pulmonary atresia. JAMA 1945; 128:189.

Burroughs JT, Kirklin JW: Complete correction of total anomalous pulmonary venous correction: Report of three cases. Mayo Clin Proc 1956; 31:182.

Cooley DA, McNamara DG, Jatson JR: Aortico-pulmonary septal defect: Diagnosis and surgical treatment. Surgery 1957; 42:101.

Crafoord C, Nylin G: Congenital coarctation of the aorta and its surgical treatment. J Thorac Surg 1945; 14:347.

Ellis FH Jr, Kirklin JW: Congenital valvular aortic stenosis: Anatomic findings and surgical techniques. J Thorac Cardiovasc Surg 1962; 43:199.

Filler, RM, and Crocker, D: Conjoined Twins. In: *Pediatric Surgery*, Ravitch, MM, Welch, KJ, Benson, CD, Aberdeen, E and Randolph, JG, eds., Year Book Medical Publishers, Inc., Chicago, IL, 1979, pp 809-814.

Fontan F, Baudet E: Surgical repair of tricuspid atresia. Thorax 1971; 26:240.

Gibbon JH Jr.: Application of a mechanical heart and lung apparatus to cardiac surgery. Minn Med 1954; 37:171.

Graybiel A, Strieder JW, Boyer NH: An attempt to obliterate the patent ductus in a patient with subacute endarteritis. Am Heart J 1938; 15:621.

Gross RE, Hubbard JH: Surgical ligation of a patent ductus arteriosus: Report of first successful case. JAMA 1939; 112:1979.

Gross RE: Surgical relief for tracheal obstruction from a vascular ring. N Engl J Med 1945; 233:586.

Hardy KL, May IA, Webster CA, Kimball KG: Ebstein's anomaly: A functional concept and successful definitive repair. J Thorac Cardiovasc Surg 1964; 48:927.

Horiuchi T, AbeT, Okada Y, et al: Feasibility of total correction for single ventricle: A report of total correction in a six-year-old girl. Jpn J Thorac Surg 1970; 23:434. (In Japanese)

Jatene AD, Fontes VF, Paulista PP, et al: Anatomic correction of transposition of the great vessel. J Thorac Cardiovasc Surg 1976; 72:364.

Kirklin JW, DuShane JW, Patrick RT, et al: Intracardiac surgery with the aid of a mechanical pump-oxygenator system (Gibbon type): Report of eight cases. Mayo Clin Proc 1955; 30:201.

Kirklin JW, Harp RA, McGoon DC: Surgical treatment of origin of both vessels from right ventricle including cases of pulmonary stenosis. J Thorac Cardiovasc Surg 1964; 48:1026.

Konno S. Iami Y, Iida Y, et al: A new method for prosthetic valve replacement in congenital aortic stenosis associated with hypoplasia of the aortic valve ring. J Thorac Cardiovasc Surg 1975; 70:909.

Lillehei CW, Cohen M, Warden HE, et al: The direct vision intracardiac correction of congenital anomalies by controlled cross circulation. Surgery 1955; 38:11.

Lillehei CW, Cohen M, Warden HE, et al: The results of direct vision closure of ventricular septal defects in eight patients by means of controlled cross circulation. Surg Gynecol Obstet 1955; 101:446.

McGoon DC, Edwards JE, Kirklin JW: Surgical treatment of ruptured aneurysm of aortic sinus. Ann Surg 1958; 147:387.

McGoon DC, Rastelli GC, Ongley PA: An operation for the correction of truncus arteriosus. JAMA 1968; 205:59.

Norwood WI, Lang P, Hansen DD: Physiologic repair of aortic atresia-hypoplastic left heart syndrome. N Engl J Med 1983; 308:23.

Ross DN, Somerville J: Correction of pulmonary atresia with a homograft aortic valve. Lancet 1966; 2:1446.

Saxena NC: Personal communication, July 1976, and Pediatric News, 10:3, 1976.

Senning A: Surgical correction of transposition of the great vessels. Surgery 1959; 45:966.

Swan H, Wilson JH, Woodwork G, Blount SE: Surgical obliteration of a coronary artery fistula to the right ventricle. Arch Surg 1959; 79:820.

## Chapter Eight
### Coronary Artery Disease and Treatment Options

Bailey CP, Hirose T: Successful internal mammary-coronary arterial anastomosis using a "minivascular" suturing technique. Int Surg 1968; 49:416.

Beck CS: Coronary sclerosis and angina pectoris: Treatment by grafting a new blood supply upon the myocardium. Surg Gynecol Obstet 1937; 64:270.

Beck CS: The development of a new blood supply to the heart by operation. In: *Disease of the Coronary Arteries and Cardiac Pain*, Levy IL, ed. Macmillan, New York, 1936, Chap 17.

Carrel A: On the experimental surgery of the thoracic aorta and the heart. Ann Surg 1910; 52:83.

Demikhov VP: Experimental transplantation of vital organs. Authorized translation from the Russian by Basil Haigh. Consultants Bureau, New York, 1962.

Favaloro RG: Saphenous vein autograft replacement of severe segmental coronary artery occlusion. Ann Thorac Surg 1968; 5:334.

Garrett EH, Dennis EW, DeBakey ME: Aortocoronary bypass with saphenous vein grafts: Seven-year follow-up. JAMA 1973; 223:792.

Green GE, Stertzer SH, Reppert EH: Coronary arterial bypass grafts. Ann Thorac Surg 1968; 5:443.

Johnson WD, Glemma RJ, Lepley D Jr, Ellison EH: Extended treatment of severe coronary artery disease: A total surgical approach. Ann Surg 1969; 171:460.

Kolessov VI: Mammary artery-coronary artery anastomosis as a method of treatment for angina pectoris. J Thorac Cardiovasc Surg 1967; 54:535.

Leriche R, Fontaine R: Essai experimental de traitement de certains infarctus du myocarde et de l'aneuvrisme du coeur par une griffe de muscle strie. Bill Soc Nat Chir 1933; 59:229.

Sabiston, David. Johns Hopkins Medical Journal 1974; 134:314.

Sones FM, Shirey EK: Cine coronary arteriography. Mod Concepts Cardiovasc Dis 1962; 31:735.

Vineberg AM: Development of an anastomosis between the coronary vessels and a transplanted internal mammary artery. Can Med Assoc J 1946; 55:117.

### Women, Race, and Coronary Artery Surgery
#### *by Dr. Reneé Hartz*

Bypass Angioplasty Revascularization Investigation (BARI). Comparison of coronary bypass surgery with angioplasty in patients with multivessel disease. N Engl J Med 1996:335:217-25.

Bypass Angioplasty Revascularization Investigation (BARI). Medical care costs and quality of life after randomization to coronary angioplasty or coronary bypass surgery. N Engl J Med 1997;336:92.

Chistakis G, Weisel R, Buth K, et al. Is body size the cause for poor outcomes of coronary artery bypass operations in women? J Thorac Cardiovasc Surg 1995;110:1344-58.

Edwards FH, Carey JS, Grover FL, et al. Impact of gender on coronary bypass operative mortality. Ann Thorac Surg 1998;66:125-31.

Goldberg KC, Hartz ZJ, Jacobsen SJ, et al. Racial and community factors influencing coronary artery bypass graft surgery rates for all 1986 Medicare patients. JAMA 1992;267:1473-7.

Kennedy, JW, Kaiser GC, Fisher LD, et al. Clinical and angiographic predictors of operative mortality for the Collaborative Study in Coronary Artery Surgery (CASS). Circulation 1981;63:793-802.

Mickleborough J, Takagi Y, Murayama H, et al. Is sex a factor in determining operative risk for aorto-coronary bypass graft surgery? Circulation 1995;90 (Suppl II):80-4.

Society of Thoracic Surgeons Cardiac Surgery National Database Analysis: Summit Medical, Minneapolis, 1996.

Sullivan JM, El-Zeky F, Vander Zwaag R, Ramanathan KB. Estrogen replacement therapy after coronary bypass surgery: effect on survival. J Am Coll Cardiol 1994;23:7A.

254

## Chapter Nine
### The Coronary Bypass: Operation and Recovery

#### Strokes, Carotid Artery Disease, and Coronary Bypass Surgery
*by Dr. Cary Akins*

Akins CW, Moncure AC, Daggett WM, et al: Safety and efficacy of concomitant carotid and coronary artery operations. Ann of Thoraci Surg 1995;60:311.

Daily PO, Freeman RK, Dembitsky WP, et al: Cost reduction by combined carotid endarterectomy and coronary artery bypass grafting. J Thoraci Cardiovasc Surg 1996;111:1185.

European Carotid Surgery Trialists' Collaborative Group: MRC European Carotid Surgery Trial: Interim results for symptomatic patients with severe (70 to 99 percent) or with mild (0 to 29 percent) carotid stenosis. Lancet 1991;337:1235.

Executive Committee for the Asymptomatic Carotid Atherosclerosis Study: Endarterectomy for asymptomatic carotid stenosis. JAMA 1995;273:1421.

Hobson RW, Weiss DG, Fields WS, et al: Efficacy of carotid endarterectomy for asymptomatic carotid stenosis. N Engl J of Med 1993;328:221.

North American Symptomatic Carotid Endarterectomy Trial Collaborators: Beneficial effect of carotid endarterectomy in symptomic patients with high-grade carotid stenosis. N Eng J Med 1991;325:445.

## Chapter Ten
### Heart Valve Problems

Acierno LJ: *The History of Cardiology.* Parthenon Publishing Group, New York, 1994, p. 635.

Arbulu A, Holmes RJ, Asfaw I: Surgical treatment of intractable right-sided infective endocarditis in drug addicts: 25 years experience. J Heart Valve Dis 1993; 2:129.

Bailey CP: The surgical treatment of mitral stenosis. Dis Chest 1949; 15:377.

Baker C, Brock RC, Campbell M: Valvulotomy for mitral stenosis: Report of six successful cases. Br Med J 1950; 1:1283.

Binet JP, Carpentier A, Langlois J, et al: Implantation de valves heterogenes dans le traitement de cardiopathies aortiques. C R Acad Sci Paris 1965; 261:5733.

Borman JB, Applebaum A, Hirsch M, et al: Quadruple valve commissurotomy. J Thorac Cardiovasc Surg 1975; 70:713.

Campbell JM: Artificial aortic valve. J Thorac Cardiovasc Surg 1958; 19:312.

Cutler EC, Levine SA: Cardiotomy and valvulotomy for mitral stenosis. Boston Med Surg J 1923; 188:1023.

Harken DE, Soroff HS, Taylor WJ, et al: Partial and complete prostheses in aortic insufficiency. J Thorac Cardiovasc Surg 1960; 40:744.

Heimbecker, RO, Baird RJ, Lajos RJ, et al: Homograft replacement of the human valve. A preliminary report. Canad Med Ass J 1962; 86:805-9.

Hufnagel CA: Aortic plastic valvular prostheses. Bull Georgetown Med Cent 1951; 4:128.

Hufnagel CA, Harvey WP, Rabil PJ, et al: Surgical correction of aortic insufficiency. Surgery 1954; 35:673.

Kaiser GA, Hancock WD, Lukban SB, Litwak RS: Clinical use of a new design stented xenograft heart valve prosthesis. Surg Forum 1969; 20:137.

Naef AP: *The Story of Thoracic Surgery.* Hogrefe & Huber, New York, 1990, p 94.

Reyes VP, Raju BS, Raju AR, Wynne J, Stephenson LW, Raju R, Fromm BS, Rajagopal R, Mehta P, Singh S, Rao P, Satyanarayana PV, Turi A: Petcutaneous Balloon Versus Open Surgical Commissurotomy for Mitral Stenosis: A randomized trial. N. Engl. J. Med. 1994; 331:15:961-967.

Ross DN: Replacement of aortic and mitral valves with a pulmonary autograft. Lancet 1967; 2:956.

Sellors TH: Surgery of pulmonary stenosis: A case in which the pulmonary valve was successfully divided. Lancet 1948; 1:988.

Spencer FC: Intellectual creativity in thoracic surgeons. J Thorac Cardiovasc Surg 1983; 86:168.

Starr A, Edwards ML, McCord CW, et al: Multiple valve replacement. Circulation 1964; 29:30.

Starr A, Edwards ML: Mitral replacement: Clinical experience with a ball-valve prosthesis. Ann Surg 1961; 154:726.

Tuffier, T: Etat actuel de la chirurgie intrathoracique. Trans Int Congr Med 1913 (London 1914), 7; Surgery 1914; 2:249.

Turi ZG, Reyes VP, Raju BS, et al.: Percutaneous balloon versus surgical closed commissurotomy for mitral stenosis: a prospective, randomized trial. Circulation 1991; 83:1179-85.

## Chapter Eleven
### Advanced Heart Failure: Transplants, Heart Assist Devices and the Future

Akutsu T, Kolff WJ: Permanent substitutes for valves and hearts. Trans ASAIO 1958; 4:230.

Barnard CN: A human cardiac transplant: An interim report of a successful operation performed at Groote Schuur Hospital, Cape Town. S Afr Med J 1967; 41:1271.

Brock R: Heart excision and replacement. Guys Hosp Rep 1959; 108:285.

Carrel A, Guthrie CC: The transplantation of veins and organs. Am Med 1905; 10:101.

Cooley DA, Liotta D, Hallman GL, et al: Orthotopic cardiac prosthesis for two-staged cardiac replacement. Am J Cardiol 1969; 24:723.

Demikhov VP: Experimental transplantation of an additional heart in the dog. Bull Exp Biol Med (Russia) 1950; 1:241.

Demikhov VP: Experimental Transplantation of Vital Organs. Authorized translation from the Russian by Basil Haigh. Consultants Bureau, New York, 1962.

DeVries WC, Anderson JL, Joyce LD, et al: Clinical use of total artificial heart. N Engl J Med 1984; 310:273.

Hardy JD, Chavez CM, Hurrus FD, et al: Heart transplantation in man and report of a case. JAMA 1964; 188:1132.

Harken DE: Presentation at the meeting of the International College of Cardiology, Brussels, 1958.

Hill JD, Farrar DJ, Hershon JJ, et al: Use of a prosthetic ventricle as a bridge to cardiac transplantation for postinfarction cardiogenic shock. N Engl J Med 1986; 314:626.

Kantrowitz, A: Heart, heart-lung and lung transplantation. In: *Heart Surgery Classics*. Stephenson LW, Ruggiero R eds, Adams Publishing Group, Boston, 1994, p 314.

Kantrowitz A, Tjonneland S, Freed PS, et al: Initial clinical experience with intraaortic balloon pumping in cardiogenic shock. JAMA 1968; 203:135.

Lower RR, Shumway NE: Studies on orthotopic homotransplantation of the canine heart. Surg Forum 1960; 11:18.

Moulopoulos SD, Topaz S, Kolff WJ: Diastolic balloon pumping in the aorta: Mechanical assistance to the failing heart. Am Heart J 1962; 63:669.

Reitz BA, Burton NA, Jamieson SW, et al: Heart and lung transplantation: Autotransplantation and allotransplantation in primates with extended survival. J Thorac Cardiovasc Surg 1980; 80:360.

Reitz BA, Wallwork JL, Hunt SA, et al: Heart-lung transplantation: Successful therapy for patients with pulmonary vascular disease. N Engl J Med 1982; 30:557.

Ruggiero, R, Commentary on Barnard CN: A human cardiac transplant: An interim report of a successful operation performed at Groote Schuur Hospital, Cape Town. S Afr Med J 1967; 41:1271. In: *Heart Surgery Classics*. Stephenson LW, Ruggiero R eds, Adams Publishing Group, Boston, 1994, p 327.

Shumacker HB Jr.: The Evolution of Cardiac Surgery. Indiana University Press, Indianapolis. 1992, p 141.

Starnes VA, Oyer PE, Portner PM, et al: Isolated left ventricular assist as bridge to cardiac transplantation. J Thorac Cardiovasc Surg 1988; 96:62.

### Gene Therapy
### by Dr. Todd Rosengart

Crystal RG, McElvaney NG, Rosenfeld MA, et al: Administration of an adenovirus containing the human CFTRcDNA to the respiratory tract of individuals with cystic fibrosis. Nat Genet 1994;8:42-51.

Mack CA, Patel SR, Schwartz EA, et al: Biological bypass utilizing adenovirus-mediated gene transfer of the cDNA for vascular endothelial growth factor121 improves myocardial perfusion and function in the ischemic porcine heart. J Thor Cardiovasc Surg 1998; 115; 168-177.

Rosengart TK, Patel SR, Lee LY: Safety of direct myocardial VEG121 cDNA adenovirus-mediated angiogenesis gene therapy in conjunction with coronary bypass surgery. Circulation 1998:98 (17 Suppl.):I-321.

### Chapter Thirteen
### Aneurysms and Other Blood Vessel Problems

Cooley DA, DeBakey ME: Resection of entire ascending aorta in fusiform aneurysm using cardiac bypass. JAMA 1956; 165:1158.

DeBakey ME, Cooley DA, Creech O Jr: Surgical consideration of dissecting aneurysm of the aorta. Ann Surg 1955; 142:586.

DeBakey ME, Cooley DA: Successful resection of aneurysm of thoracic aorta and replacement by graft. JAMA 1953; 152:673.

DeBakey ME, Crawford ED, Cooley DA, Morris GC Jr: Successful resection of fusiform aneurysm of aortic arch with replacement by homograft. Surg Gynecol Obstet 1957; 105:657.

DeBakey ME, Creech O Jr, Morris GC Jr: Aneurysm of the thoracoabdominal aorta involving the celiac superior mesenteric and renal arteries: Report of four cases treated by resection and homograft replacement. Ann Surg 1956; 144:549.

Dubost C, Allary M, Oeconomos N: Resection of an aneurysm of the abdominal aorta: Reestablishment of the continuity by a preserved human arterial graft, with results after five months. Arch Surg 1952; 62:405.

Spencer FC: Intellectual creativity in thoracic surgeons. J Thorac Cardiovasc Surg 1983; 86:164.

Voorhees AB Jr, Janetzky A III, Blakemore AH: The use of tubes constructed from Vinyon "N" cloth in bridging defects. Ann Surg 1952; 135:332.

### Surgery of the Thoracic Aorta
### by Dr. Nicholas Kouchoukos

Downing, SW, Kouchoukos, NT, Ascending Aortic Aneurysm. In: *Cardiac Surgery In the Adult*, Edmunds, L.H. Jr. ed., McGraw Hill, New York, 1997, pp 1165-1195.

Kouchoukos, NT, Daily BB, Rokkas, CK, et al: Hypothermic bypass and circulatory arrest for operations of the descending thoracic and thoracoabdominal aorta. Ann of Thoraci Surg 1995;60:67-77.

Kouchoukos, NT and Dougenis, D: Medical progress: surgery of the thoracic aorta. N Eng J Med 1997; 336: 1876-88.

### Chapter Fourteen
### Heart Surgery in the Elderly

Edmunds LH Jr, Stephenson LW, Edie RN, Ratcliffe MB: Open heart surgery in octogenarians. N Engl J Med 1988; 319:131-36.

Stason WB, Sanders CA, Smith HC: Cardiovascular care of the elderly: Economic considerations. J Am Coll Cardiol 1987; 10(Suppl A):18A-21A.

Stephenson LW, Mac Vaugh H III, Edmunds LH Jr: Surgery using cardiopulmonary bypass in the elderly. Circulation 1978; 58; 2:250-254.

Vidne B, Levy MJ: Heart valve replacement in the elderly patient. Geriatrics 1970; 25: 136.

Wenger NK, Marcus FI, O'Rourke RA: Cardiovascular disease in the elderly. J Am Coll Cardiol 1987;10 (Suppl A):80A-87A.

# Common Drugs for Heart Patients

**Courtesy of Detroit Medical Center/Harper Hospital**

*(This is intended for informational purposes only. It does not cover all possible side effects, interactions or uses of the drug. If you develop symptoms not mentioned on this sheet or if you have questions concerning your medications, contact your doctor, nurse, or pharmacist and follow their instructions. Also, keep these and all medications away from children.)*

## Ace-Inhibitors

**Profile:**
This medicine is taken orally and used to help the heart work better. It is also used to treat high blood pressure.

**Conditions:**
♥Tell your doctor if you are taking a salt substitute.
♥Tell your doctor if you are taking potassium.
♥Tell your doctor if you have had a problem with any other ACE inhibitor, such as swelling or sudden trouble breathing.
♥Tell your doctor about all the medicines you take or use.
♥Do not stop taking this medicine without talking to your doctor.
♥Do not take a missed dose if it is almost time to take your next dose.

**Common Side Effects:**
Dizziness or lightheadedness. A dry continuing cough and no other signs of a cold. Nausea, headache.

**Call the Doctor If...**
♥You have fainting spells, skin rash, hoarseness, a sudden swelling of the face, mouth, hands or feet, or sudden trouble swallowing or breathing.

## Amiodarone (Cordarone)

**Profile:**
This medicine is taken orally and used to help heartbeat.

**Conditions:**
♥Tell your doctor about all the medicines you take or use.
♥Tell your doctor about all medical problems, especially thyroid conditions.
♥Take a missed dose as soon as you remember, but do not double the dose.

♥Continue to take the medication even when you feel better.
♥Be careful in the sunlight when you take this medicine. If you must be in sunlight, cover up, wear a hat or wear sunscreen.
♥Do not stop taking this medicine without asking your doctor.

**Common Side Effects:**
Constipation. Taste may be bitter or metallic. Decreased appetite.

**Call the Doctor If...**
♥You develop painful breathing, coughing or shortness of breath.
♥You experience numbness or tingling in the fingers or toes, or shaking of the hands.
♥You have trouble walking, or unusual body movements you cannot control.
♥You develop a blue-gray coloring of the skin on the upper body.

## Aspirin

**Profile:**
Aspirin is taken orally and used to help thin the blood. It may help prevent heart attack. It is also used for fever, aches or pain.

**Conditions:**
♥Tell your doctor if you are taking blood thinners.
♥Tell your doctor if you are taking other pain or arthritis medicines.
♥Take a missed dose as soon as you remember, but do not take a missed dose if it is almost time for the next aspirin.

**Common Side Effects:**
Mild stomach upset or heartburn.

**Call the Doctor If...**
♥Unusual bleeding or bruises.
♥Skin rash or hives.
♥Dark, tar-looking stool.

### Beta Blockers

**Profile:**

This medicine is oral and is used to help the heart work better. It can also slow the heartbeat, treat high blood pressure, and prevent heart attack or chest pain.

**Conditions:**

♥Tell your doctor about all medicine you are taking.

♥Tell your doctor if you have sugar diabetes or suffer from depression.

♥Take a missed dose as soon as possible unless it is close to your next dose.

♥Do not stop taking this medicine without first asking your doctor.

**Common Side Effects:**

Dizziness or lightheadedness when getting up from lying or sitting; decreased sexual ability.

**Call the Doctor If...**

♥You experience difficulty breathing, wheezing.

♥There is an unusually slow heartbeat.

♥You experience confusion or vivid dreams.

♥You faint.

### Calcium Channel Blockers
### (Adalat, Adalat CC, Calan, Calan SR,
### Cardizem, Cardizem CD, Procardia, Procardia XL)

**Profile:**

This medicine is taken orally. Some calcium channel blockers (CCBs) are used to control the heart beat, others are used to treat angina. CCBs can also be used to treat high blood pressure.

**Conditions:**

♥Tell your doctor if you have any other heart or blood vessel problems, or kidney problems.

♥Tell your doctor about all the medicine you take.

♥Tell your doctor if you have had a bad reaction to this medicine before.

♥Take a missed dose as soon as you remember, but do not take a missed dose if it is almost time for your next dose.

♥Do not stop taking this medicine without asking your doctor.

♥Do not crush or chew any products having parts to their names like CD, SR, XL, or CC. Swallow these whole.

**Common Side Effects:**

Mild headache (this often goes away with time). Mild dizziness, lightheadedness.

**Call the Doctor If...**

♥You experience breathing difficulty or wheezing.

♥You have swelling of the ankles, feet or lower legs.

♥You have an unusual heart beat or chest pain.

♥There is fainting.

### Clopidogrel (Plavix)

**Profile:**

This medication is shown to cut your risk of having a heart attack or stroke. If you have a stent, it is used to keep the stent from clotting.

**Conditions:**

♥Take the medicine even if you are beginning to feel better. Even though you may not feel differently once you start Plavix, it is working.

♥Get your blood check occasionally if recommended by your doctor.

♥Take a missed dose as soon as you remember, but DO NOT take a missed dose if it is almost time for your next one and DO NOT stop taking Plavix unless told to by your doctor.

♥Tell your doctor and dentist you are taking Plavix before any surgery is scheduled or before any new drug is taken.

**Common Side Effects:**

Stomach pain or upset, diarrhea. Rash.

**Call the Doctor If...**

♥You have unusual bleeding that does not stop.

♥You have stomach pain or upset, or diarrhea you cannot tolerate.

### Digoxin (Lanoxin)

**Profile:**

This is taken orally or administered with a shot. It is used to strengthen the heart and control the heart.

**Conditions:**

♥Tell your doctor if you are taking cholesterol drugs.

♥Tell your doctor if you are taking potassium drugs.

♥Ask your doctor about checking your pulse rate.

♥Do not take a missed dose if it is almost time to take your next dose and do not double dose.

♥Tell your doctor about all prescription or nonprescription medications you take or use.

♥Do not stop taking this medicine without asking your doctor.

**Common Side Effects:**

Mild nausea, loss of appetite.

**Call the Doctor If...**

♥You have skin rash or hives.

♥You experience an unusual or extreme loss of appetite, nausea or vomiting.

♥You are unusually tired, weak, drowsy or confused.

♥You have a slow or irregular heartbeat or blurred vision.

♥You experience an unusual or bad headache or fainting spells.

### Furosemide (Lasix)

**Profile:**

This medication is administered orally or with a shot. Known as the "water pill," it decreases the amount of water in the body, causing your kidneys to make more water and you lose potassium. It can also be used to lower blood pressure.

**Conditions:**

♥Tell your doctor if you have sugar diabetes, gout or problems holding your urine.

♥Tell your doctor if you had any allergy to any other water pill.

♥Tell your doctor about any medicine you take or use.

♥Take a missed dose as soon as you remember, but DO NOT take a missed dose if it almost time for the next one and DO NOT stop taking it without advice from your doctor.

**Common Side Effects:**
Dizziness, lightheadedness when getting up from lying down or sitting.

**Call the Doctor If...**
♥You have muscle cramps or pain; nausea or vomiting; unusual weakness. These are signs of too much potassium loss.
♥You have skin rash or fainting.

### Hydralazine (Apresoline)

**Profile:**
This medicine is taken orally and used to help the heart work better. It can also be used to lower high blood pressure.

**Conditions:**
♥Tell your doctor about all the medicines you take or use.
♥Tell your doctor about all medical problems, including stroke or kidney problems.
♥Take a missed dose as soon as you remember, but do not take a missed dose if it is almost time for your next dose.
♥Do not stop taking this medicine without talking to your doctor.

**Common Side Effects:**
Decreased appetite. Fast, or "jumpy" heartbeat. Dizziness, lightheadedness or flushing.

**Call the Doctor If...**
♥You have a pounding heartbeat, chest pain or skin rash.
♥You experience unusual swelling of feet or lower legs.
♥You have fainting spells.

### Nitroglycerin (Nitro-Bid)

**Profile:**
This medicine is taken orally. It is used to help the heart by increasing its supply of blood and oxygen. It is also used to prevent angina.

**Conditions:**
♥Tell your doctor about any medicine you take or use.
♥Do not break, crush or chew the tablets.
♥Take a missed dose as soon as you remember, but not if it is almost time to take your next dose.
♥Continue to take this medication even when you feel better.
♥Do not stop taking it without asking your doctor.

**Common Side Effects:**
Dizziness or lightheadedness. Headache. Flushing of the face or neck.

**Call the Doctor If...**
♥You have severe prolonged headache or pressure in the head.
♥There is extreme dizziness or fainting.
♥You have a weak or fast heartbeat.

### Potassium (K-Dur, Slow-K, K-Lyte)

**Profile:**
This is used to add potassium to your body. Potassium is important to the heart and muscles. It comes in a pill, liquid or flat tablet to fizz in water or juice.

**Conditions:**
♥Tell your doctor if you take a salt substitute.
♥Tell your doctor if you are on a special diet.
♥Tell your doctor if you are taking a water pill or ace-inhibitor drug.
♥Take a missed dose as soon as you remember, but DO NOT take the dose if it is almost time for your next one.
♥DO NOT stop taking this without permission from your doctor.
♥Tell your doctor about all the medicines you take.
♥Do not crush the potassium pill. Do put the potassium fizz tablet or liquid in water or juice.

**Common Side Effects:**
Mild stomach upset or heartburn. Bad taste in the mouth.

**Call the Doctor If...**
♥You have severe stomach pain.
♥You have a dark, tar-looking stool.
♥You experience muscle weakness, unusual heart beat or pulse, confusion.

### Ticlopidine (Ticlid)

**Profile:**
TICLID has been shown to cut the risk of having a stroke or heart attack. If you have a stent, it is used to keep the stent from clotting.

**Conditions:**
♥Take the medicine even if you begin to feel better.
♥Have your blood monitored regularly once you start TICLID. You will need to have blood drawn every two weeks for the first three months. Do not skip any of these appointments.
♥Take a missed dose as soon as you remember, but do not take a missed dose if it is almost time for the next dose.
♥Do not stop taking TICLID unless told to do so by your doctor. If you are told to stop taking TICLID, you will still have to have your blood drawn. This will only be for two weeks after you stop.

**Common Side Effects:**
Stomach pain or upset, diarrhea.

**Call the Doctor If...**
♥You develop a rash.
♥You have stomach pain or upset, or diarrhea you cannot stand.
♥Signs of infection such as fever, chills or sore throat.

### Warfarin (Coumadin)

**Profile:**
Warfarin is an oral anticoagulant that prevents harmful blood clots from forming or getting larger. It is

sometimes called a blood thinner, although it does not actually thin the blood.

**Conditions:**

♥Tell your doctor if you are pregnant or plan on becoming pregnant.

♥Keep all doctor appointments, especially involving blood work.

♥Avoid activities that have a risk of injury since warfarin affects the body's ability to stop bleeding.

♥Alert your doctor to missed doses.

♥Take a missed dose as soon as possible, but do not double the dose to make up for the missed dose.

♥Let your doctor know about all the medication you are taking, including nonprescription.

♥Tell your dentist and any other doctors you are taking warfarin.

**Common Side Effects:**

Minor bleeding from the gums, occasional nose bleeds, easy bruising.

**Call the Doctor If...**

♥There is unexplained or excessive bruising, nosebleeds or menstrual bleeding.

♥There is excessive bleeding or oozing from gums, cuts or wounds.

♥You experience tar colored stools or blood in the urine.

♥There is unexplained stomach pain, abdominal swelling, back pain or back aches.

♥You experience excessive fatigue, chills, fever, sore throat, unexplained mouth sores.

♥There is dizziness, severe headache, unexplained joint pain, stiffness or swelling.

# GLOSSARY

**ablation**: Removal or elimination of tissue, usually because it is harmful.

**ACE inhibitors (angiotensin-converting enzyme inhibitors)**: Drugs that dilate blood vessels and improve blood flow. By dilating the blood vessels, these chemicals cause resistance in the circulatory system to be less so the heart does not have to work as hard. They are used to treat patients with heart failure and/or coronary artery disease and can also be used for other purposes.

**adventitia**: The outermost layer of the artery's wall.

**aerobic capacity**: When someone is exercising, this is the maximal amount of oxygen that can be taken up by the body.

**allograft**: *See* homograft.

**alveoli**: Small air sacs in the lung that collect oxygen, which is then absorbed by the blood vessels. When the blood vessels release carbon dioxide, it passes back through the alveoli and is exhaled during respiration.

**anasarca**: A generalized swelling of the body tissues due to excessive fluid, usually from failure of an organ like the heart, kidney, or liver.

**anastomosis**: When two blood vessels are connected. Usually done with stitching but can be done with stapling or other methods. Could also be the joining of an artificial blood vessel graft to a native blood vessel, the joining of two pieces of intestine together, or the joining of other hollow lumen-type tissues.

**aneurysm**: An abnormal dilatation, or ballooning, of a blood vessel. Also, if the heart muscle is damaged and a wall of the heart itself dilates, it is referred to as an aneurysm of the ventricle or a ventricular aneurysm.

**angina pectoris**: Chest pain that occurs when the heart is not getting enough blood. Often described as pressure, like a band tightening around the chest, or a dull, aching pain over the front left side of the chest. Can also be a pain radiating down the left arm or, occasionally, it can radiate into the neck or jaw. It can be associated with shortness of breath.

**angiography**: The process of making a blood vessel visible by injecting a substance that can be seen under x-ray.

**angioplasty**: Repair of a blood vessel, usually done with some form of surgery. Also refers to the widening of a narrowed blood vessel with a balloon catheter.

**anticoagulant**: A drug that prevents or slows the blood clotting process. Also referred to as a blood thinner. Common examples include heparin and coumadin-type drugs.

**antiplatelet drug**: A drug that prevents blood platelets from clumping together, thereby slowing the blood clotting process. Aspirin is the most common example.

**aorta**: The main artery that supplies the body with oxygenated blood. It originates at the top of the heart and begins with the aortic valve. It gives off branches that divide into smaller arterial branches.

**aortic arch**: The portion of the aorta at the top of the heart where it makes a U-turn. It gives off three important blood vessels: the innominate artery, the left carotid artery, and the left subclavian artery.

**aortic insufficiency**: Also called aortic valve regurgitation or aortic valve incompetence. Occurs when the three leaflets, or flaps, of the aortic valve do not come together when the valve is closed and blood leaks backwards into the left ventricle.

**aortic stenosis**: An abnormal narrowing of the aortic valve. This can be a condition a person is born with, or it can be related to scarring of the aortic valve leaflets, or flaps, due to rheumatic fever or other causes.

**aortic valve**: One of the four heart valves. The aortic valve is a one-way valve located between the left ventricle and the aorta. It typically has three leaflets, or flaps. It allows for blood to pass from the left ventricle into the aorta.

**aortography**: The process of making the aorta visible through x-ray using a radiopaque dye.

**arrhythmia**: Any abnormal heart rhythm. Also called dysrhythmia.

**arteriogram**: X-ray picture of an artery.

**arteriography**: Technique used for taking a picture of an artery.

**arterioles**: Very small arteries.

**arteriosclerosis**: Literally means "hardening of the arteries." It is usually caused by deposits of cholesterol and other fatty substances on and in the artery lining, resulting in narrowing, blockages, scarring, and eventually hardening of the arteries.

**artery**: A blood vessel that carries blood from the heart to the body or from the heart to the lungs.

**ascending aorta**: The portion of the aorta between the heart and the aortic arch.

**ascites**: An abnormal accumulation of serum-like fluid in the abdomen.

**assist device**: A mechanical device used to aid the failing heart's left or right ventricle.

**atelectasis**: Collapse of the tiny air sacs in the lung, common after major operations. Atelectasis can lead to pneumonia.

**atheromatous plaque**: Similar to atherosclerosis but referring to a specific area of plaque.

**atherosclerosis**: The most common form of arteriosclerosis. Lipids, cholesterol, and other fatty deposits are located on the inner surface and wall of the artery. It can cause coronary blockages and heart attack.

**atresia**: Absence of a normal opening.

**atria**: Plural of atrium.

**atrial fibrillation**: When the atria contract in an irregular rhythm and no longer help pump blood into the ventricles. This condition allows an uncontrolled amount of blood to flow through the tricuspid valve into the right ventricle and through the mitral valve into the left ventricle.

**atrial septal defect**: An abnormal hole in the common wall between the right and left atria, usually a congenital heart defect.

**atrioventricular node (also A-V node)**: A specialized nerve-type tissue located in the wall of the right ventricle. It receives electrical impulses from the sinoatrial node.

**atrium**: A filling chamber of the heart. The right atrium furnishes blood for the right ventricle, and the left atrium furnishes blood for the left ventricle.

**atrophy**: A wasting away of tissue.

**auricle**: Synonymous with atrium.

**auscultation**: Listening to the heart or lungs, usually with a stethoscope. Auscultation can also be done over arteries or the abdomen.

**autograft**: Using tissue from one's own body as a graft.

**bacterial endocarditis**: An infection involving the heart, caused by bacteria.

**beta-blockers**: Drugs used to slow the heart rate and the force of contraction, thereby reducing workload and oxygen requirements of the heart. Most commonly used for treatment of coronary artery disease.

**bicuspid valve**: A valve with two leaflets. The mitral valve is naturally bicuspid, while the pulmonary valve, the aortic valve, and the tricuspid valve normally have three leaflets.

**bifurcation**: When an artery or vein separates into two branches.

**biopsy**: Either the process of removing tissue from a patient for examination or the specimen obtained from such a procedure.

**blue baby**: A baby born with congenital heart defects that cause the unoxygenated blood returning to the heart to be pumped out through the aorta. This abnormality gives the child a bluish skin color from unoxygenated blood.

**board certified physician**: After physicians finish their training in a specialty in the United States, they take a series of tests. These tests are administered by the American board of each specialty, for example, the American Board of Internal Medicine, the American Board of Surgery, etc. The physicians that pass these tests receive a certificate stating that they are board certified in that specialty. Most board certified physicians must periodically take recertification tests. For example, cardiac and thoracic surgeons must retake their board examinations every ten years.

**bradycardia**: An abnormally slow heart rate.

**brain death**: A condition in which the brain no longer functions while the body is still living. This is determined both by an electroencephalogram, which shows a "flat line" indicating no electrical activity in the brain, and by physical examination showing no brain response under any conditions.

**bundle of His**: A special nerve-type tissue extending from the atrioventricular node (A-V node) along the ventricular septum. They help conduct electrical impulses from the A-V node into the ventricles.

**calcification**: A condition in which calcium abnormally builds up in the tissues, for instance in a heart valve or an artery.

**cannula**: A hollow tube that is inserted into a blood vessel, the heart, or another body cavity.

**capillaries**: The smallest blood vessels, connecting the smallest arteries or arterioles to the smallest veins, called venules. In the capillaries, oxygen is given off by the red blood cells to the tissues, and waste products are picked up.

**carbon dioxide**: A waste product of cell function. This gas is picked up by the capillaries and transported to the lungs, where it is exhaled.

**cardiac**: Referring to the heart.

**cardiac arrest**: When the heart either stops beating or goes into an abnormal heart rhythm, in which the ventricles can no longer effectively pump blood. This is a serious condition and often results in unconsciousness within seconds.

**cardiac catheterization**: When catheters are inserted into the heart. They can be used to measure pressures in the heart, inject radiopaque dyes, detect coronary artery blockages, or learn more about the heart and possible abnormalities.

**cardiac output**: The amount of blood the heart pumps per minute.

**cardiac rehabilitation**: A formal or informal program for patients who have had a heart attack or heart surgery. It often includes diet modification, exercise, and education on heart medications. The aim of a cardiac rehabilitation program is to get patients back to a relatively normal lifestyle.

**cardiac surgeon**: Also referred to as a heart surgeon, cardiothoracic surgeon, cardiovascular surgeon, chest surgeon, or thoracic surgeon. A surgeon who, in the United States, has spent five or six years in a training program (residency) in general surgery, followed frequently by a year or two in the research laboratory, and then spends two to three years in a training program in surgery of the chest, including surgery of the heart and lungs.

**cardiac tamponade**: A process in which fluid or blood clots build up between the heart and the pericardium. It can interfere with heart function and may eventually cause the heart to fail and may possibly even cause death.

**cardiac transplantation**: Replacement of a heart with a donor heart.

**cardiogenic shock**: A very serious condition in which the heart is unable to pump enough oxygenated blood to supply the body's tissues and organs. It is usually related to the heart muscle failing as a result of a heart attack and must be treated immediately.

**cardiologist**: A physician who has completed training in internal medicine and then typically spends another three or four years specializing in heart disease. A cardiologist is an internist who has specialized in heart disease, whereas a cardiac surgeon is a surgeon who specializes in operations on the heart and other structures in the chest. Some cardiologists, called interventional cardiologists, perform cardiac catheterizations.

**cardiology**: The study of the heart and related structures.

**cardiomyopathy**: A condition in which the heart muscle is not able to contract or function properly.

**cardiomyoplasty**: A surgical procedure using a muscle, usually the latissimus dorsi muscle in the back, to wrap around a failing heart. The muscle is then electrically stimulated so it will contract in synchrony with the failing heart and hopefully improve the signs and symptoms of heart failure.

**cardioplegia solution**: A solution that stops the heart from beating and reduces its oxygen consumption, thus allowing surgery to take place.

**cardiopulmonary bypass**: Using the heart-lung machine to temporarily bypass the heart and lungs, usually during open heart surgery. While on cardiopulmonary bypass, the patient's body is supported by the heart-lung machine.

**cardiopulmonary resuscitation (CPR)**: The act of attempting to revive a patient, usually unconscious and no longer breathing, after the heart has stopped or gone into a serious, fatal rhythm. It involves mouth-to-mouth breathing and external massage or pressing on the chest to help the heart pump blood. If this is done in a hospital or by emergency medical technicians, electrode paddles are often used to shock the heart back into a more normal rhythm.

**cardiothoracic surgeon**: *See* cardiac surgeon.

**cardiovascular**: Referring to the heart and blood vessels.

**cardiovascular surgeon**: *See* cardiac surgeon.

**cardioversion**: Changing the heart rhythm. This can be done with an electric shock or drugs.

**cardioverter/defibrillator**: A cardioverter or defibrillator is usually used with electrode paddles to electrically shock the heart into a more normal or normal rhythm. There are also implantable versions of this device.

**carotid arteries**: Two arteries that supply the head and brain with oxygenated blood.

**CAT scan**: *See* computed tomography.

**catheter**: A long, thin, hollow tube that is inserted into the body.

**catheterization**: The process of inserting the catheter into the body.

**CCU**: Cardiac care unit or, in some cases coronary care unit, where patients with conditions such as heart attacks and other types of heart conditions are placed for close monitoring.

**cholesterol**: A fat-like substance, both produced in the body and present in certain types of foods that are made from animals.

**cholesterol ratio**: Ratio of the total cholesterol measured in the blood to the amount of high-density lipoproteins (HDL). A high ratio of total cholesterol to HDL-cholesterol usually indicates greater risk for having coronary disease or a more rapid progression of existing coronary artery disease.

**chordae tendineae**: Stringlike attachments that are part of a mitral and tricuspid valve apparatus which connect the valve leaflets, or flaps, to the papillary muscles on the ventricular wall.

**cineangiography**: Similar to an arteriography or an angiography. It is the process of making a "movie" of the blood vessel as radiopaque dye moves through the vessel and helps to identify blockages. This is commonly done in the coronary arteries and referred to as a coronary cineangiogram.

**circulation**: The circulation of blood through the heart, lungs, and blood vessels.

**circumflex coronary artery**: A branch of the left main coronary artery.

**claudication**: Pain, numbness, or tiredness in the leg caused when the muscles are not getting enough oxygenated blood. It is usually due to a blockage in one of the arteries supplying the leg muscles with blood.

**coarctation of the aorta**: A birth defect in which there is a segment of the aorta that is abnormally narrowed. Typically, this coarcted area is in the descending aorta just after the aortic arch.

**collateral circulation**: Referring to tiny blood vessels that are used to carry blood around blockages in arteries or veins.

**commissurotomy**: A procedure to open a heart valve after its leaflets, or flaps, have become stuck together, usually because of rheumatic fever. This procedure is also called valvulotomy. It can be done during a heart operation or with balloon-tipped catheters.

**computed tomography**: Also referred to as CT scans or CAT scans. A special type of three-dimensional x-ray picture that yields more information than can be obtained with a regular x-ray.

**conduit**: In heart surgery, this usually refers to any tube used to channel blood. It can be the patient's own artery or vein, taken from one area of the body and moved to another. It can also be made from synthetic material, taken from another human, or in some cases, taken from an animal.

**congenital cardiac anomaly**: Also referred to as a congenital heart defect. This is an abnormality of the heart or the blood vessels surrounding the heart. A person is born with it.

**congestive heart failure**: When the heart does not pump an adequate amount of blood, the blood backs up into the veins so that they become engorged and swollen with fluid.

**coronary arteries**: Arteries that supply the heart muscle with oxygenated blood.

**coronary arteriography**: Same as coronary cineangiography. The process of obtaining a coronary arteriogram or an x-ray picture of the arteries of the heart. This is done by injecting a radiopaque dye that shows up on x-ray.

**coronary artery bypass grafting (CABG)**: A surgical technique in which one's own veins or other arteries are used to move blood around a blocked area in a coronary artery.

**coronary artery disease**: Referring to atherosclerotic heart disease, or a buildup of fatty substances or cholesterol in the walls of the coronary artery causing blockages and possibly even a heart attack.

**coronary insufficiency**: Refers to coronary artery disease or a condition in which the coronary arteries do not supply a sufficient amount of blood.

**coronary occlusion**: A partial or total blockage of a coronary artery.

**coronary thrombosis**: A clot in one of the coronary arteries, typically an artery that is already partially blocked from cholesterol buildup or other fatty deposits.

**CPR**: *See* cardiopulmonary resuscitation.

**cyanosis**: A condition in which there is a lack of oxygenated blood, causing the blood to turn a dark bluish or purple color, which will make the skin appear bluish. In darker skinned people, the tissue under the fingernails will be bluish.

**cyclosporine**: A drug used to help prevent organ rejection in patients who have had transplants.

**defibrillation**: A process usually using an electric shock to the heart to stop the atria and/or ventricles from beating chaotically and convert the heart to a more normal rhythm.

**descending aorta**: The portion of the aorta between the aortic arch and the abdomen.

**diastole**: The portion of the cardiac cycle of beating and resting in which the heart is relaxed.

**digitalis**: A drug made from the foxglove plant. It is believed to help the heart contract more forcefully and efficiently and also help the failing heart contract more normally.

**dissection**: When tissues in the body are separated.

**distal**: Meaning beyond or the farther end. When referring to a blood vessel, it's the portion that's farthest from the heart.

**diuretic**: This is a drug or other substance used to stimulate the kidneys to produce more urine and remove excess fluid from the body.

**Doppler ultrasonography**: A technique using high frequency sound waves to detect blood flow through the heart and blood vessels. It is somewhat like the sonar used to detect submarines.

**ductus arteriosus**: A tube connecting the pulmonary artery to the aorta. After birth, when the lungs begin to function, this tube normally closes. If it stays open, it's known as patent ductus arteriosus. Over time, this can cause problems such as heart failure and may need to be surgically closed.

**dyspnea**: The sensation of being short of breath.

**echocardiogram**: A movie of your heart functioning using a technique whereby high frequency sound waves develop images of the beating heart.

**edema**: Swelling of tissues due to excessive fluid.

**ejection fraction**: Referring to the percentage of blood ejected out of the heart ventricles, usually the left ventricle, during a single contraction. With a single normal heartbeat, about 50 percent to 60 percent of the blood in the left ventricle is ejected. With some degree of heart damage due to a heart attack or other causes, the amount of blood ejected may be only 30 percent or 40 percent. When the left ventricle is significantly damaged, only 20 percent or even less may be ejected.

**electrocardiogram**: Also called an ECG or EKG. A recording of the heart's electrical activity. EKG is a historical spelling used because much of the original work on the electrocardiogram was done in Holland.

**electrophysiologic study**: A mapping out of the heart's electrical conduction system, done with special catheters that are passed through the bloodstream to the heart.

**embolectomy**: A surgical procedure in which an embolus is removed from the bloodstream.

**embolism**: The complete blocking or partial blocking of a blood vessel by an embolus.

**embolus**: An object (usually a blood clot) traveling through the bloodstream that should not be in the bloodstream. It frequently blocks off a blood vessel.

**endarterectomy**: A surgical procedure in which atherosclerotic material in an artery is removed and the artery is either sewn back together or a patch is placed over the surgical incision.

**endocardium**: The inner lining of the heart.

**endothelium**: The inner lining of the blood vessel.

**epicardium**: The outer lining of the heart. It is in contact with the pericardium.

**erectile dysfunction**: Also referred to as impotence. It is the inability to achieve or maintain an erection for sexual intercourse.

**erythrocyte**: A red blood cell that contains hemoglobin. Its main function is to carry oxygen through the bloodstream.

**etiology**: The study of the cause or origin of a problem, usually a disease. Also the factor causing the problem.

**excision**: Surgical removal of a piece of tissue.

**exercise stress test**: A test during which a patient is connected to an electrocardiogram, or possibly other types of monitoring machines, and asked to walk on a treadmill or possibly pedal a stationary bicycle while being monitored.

**extracorporeal circulation**: Process in which the blood is routed outside of the body and then back into the body. It is usually done with a machine, such as a heart-lung machine.

**femoral arteries**: The main arteries in the upper portion of the leg.

**fibrillation**: A chaotic beating pattern of the heart.

**fluoroscope**: A type of x-ray device that enables a physician to see images, such as the heart beating, as they are actually happening as opposed to a one-time picture.

**foramen ovale**: A hole between the left and the right atrium in the atrial septum present in the fetus. If it remains open after birth, it is called a patent foramen ovale.

**guanosine monophosphate (cyclic GMP)**: A chemical neuromediator that helps to transmit messages through the nervous system.

**graft**: Insertion of one thing into another, and making it an integral part of the latter. An example is grafting a living branch onto a tree until it becomes part of the host tree. In heart surgery, it refers to attaching vessel grafts onto arteries.

**HDL, high-density lipoprotein**. This is known as the good type of cholesterol. A higher HDL level is good and indicates one is less likely to suffer from a heart attack.

**heart attack**: When a portion of the heart muscle dies. Doctors refer to this as a myocardial infarction, infarction, or MI.

**heart block**: When the electrical impulse that originates in the S-A node is blocked from getting through the A-V node to pace the ventricles.

**heart block, complete**: When none of the S-A electrical activity is getting through the A-V node to the ventricles.

**heart block, first-degree**: When the S-A node's electrical activity arriving at the A-V node is slowed, causing an abnormality on the electrocardiogram.

**heart block, second-degree**: When only some of the beats from the S-A node are getting through to pace the ventricle.

**heart block, third-degree**: The same as complete heart block.

**heart disease**: A term used to indicate any type of abnormal heart condition, whether acquired or congenital.

**heart failure**: When the heart is weakened and cannot pump enough blood.

**heart-lung machine**: A machine used to bypass the function of the heart and lungs.

**heart massage** (*see also* CPR): A rhythmic compression on the chest to force blood through a heart that has stopped pumping. If the chest is already open, the heart surgeon may squeeze the heart in a rhythmic fashion so blood will be forced through the heart. This is called internal heart massage.

**heart surgeon**: *See* cardiac surgeon.

**hemodynamics**: The circulation and the function of the heart, blood, and blood vessels.

**hemoglobin**: A protein in the red blood cell that helps transport oxygen and carbon dioxide.

**heparin**: A powerful chemical that prevents blood from clotting, used as an anticoagulant.

**heterograft**: *See* xenograft.

**heterotopic transplant**: The transplant of an organ or tissue, usually from one person to another, when the organ or tissue is not put in the location where it normally resides.

**homograft**: A donor graft, or piece of tissue, taken from a donor and placed into a recipient of the same species.

**hypertension**: Abnormally high blood pressure.

**hypertrophy**: Abnormally enlarged organs or tissues.

**hyperventilation**: Breathing fast in such a manner that the carbon dioxide level in the blood falls to an abnormal level.

**hypoplasia**: Underdeveloped tissues or organs.

**hypothermia**: Lowering the body temperature. This technique is used in heart surgery, usually with the heart-lung machine, so the body's demand for oxygen will be less during certain types of surgical procedures.

**hypoxia**: Abnormally low oxygen levels in the blood and tissues of the body.

**iatrogenic**: Caused by the doctor.

**idiopathic**: Of unknown cause.

**iliac arteries**: The two main terminal branches of the aorta as it ends in the lower abdomen. They carry blood to the pelvis and the legs.

**incompetent valve**: A leaking heart valve.

**infarction**: Death of tissue.

**inferior vena cava**: The large vein that brings blood from the lower body back to the heart.

**innominate artery**: The first main branch off the aortic arch, which in turn divides into the right carotid artery, supplying blood to the head and neck, and the right subclavian, supplying blood to the right arm.

**innominate vein**: A large vein in the upper portion of the chest near the neck that channels venous blood back into the superior vena cava.

**insulin**: A hormone produced in the pancreas that promotes use of glucose by the cells and protein formation. Insulin is also responsible for the formation and storage of fats (lipids).

**intima**: The inner lining of a blood vessel that is in contact with the blood. It includes the endothelial cell layer.

**intra-aortic balloon pump**: A pump that is threaded into the aorta, usually through an artery in the groin, and connected to an external power source. There is a balloon on the tip of a catheter that inflates and deflates in synchrony with the heart, helping the heart to pump blood through the early postoperative period.

**ischemia**: When a portion of the body, an organ, or a tissue is not getting enough oxygenated blood. It is usually related to a blockage in one of the arteries delivering blood to that area.

**jugular vein**: Large vein in the neck that returns blood from the head and neck.

**LDL-cholesterol**: Low-density lipoprotein cholesterol. Although it is necessary for the body to function, it is considered the bad type of cholesterol. An excess amount may make a person more prone to develop coronary artery and other types of atherosclerotic diseases.

**left anterior descending coronary artery**: One of the two major branches of the left main coronary artery that supply blood to the left ventricle. The other major branch is the circumflex coronary artery.

**Leriche's syndrome**: A condition involving blockages of the arteries coming off the lower aorta, including the iliac arteries, that is characterized by claudication. It is associated with erectile dysfunction.

**lesion**: An abnormality of any body tissue or part.

**leukocyte**: White blood cell. They are part of the blood and are primarily involved in protecting the body against infections.

**licensed physician**: A physician who has been granted a license by a state to practice medicine in that state. All practicing physicians in the United States must be licensed, but they need not all be board certified (*see* board certified physician).

**lipid**: The fats circulating in the bloodstream, including cholesterol, triglycerides, and phospholipids.

**lipid profile**: The percentage of the different types of lipids in the bloodstream.

**lipoprotein**: Identical to LDL except for the addition of certain other proteins.

**low-density lipoprotein cholesterol**: *See* LDL cholesterol.

**lumen**: Inner open area of the blood vessel through which blood flows.

**magnetic resonance imaging**: Also called MRI. Radio waves and magnetic fields are used to form images of the internal portions of the body. The MRI is particularly good for studying blood vessels and blood flow through the heart.

**media**: Middle layer of the wall of an artery. It includes elastic tissue, collagen, and muscle.

**MI**: Myocardial infarction, or heart attack.

**mitral valve**: A one-way valve located between the left atrium and the left ventricle. The mitral valve has two leaflets, or flaps.

**mitral valve prolapse**: A common condition characterized by the two leaflets, or flaps, of the mitral valve not coming together completely when the mitral valve closes. There is usually some leakage of blood back into the atrium. This has also been called the "click murmur syndrome."

**mitral valve regurgitation (or incompetence)**: Leakage of blood backwards through the mitral valve when it should be closed while the left ventricle is contracting.

**mitral valve stenosis**: Abnormal narrowing of the mitral valve, causing difficulty in blood flow through the valve.

**murmur**: A noise produced from blood flowing through the heart, other blood vessels, or lungs.

**myocardial infarction**: *See* heart attack or MI.

**myocarditis**: An inflammation of the heart muscle.

**myocardium**: The heart muscle.

**myxoid degeneration**: Degeneration of the middle layer of tissue in blood vessels and heart valves.

**necrosis**: Death of tissue.

**neonate**: A newborn child within the first few weeks of life.

**nitroglycerin**: A drug used to dilate coronary arteries so more oxygenated blood can reach the heart muscle. This drug is generally used by patients with atherosclerotic coronary artery disease.

**occlusion**: Narrowing or blockage of a blood vessel.

**open heart surgery**: Heart operations in which the heart-lung machine is used and the heart is opened so various structures can be repaired or replaced. However, many people also use the term to refer to any heart operation in which the heart-lung machine is used, including coronary bypass surgery, in which only the surface of the heart is worked on.

**pacemaker**: A small, battery-powered device implanted in the chest to send electrical impulses to the heart, causing it to contract in a rhythmic fashion. Electrical pacemakers are used when the body's natural pacemaker, the sinoatrial node, is not functioning properly.

**palliative**: A treatment that improves a condition but does not cure it. A palliative heart procedure would be one that would improve the patient's condition but not cure the heart disease.

**papillary muscles**: Tiny muscles located in the left and right ventricles that are attached with stringlike structures called chordae tendineae to the mitral and tricuspid valves. These muscle structures help control the valve function.

**patent**: Patent means open. Usually it means that a blood vessel is open.

**patent ductus arteriosus**: *See* ductus arteriosus.

**pediatric cardiologist**: A physician who specializes in heart diseases of children.

**pediatric heart surgeon**: A heart surgeon who specializes in heart surgery in children.

**percutaneous transluminal coronary angioplasty (PTCA)**: A procedure using a balloon-tipped catheter that is inflated and crushes atherosclerotic plaque or other material against the inside wall of the coronary artery, opening the blockage and allowing more blood flow to the heart muscle. This is done by introducing a catheter through a needle stick in the skin (percutaneous). The catheter is threaded up through the arteries and into the coronary lumen across the area of the blockage (transluminal coronary), and the balloon is inflated (angioplasty).

**pericardial tamponade**: *See* cardiac tamponade.

**pericarditis**: Inflammation of the pericardium.

**pericardium**: The fibrous sac that surrounds the heart.

**phlebitis**: An inflammation of a vein, usually associated with a blood clot forming in the vein.

**phospholipid**: One of the types of lipids present in the bloodstream. Phospholipids are a necessary part of a cell membrane. They are also thought to be important in keeping cholesterol and triglycerides in solution in our circulation.

**physicians in training**: Physicians training in a specialty used to be known as interns during the first year after medical school, and residents while training after that. In recent years, however, the term intern is used less commonly in the United States. Most physicians are known as residents from the day they start a training program after medical school. In some cases, if they obtain additional training in a subspecialty, they are known as a fellow during that period of training.

**plaque**: A raised, abnormal area. In the bloodstream, these are typically referred to as atheromatous plaques, and they're composed of cholesterol and other lipid material. As the plaque enlarges, it obstructs blood flow in various arteries including the coronary arteries to the heart.

**platelets**: Tiny disc-shaped structures in the bloodstream that help the blood to clot.

**pleural effusion**: A condition in which a serum-like fluid floods into the space between the inner lining of the chest cavity and the outer lining of the lung (pleura). It can be treated by drawing the fluid off with a needle that is inserted through the chest wall. If it is caused by heart failure, it can be treated by treating the underlying cause of the heart failure. In some cases, a small plastic tube has to be inserted through the chest wall and left in place for a few days or longer to treat this condition.

**pleurocentesis**: Also referred to as a "chest tap." A procedure in which a hollow tube is inserted through the skin into the chest cavity. This is usually done by attaching a needle to a syringe so that fluid abnormally present in the space between the inner chest wall and lung can be removed.

**pneumothorax**: Collapse of the lung.

**prosthesis**: Artificial material or an artificial device used to replace a body part.

**proximal**: A point closer to the point of reference. When referring to a blood vessel, it's the portion that's closest to the heart.

**pulmonary artery**: Artery that carries blood from the right ventricle to the lungs.

**pulmonary circulation**: The portion of circulation in which blood is pumped from the right ventricle to the lungs, where it is oxygenated and returned through the pulmonary veins to the left atrium.

**pulmonary edema**: A condition in which the lungs become congested with fluid, usually related to a back-up of blood due to either mitral or aortic heart valve malfunction or to heart failure.

**pulmonary embolism**: This happens when an abnormal piece of material, such as a blood clot, lodges in one of the blood vessels in the lungs, usually causing damage and possible shortness of breath. A large lung embolism can cause sudden death.

**pulmonary hypertension**: A condition in which blood pressure in the vessels of the lung is abnormally elevated.

**pulmonary insufficiency**: A leaking pulmonary valve, or can mean the lungs are not functioning properly.

**pulmonary valve**: One-way heart valve at the junction of the right ventricle and the pulmonary artery.

**pulse**: With each contraction of the left ventricle, the arteries throughout the body expand. This can be felt by placing the fingers on the wrist next to an artery and is known as the pulse.

**pulse pressure**: The difference between the pressure in the arteries when the heart is contracting and the pressure when the left ventricle is relaxing. For example, blood pressure may increase to a peak of 120 millimeters of mercury when the left ventricle is contracting and be as low as 80 millimeters of mercury while the heart is relaxing. That blood pressure would be written as 120/80.

**radionuclide**: A small amount of a nuclear substance that is used during some diagnostic tests to help physicians better see the heart and blood vessels.

**red blood cell**: *See* erythrocyte.

**rejection**: When the body's immune system recognizes a tissue as foreign, such as a transplant from one person to another, and mounts a defense against that tissue. If appropriate measures, such as antirejection drugs, are not administered, the body will probably reject the foreign tissue.

**retrograde coronary perfusion catheter**: A catheter that is inserted through the right atrium into the coronary sinus, a vein that drains the heart itself. This catheter is usually used to administer cardioplegia solution.

**rheumatic fever**: Usually associated with streptococcus infections, although not actually an infection itself. It usually comes on weeks after the infection and may be an allergic reaction to the infection. It can affect the heart, the heart valves, the joints, and the nervous system.

**rheumatic heart disease**: Specifically referring to the heart's involvement with rheumatic fever.

**rubella**: Commonly known as the German measles.

**saphenous vein**: A greater saphenous vein runs from the groin down to about the ankle. A lesser saphenous vein runs behind the leg in the calf area. These veins generally run right under the skin and are not critical veins. They are frequently used for coronary bypass operations and for various other types of blood vessel grafts in the legs and other areas in the body.

**sclerosis**: Hardening or scarring of arteries. Arteriosclerosis is usually associated with coronary artery disease due to buildup of lipids in the arteries.

**septicemia**: An infection in the bloodstream.

**septum**: A wall that separates two chambers, such as two chambers of the heart. The atrial septum separates the right atrium and the left atrium, and the ventricular septum separates the right and the left ventricles.

**shock**: Refers to a sudden or relatively sudden collapse of the cardiovascular system. Cardiogenic shock refers to a type of shock in which the heart is failing significantly and the blood pressure is usually very low, causing the skin to be cool and clammy. Urine output is low, and the patient may be barely responsive.

**shunt**: Usually an abnormal communication between two blood vessels or portions of the heart itself so blood is not routed through its normal path. Shunts are sometimes created by surgeons for the treatment of various heart conditions.

**sinoatrial node**: Also sinus node and S-A node. This is the true pacemaker of the heart, located at the junction of the right atrium and superior vena cava. These cells rhythmically discharge electrical impulses that cause the heart to contract. This impulse also travels to the A-V node, causing the ventricles to contract.

**sinus rhythm**: The normal rhythm of the heart that is stimulated by the sinoatrial node.

**sphygmomanometer**: Also called the blood pressure cuff because it is used to measure blood pressure. The cuff portion of this device is wrapped around the arm and tightened by squeezing a bulb. A column of mercury rises as the pressure increases, and as it slowly falls, the blood pressure is measured through the pulse in the wrist and by listening to the sounds just below the blood pressure cuff in the arm.

**stenosis**: An abnormal narrowing of a blood vessel, heart valve, or any other orifice or tube-like structure in the body.

**stent**: A device usually made from metal or other material that is placed in a blood vessel to help keep it open.

**sternotomy**: An incision usually made from near the neck to the lower portion of the chest through the middle of the sternum (breastbone). The sternum is then opened so the heart is exposed.

**stethoscope**: A device used for listening to the inner workings of the body, including the chest, intestines, abdomen, and blood vessels.

**stress test**: *See* exercise stress test.

**stroke**: Also referred to as a cerebral vascular accident, or CVA. It can be caused by a blood vessel in the brain becoming blocked or rupturing, a blood clot or other material traveling to the brain and lodging in a blood vessel, or a tumor causing an expansion or pressure in the brain. This will often result in some type of a neurological deficit such as impaired speech, reduced function of an arm or leg, or possible loss of vision, coma, or even death.

**subclavian artery**: An artery that arises from the aortic arch and supplies the upper chest and left arm with blood. The right subclavian artery arises from the innominate artery and supplies the upper chest and right arm with blood.

**superior vena cava**: The main vein that drains the unoxygenated blood from the upper portion of the body, head, and neck, and channels blood back into the right atrium.

**Swan-Ganz catheter**: A catheter that is usually guided through the heart into the pulmonary artery, where it can be used to measure pressures in the heart and pulmonary artery, as well as take blood samples, administer intravenous drugs, and measure cardiac output.

**syncope**: Temporary loss of consciousness. Also referred to as fainting, blacking out or passing out.

**syndrome**: A group of signs and symptoms that collectively indicate a certain type of abnormality or disease process.

**systemic circulation**: The portion of the blood circulating throughout the body except for the blood that's being pumped to the lungs and is returning. This is called the pulmonary circulation.

**systole**: Means the heart is contracting. It usually means the ventricles are contracting, but it can also refer to atrial contraction.

**tachycardia**: An abnormally fast heart rate, usually referring to a heart rate of more than one hundred beats per minute.

**tachycardia, ventricular**: A rapid heart rate originating in the ventricles. It is a regular, fast rhythm that can be life threatening.

**tachypnea**: Abnormal rapid breathing.

**tetralogy of Fallot**: A congenital heart defect that consists of four different abnormalities. The four defects are: 1. Abnormal opening between the right and left ventricles, or ventricular septal defect; 2. Abnormal position of the aorta, which partially overrides the right and left ventricular hole or defect; 3. Obstruction of blood flow to the lungs. Sometimes this is a buildup of muscle tissue in the right ventricle, or it can be an obstruction of the pulmonary valve; 4. Abnormal thickening of the right ventricle.

**thallium scanning**: A type of a nuclear perfusion test using a tiny number of radioactive particles that is injected into the bloodstream. This test is used to determine blood flow to various portions of the heart muscle. It is frequently done with some type of an exercise test so physicians can better determine which areas of the heart muscle are getting adequate amounts of blood.

**thoracic**: Pertaining to the chest.

**thoracic surgeon**: *See* cardiac surgeon.

**thromboembolism**: A blood clot that has broken loose from one area of the blood vessels or heart and traveled to another area.

**thrombolytic agents**: Drugs used to dissolve blood clots.

**thrombolytic therapy**: The procedure by which drugs are administered to help dissolve blood clots.

**thrombosis**: The development of a blood clot in the blood vessels or heart.

**thrombus**: A blood clot, usually in an artery or the heart.

**transesophageal echocardiogram**: A form of echocardiogram, or diagnostic test, using a special small tube that is passed through the mouth into the throat and down into the esophagus. This differs from the transthoracic echocardiogram, in which the echo probe is placed on the chest over the heart and moved around so that pictures can be obtained from various angles. With the transesophageal echocardiogram, the probe is very close to the heart, and certain structures can be better seen.

**transient ischemic attack**: Also referred to as a TIA. A condition in which a portion of the brain temporarily does not get enough oxygenated blood. It may result in temporary conditions such as slurred speech, partial loss of vision, weakness of an arm or a leg, or other neurologic conditions.

**transposition of the great arteries**: A severe form of congenital heart defect in which the aorta, which normally comes off the left ventricle, instead originates from the right ventricle, and the pulmonary artery, which normally originates from the right ventricle, originates from the left ventricle. As a result of this condition, children are usually cyanotic or bluish in color. This condition requires heart surgery to correct it.

**transvenous**: Through a vein.

**tricuspid valve**: The one-way heart valve located between the right atrium and the right ventricle. Tricuspid can also refer to the aortic valve and the pulmonary valve, which each have three cusps, or flaps.

**triglyceride**: A form of lipid that is obtained in the diet through animal fat and certain vegetables. Triglycerides can also be produced by the body. If triglyceride levels are abnormally elevated, there may be an increased risk of developing coronary artery disease.

**truncus arteriosus**: A congenital heart defect in which the aorta and pulmonary artery are one artery instead of two. There are various forms of this defect.

**ultrasonography**: An imaging test using sound waves to outline various internal structures and organs, used to determine potential abnormal conditions.

**vagus nerve**: A nerve running from the base of the skull into the abdomen. It gives off branches to various structures, and its main effect on the heart is to slow heart rate.

**valves**: Structures in the heart and blood vessels that control blood flow. When working properly, they direct the blood flow so it can only go in one direction.

**valvular insufficiency**: When a heart valve allows blood to leak backwards.

**valvuloplasty**: *See* commissurotomy.

**valvulotomy**: *See* commissurotomy.

**varicose veins**: Veins that are abnormally dilated and engorged. Often these veins are visible under the skin in the legs.

**vascular**: Referring to blood vessels.

**vascular ring**: A birth defect of the aortic arch and its branches whereby these branches form a ring around the esophagus and the trachea (windpipe) and compress them. These abnormalities can be so severe as to cause the death of an infant. Fortunately, if necessary vascular ring abnormalities can be corrected with surgical procedures.

**vascular surgeon**: Also peripheral vascular surgeon. A physician who specializes in surgery of the blood vessels, usually those in the head and neck, the abdomen, the arms, and the legs, and to some extent of the chest. There is some overlap between the areas of expertise of cardiovascular surgeons and peripheral vascular surgeons.

**vascular tree**: Refers to the blood vessels with their various branches. The arterial branches become smaller arterioles and eventually tiny capillaries. From there, unoxygenated blood is transferred into small venules, then to the larger veins as they return to the heart.

**vein**: Vessels that channel unoxygenated blood from the capillaries back to the heart.

**ventricles**: The two main pumping chambers of the heart. There are right and left ventricles.

**ventricular fibrillation**: A fatal heart rhythm in which the ventricles contract in a chaotic manner, and the heart cannot pump blood. It is a very dangerous condition that results in death if not treated immediately.

**ventricular septal defect**: A hole in the wall between the right and left ventricles. It can be a congenital heart defect or it can occur as a result of either a heart attack or possible trauma to the heart.

**vertebral arteries**: Two arteries that supply blood to the brain. They originate at the right and left subclavian arteries.

**white blood cell**: *See* leukocyte.

**xenograft**: Same as heterograft. Graft tissue taken from an animal of one species and used in another species. Pig heart valves, which are commonly used to replace heart valves in humans, are one form of xenograft. If a pig valve is put back in another pig, it is called an allograft. If the pig valve is put back in the same pig (usually to replace one of the heart valves), it is called an autograft.

# INDEX

# To order additional books, photocopy this form and fax it to 954-463-2220 or call toll-free and order direct 1-800-900-Book! (1-800-900-2665).

Visit our website at **www.writestuffbooks.com** to order books online.

<u>State of the Heart</u>: *The Practical Guide to Your Heart and Heart Surgery* is available at $39.95 (hardcover) or $29.95 (softcover).

## Quantity Discounts Available:

- ♥ 5-24 Copies 25% Discount
- ♥ 25-99 Copies 35% Discount
- ♥ 100-999 Copies 45% Discount
- ♥ Larger Quantities: Call for Special Price

My Name: _____ Phone: ( ___ )_____

Street: _____

City/State/Zip:_____

Visa ___ MC ___ AMEX ___ # _____ Expires _____

VISA  MasterCard  AMERICAN EXPRESS  Signature _____

| Qty. | Title (hardcover) | Price | Total |
|------|-------------------|-------|-------|
| | *State of the Heart* | $39.95 | |
| | Shipping/Handling (per book) | 7.25* | |

| Qty. | Title (softcover) | Price | Total |
|------|-------------------|-------|-------|
| | *State of the Heart* | $29.95 | |
| | Shipping/Handling (per book) | 7.25* | |

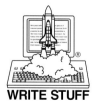

**WRITE STUFF SYNDICATE, INC.**
1001 S. Andrews Avenue,
Second Floor
Fort Lauderdale, FL
33316

Subtotal _____.____

Florida residents add 6% sales tax _____.____

Grand Total _____.____

**Canada and International orders:**
**Additional shipping required. Call (954) 462-6657**

*Shipping/handling accurate at time of printing and is subject to change.

Three Easy Ways to Buy
# *State of the Heart*

1. Call **1-800-900-BOOK**
2. Order online at: **www.writestuffbooks.com**
3. Drop this card in the mail

My Name _____

Street _____

_____

City/State/Zip _____

Phone: ( ) _____

Visa/MC/AMEX_____ Exp._____

| QTY | TITLE | PRICE | SUBTOTAL |
|-----|-------|-------|----------|
|  | State of the Heart - Hardcover | **$39.95** |  |
|  | State of the Heart - Paperback | **$29.95** |  |
|  | SHIPPING | **$7.25** | + |
|  |  | TOTAL | $ |

Three Easy Ways to Buy
# *State of the Heart*

1. Call **1-800-900-BOOK**
2. Order online at: **www.writestuffbooks.com**
3. Drop this card in the mail

My Name _____

Street _____

_____

City/State/Zip _____

Phone: ( ) _____

Visa/MC/AMEX_____ Exp._____

| QTY | TITLE | PRICE | SUBTOTAL |
|-----|-------|-------|----------|
|  | State of the Heart - Hardcover | **$39.95** |  |
|  | State of the Heart - Paperback | **$29.95** |  |
|  | SHIPPING | **$7.25** | + |
|  |  | TOTAL | $ |

Three Easy Ways to Buy
# *State of the Heart*

1. Call **1-800-900-BOOK**
2. Order online at: **www.writestuffbooks.com**
3. Drop this card in the mail

My Name _____

Street _____

_____

City/State/Zip _____

Phone: ( ) _____

Visa/MC/AMEX_____ Exp._____

| QTY | TITLE | PRICE | SUBTOTAL |
|-----|-------|-------|----------|
|  | State of the Heart - Hardcover | **$39.95** |  |
|  | State of the Heart - Paperback | **$29.95** |  |
|  | SHIPPING | **$7.25** | + |
|  |  | TOTAL | $ |

Three Easy Ways to Buy
# *State of the Heart*

1. Call **1-800-900-BOOK**
2. Order online at: **www.writestuffbooks.com**
3. Drop this card in the mail

My Name _____

Street _____

_____

City/State/Zip _____

Phone: ( ) _____

Visa/MC/AMEX_____ Exp._____

| QTY | TITLE | PRICE | SUBTOTAL |
|-----|-------|-------|----------|
|  | State of the Heart - Hardcover | **$39.95** |  |
|  | State of the Heart - Paperback | **$29.95** |  |
|  | SHIPPING | **$7.25** | + |
|  |  | TOTAL | $ |

**BUSINESS REPLY MAIL**

FIRST-CLASS MAIL PERMIT NO. 5437 FT. LAUDERDALE, FL

POSTAGE WILL BE PAID BY ADDRESSEE

**WRITE STUFF ENTERPRISES INC.**
1001 S ANDREWS AVE 2ND FLR
FT LAUDERDALE FL 33316

NO POSTAGE
NECESSARY
IF MAILED
IN THE
UNITED STATES

---

**BUSINESS REPLY MAIL**

FIRST-CLASS MAIL PERMIT NO. 5437 FT. LAUDERDALE, FL

POSTAGE WILL BE PAID BY ADDRESSEE

**WRITE STUFF ENTERPRISES INC.**
1001 S ANDREWS AVE 2ND FLR
FT LAUDERDALE FL 33316

NO POSTAGE
NECESSARY
IF MAILED
IN THE
UNITED STATES

---

**BUSINESS REPLY MAIL**

FIRST-CLASS MAIL PERMIT NO. 5437 FT. LAUDERDALE, FL

POSTAGE WILL BE PAID BY ADDRESSEE

**WRITE STUFF ENTERPRISES INC.**
1001 S ANDREWS AVE 2ND FLR
FT LAUDERDALE FL 33316

NO POSTAGE
NECESSARY
IF MAILED
IN THE
UNITED STATES

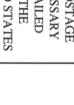

---

**BUSINESS REPLY MAIL**

FIRST-CLASS MAIL PERMIT NO. 5437 FT. LAUDERDALE, FL

POSTAGE WILL BE PAID BY ADDRESSEE

**WRITE STUFF ENTERPRISES INC.**
1001 S ANDREWS AVE 2ND FLR
FT LAUDERDALE FL 33316

NO POSTAGE
NECESSARY
IF MAILED
IN THE
UNITED STATES

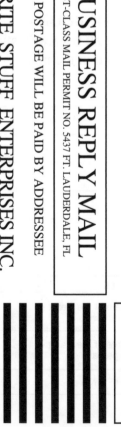